MAGNETIC RESONANCE SPECTROSCOPY

Edited by **Donghyun Kim**

Magnetic Resonance Spectroscopy
Edited by Donghyun Kim

Published by InTech

Janeza Trdine 9, 51000 Rijeka, Croatia

Publishing Process Manager Vedran Greblo

Technical Editor Teodora Smiljanic

Cover Designer InTech Design Team

Additional hard copies can be obtained from orders@intechopen.com

Magnetic Resonance Spectroscopy, Edited by Donghyun Kim
p. cm.
ISBN 978-953-51-0065-2

For EU product safety concerns:
IN TECH d.o.o., Prolaz Marije Krucifikse Kozulić 3, 51000 Rijeka, Croatia,
info@intechopen.com or visit our website at intechopen.com.

Meet the editor

Dr Dong-Hyun Kim is an associate professor of the Department of Electrical and Electronic Engineering at Yonsei University located in Seoul, Korea. He received his Bachelor's degree from Yonsei University. He obtained his M.S. and Ph.D degree from Stanford University in the Department of Electrical Engineering specializing in 'Technical developments for 1H in-vivo Magnetic Resonance Spectroscopic Imaging". After completion of his training, he joined the faculty of Radiology at the University of California, San Francisco where he continued his research on Magnetic Resonance Spectroscopy (MRS) and Magnetic Resonance Spectroscopic Imaging (MRSI). Since 2006, he has been teaching and conducting research at Yonsei University. He has worked in the field of Magnetic Resonance Imaging (MRI) and MRS/MRSI for over ten years and has published numerous peer reviewed articles on the topic.

Contents

Preface

Magnetic Resonance Spectroscopy (MRS) is a unique tool to probe the biochemistry in vivo providing metabolic information non-invasively. Applications using MRS has been found over a broad spectrum in investigating the underlying structures of compounds as well as in determining disease states. In this book, topics of MRS both relevant to the clinic and also those that are beyond the clinical arena are covered. The book consists of two sections. The first section is entitled 'MRS inside the clinic' and is focused on clinical applications of MRS. For clinical routine usage of MRS, accurate quantification methods are necessary. The first chapter starts with the various quantification methods used in 1H MRS. This is followed by an in depth coverage of MRS used in different clinical settings. Diseases that are covered include MRS for Multiple Sclerosis, Wilson's disease, kidney transplantation, chronic obstructive pulmonary disease. In addition, 13C MRS is also an important application in studying the energy metabolism in neurobiology. This is also covered in the book. In the second section of the book entitled 'MRS beyond the clinic', topics related either directly or indirectly to the clinic settings are discussed. These include a variety of NMR applications to probe chemical structures further using MRS. Our hope is that through this book, readers can understand the broad applications that NMR and MRS can offer and also that there are enough references to guide the readers for further study in this important topic.

Donghyun Kim
School of Electrical and Electronic Engineering,
Yonsei University,
Korea

Part 1

MRS Inside the Clinic

1

Quantification Improvements of ^{1}H MRS Signals

Maria I. Osorio-Garcia[1], Anca R. Croitor Sava[1], Diana M. Sima[1], Flemming U. Nielsen[2], Uwe Himmelreich[2] and Sabine Van Huffel[1]

[1]*Dept. Electrical Engineering, ESAT-SCD, Katholieke Universiteit Leuven*
IBBT - K.U. Leuven Future Health Department
[2]*Biomedical Nuclear Magnetic Resonance Unit, Katholieke Universiteit Leuven*
Belgium

1. Introduction

In vivo ^{1}H Magnetic Resonance Spectroscopy (MRS) and Magnetic Resonance Spectroscopic Imaging (MRSI) signals contain relevant metabolic information commonly used as biomarkers of diseases that can provide complementary information for the diagnosis. These signals are measured in the time domain, however, their representation in the frequency domain provides a better visualization of the metabolites in the form of resonances (peaks). In ^{1}H MRS(I), not only metabolites but also water and macromolecule/lipid resonances can be observed. In practice, the concentrations of metabolites and the presence of macromolecule/lipids contain the relevant information for diagnosis purposes.

The technique used to determine metabolic contributions is called quantification and different methods have been proposed in the time or the frequency domain. In these methods, the metabolite concentrations are estimated, *e.g.*, using a linear combination of individual peaks or a basis set of known metabolite profiles to fit the MR signal (Poullet et al., 2007; Provencher, 1993; 2001; Ratiney et al., 2004; Slotboom et al., 1998). No matter which quantification method is used, the quality of MRS signals is important for obtaining accurate estimates of the metabolite concentrations.

Although *in vivo* MRS(I) acquisitions provide non-invasively metabolic information, different limitations related to the specifications of the acquisition protocol, the localization of the voxels of interest and the homogeneity of the magnetic field in the selected region make the accurate quantification of these signals still a challenge. Therefore, advanced and efficient measurements have been developed to decrease the scanning time and to increase the spectral resolution. Nevertheless, it is essential to perform a series of preprocessing steps to improve spectral quality of MRS signals before performing quantification. Successful combinations between advanced acquisition techniques and appropriate signal processing increase the potential of integrating MR techniques in the clinical diagnosis routines (Chu et al., 2003; Devos et al., 2004; Huang et al., 2001; Ruiz-Pena et al., 2004; Vermathen et al., 2003).

In the next sections, we introduce the MRS(I) signals together with some of the most common preprocessing and quantification methods. In particular, we focus on recent methods and approaches to improve the quantification of *in vivo* MRS(I) signals, performed with the quantification method AQSES (Poullet et al., 2007): *a*) filtering of residual water, *b*) lineshape estimation, *c*) baseline estimation and *d*) inclusion of spatial constraints in MRSI quantification.

2. Description of ^{1}H MRS(I) signals and preprocessing methods

2.1 ^{1}H MRS(I) signals

These signals are measured in the time domain and have ideally a decaying shape, also called FID, which can be represented as a sum of complex-damped exponentials. They can be measured from a specific anatomical region (single voxel MRS), or from an entire organ overlaid by a grid of multiple voxels (MRSI). In order to observe the contribution of individual metabolites, MRS(I) signals are transformed to the frequency domain using the Fast Fourier Transform (FFT), producing a spectrum where the metabolite resonances can be visualized. Typically, a water suppression technique is applied as part of the acquisition protocol in order to enhance the visualization of the metabolites of interest. Additionally, an unsuppressed water signal is always measured, which is commonly used as a reference for phase, eddy currents and lineshape corrections. Depending on the acquisition protocol, single voxel signals have commonly a better signal-to-noise (SNR) ratio and thinner linewidths than multi-voxel signals, however, the advantage of multi-voxel signals is the possibility to study complete anatomical organs using one acquisition. See Fig. 1 for an example of a single and multi-voxel acquisition.

2.2 Preprocessing ^{1}H MRS(I) signals

Preprocessing of MRS signals aims at the improvement of signal quality in order to accurately extract relevant information about the metabolites via the technique called quantification. Some essential preprocessing procedures in ^{1}H MRS(I) are:

- **Time circular shift**. The digital filter and decimation in the Bruker scanners distort the beginning of the FIDs, as a consequence, the MR spectrum is filled with wiggles and the metabolite resonances are hard to identify. These first data points are initially zero and then increase, until the actual FID starts (Cobas & Sardina, 2003). A solution to this distortion is a time circular shift. This step is performed in the time domain and consists of removing data points from the beginning and adding them to the end of the signal.
- **Frequency alignment**. Due to variations in the physiological and experimental conditions (*e.g.*, temperature and pH), MR resonances experiment a frequency shift. Specially in multivariate analysis, this peak misalignment needs to be corrected. Thus, the FIDs are first transformed to the frequency domain and the spectra are shifted such that some recognizable peaks reach the desired frequency locations (Veselkov et al., 2009). In ^{1}H MRS, the resonance frequency of known metabolites can be used for shifting the full spectra. For instance, the peak of N-Acetyl-Aspartate (NAA) is known to be located at 2.01 ppm. Moreover, the displacement of individual spectral peaks from one metabolite can be corrected using advanced frequency alignment techniques, such as, quantum mechanics approaches and advanced warping algorithms (Giskeødegård et al., 2010; Lazariev et al., 2011).
- **Phase correction**. Ideally, MRS spectra should have zero-phase (*i.e.*, all peaks are pointing upwards), however, differences between the reference phase and the receiver detector

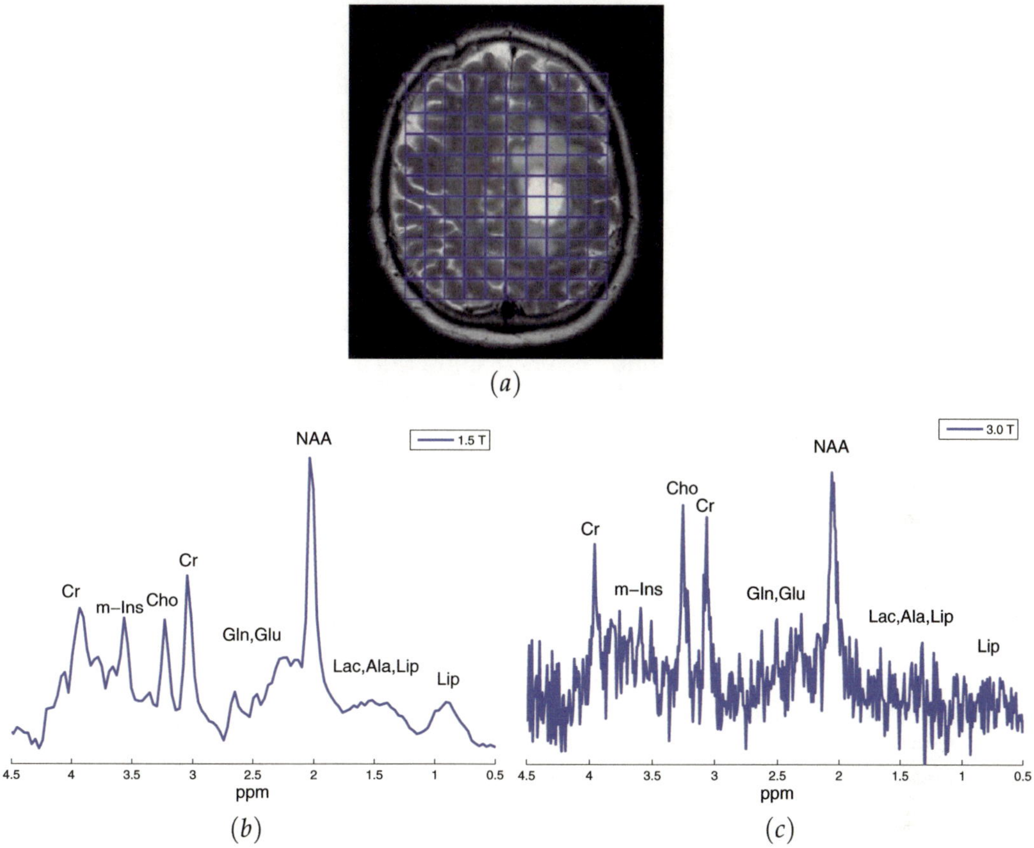

Fig. 1. (*a*) T2-weighted MRI of a brain tumor patient overlaid with a grid of voxels corresponding to an MRSI measurement. (*b*) Real part of the spectrum of a single voxel *in vivo* MRS signal acquired with a 1.5 T Philips NT Gyroscan (Philips Medical Systems, Best, The Netherlands) with acquisition parameters: PRESS sequence, repetition time (TR)=6 s, echo time (TE)=23 ms, bandwidth (SW)=1 KHz, number of points (NDP)=512 points and 64 averages. (*c*) Real part of the spectrum of a signal from a selected multi-voxel (MRS(I)) measurement acquired with a 3.0 T Philips Achieva (Philips Medical Systems, Best, The Netherlands) with acquisition parameters: PRESS sequence, TR=2 s, TE=35 ms, SW=2 KHz and NDP=2048 points and 1 average. These measurements were done at the University Hospital of the Katholieke Universiteit Leuven, Belgium.

phase, the time delay between the excitation and detection, the flip-angle variation across the spectrum, and the phase shifts from the filter employed to reduce noise outside the spectral bandwidth, produce different phase distortions (Chen et al., 2002). As a solution, phase correction approaches have been successfully used to improve the visualization of MR spectra. In practice, the phase correction consists of two components, one frequency-dependent (first order phase) and one frequency-independent (zero order phase). In particular, the zero-order phase correction consists of the multiplication of the complex spectrum by a complex phase factor equal to the initial phase of the FID (Jiru, 2008). On the other hand, adjusting the first order phase corresponds to the modification of the begin time of the MR signal (Chen et al., 2002). Although some quantification methods (Poullet et al., 2007; Provencher, 2001; Ratiney et al., 2005) are able to take into consideration phase distortions and provide accurate metabolite estimates even if the spectra are not zero-phased, other quantification methods, such as peak integration, require zero-phased spectra in order to obtain reliable metabolite estimates.

- **Eddy current corrections**. These currents are induced by the rapid switching of the magnetic field gradient in the magnet coils and surrounding metal structures (de Graaf, 1998). Because these currents are caused by the scanner and can not always be avoided, a spectral correction is necessary. Klose (Klose, 1990) has developed a method to correct eddy currents, called ECC, by point-wise dividing the water suppressed signal by the phase term of the water unsuppressed signal measured at the same location.
- **Lineshape correction/estimation**. The lineshape of MR signals is determined by the decay function (damping) of the time domain signal and refers to the shape of the peaks in the frequency domain. Ideally, it is represented by a Lorentzian, Gaussian or Voigt function, corresponding in the time domain to an exponentially decaying sinusoid. However, when magnetic field perturbations and field inhomogeneities are present, these lineshapes are disturbed (in symmetry and linewidth) and as a consequence, the ideal model used in the quantification method is unable to yield accurate metabolite estimates. Therefore, different hardware and mathematical approaches have been developed to cope with this problem. For instance, shimming techniques (*i.e.*, coils adjustment) are applied during the MR acquisition in order to correct field inhomogeneities and thus improve spectral quality (Blamire et al., 1996; Gruetter, 1993; Juchem et al., 2010). Moreover, local magnetic field susceptibility problems caused by measurements near an air cavity such as sinuses, may not always be corrected with shimming techniques making lineshape distortions unavoidable. Notwithstanding, some preprocessing methods have been successfully used based on the deconvolution of the spectra using either the unsuppressed water signal or a reference peak from the experimental signal (Bartha et al., 2000; de Graaf et al., 1990; Metz et al., 2000). Alternatively, other lineshape estimation methods based on self-deconvolution have been proposed in cases when a reference signal is not available (Maudsley, 1995; Popa et al., 2011; Sima et al., 2009).
- **Baseline correction/estimation**. ^{1}H MRS signals measured at short TE contain not only information from metabolites but also from lipids and macromolecules which may affect the baseline of the spectra. This baseline influences the quantification causing the mis-fitting of individual peaks or metabolite profiles. Therefore, different correction algorithms have been proposed to estimate and remove the baseline contribution from the spectrum (Chang et al., 2007; Cobas et al., 2006; Xi & Rocke, 2008). Alternatively, other methods have been proposed to estimate the baseline using special acquisition protocols or characterizing each macromolecule/lipid component to finally consider them in the quantification procedure (Behar & Ogino, 1993; Hofmann et al., 2001; Knight-Scott, 1999).
- **Filtering of residual water**. ^{1}H MRS signals contain a water peak thousands of units larger than those of metabolites. Therefore, in order to visualize metabolites, this water peak needs to be suppressed. Although the water resonance is partially suppressed during acquisition, the residual water requires a reliable filter for further elimination without affecting the metabolite resonances. Moreover, especially at short TE, the tail of this residual water may overlap with the baseline of macromolecule/lipids and thus, pose problems for accurate quantification. As a solution, the Hankel Lanczos Singular Value Decomposition (HLSVD) method proposed by (Pijnappel et al., 1992) parametrizes

the MR signals as a sum of complex-damped exponentials. Extensions of this method for quantification and peak suppression have been successfully applied to MR signals (Chen et al., 2004; Laudadio et al., 2004). Alternative to HLSVD, other filtering approaches have also been used for this purpose (Antoine et al., 2000; Sundin et al., 1999). Additional to the residual water, other unwanted resonances (*e.g.*, reference peaks from *in vitro* phantom solutions) may also need to be suppressed from the spectrum (Cabanes et al., 2001).

3. Quantification

Several quantification methods have been developed in the time and the frequency domain to determine metabolite concentrations. Thus, depending on the nuclei, the complexity of the signal and the *prior* information available, MR signals can be quantified with the methods listed below. An extended review of time- and frequency domain methods has been given in (Mierisová & Ala-Korpela, 2001; Vanhamme et al., 2001) and more recently in (Poullet et al., 2008).

- Time- and frequency domain fitting using a linear combination of individual peaks/profiles to fit the spectra QUEST (Ratiney et al., 2004), AQSES (Poullet et al., 2007) LCModel (Provencher, 1993; 2001)
- Time-domain estimation of parameters using *prior knowledge* (Soher et al., 1998; Young et al., 1998), AMARES (Vanhamme et al., 1997)
- Time-domain non-iterative fitting methods such as HLSVD (Barkhuijsen et al., 1987; Chen et al., 1996; Dologlou et al., 1998; Laudadio et al., 2002; Pijnappel et al., 1992; van den Boogaart, 1997)
- Iterative time- and frequency domain fitting (Slotboom et al., 1998)
- Semi-parametric fitting (Elster et al., 2005)
- Time-domain variable projection (VARPRO) (Cavassila et al., 1999; van der Veen et al., 1988)
- Time domain fitting of one peak at a time and wavelet modeling for the baseline (Dong et al., 2006; Romano et al., 2002)
- Constrained least squares (TARQUIN) (Reynolds et al., 2006; Wilson et al., 2011)
- Genetic algorithms (Metzger et al., 1996)
- Fast Padé Transform (Belkić & Belkić, 2006)
- Artificial Neural Networks (Bhat et al., 2006; Hiltunen et al., 2002)
- Sparse representation (Guo et al., 2010)
- Circular fitting (Gabr et al., 2006)
- Principal Component Analysis (PCA), Independent Component Analysis (ICA) (Hao et al., 2009; Stoyanova & Brown, 2001)

3.1 Automated Quantification of Short echo time MRS signals (AQSES)

We present in more details the method AQSES, which will be used in the next sections to illustrate several recent improvements in the field of MRS(I) signal processing. This time-domain quantification method has been especially developed for short TE MRS signals, where a mathematical model fits to a basis set of predefined metabolite profiles. From this fit, metabolite amplitudes are obtained, which represent the weighting coefficients of a linear combination of corrected metabolite profiles with Lorentzian lineshapes used for quantification. Finally, these values are proportional to the concentrations of all estimated metabolites. AQSES is available in the Java open source software AQSES GUI (De Neuter et al., 2007; Poullet et al., 2007), as a quantification method inside the Matlab® graphical user interface SPID (Poullet, 2008) and as a plug-in in the jMRUI software package (version 4.1) (Stefan et al., 2009). Fig. 2 shows the results window for a quantification made in SPID.

The model describing a short TE *in vivo* time-domain MRS signal $y(t)$ as a combination of several metabolite profiles is:

$$y(t) = \sum_{k=1}^{K} a_k e^{(j\phi_k)} e^{(-d_k t + 2\pi j f_k t)} v_k(t) + B(t) + w(t) + \epsilon(t) \quad (1)$$

where K is the number of metabolites ($k = 1, \ldots, K$), $v_k(t)$ the metabolite profile in the basis set measured as individual phantoms or simulated using quantum mechanics, a_k the amplitudes, ϕ_k the phase shifts, d_k the damping corrections, f_k the frequency shifts due to field inhomogeneity, $j = \sqrt{-1}$, $B(t)$ is the baseline due to macromolecule/lipid contamination (in AQSES it is fitted via nonparametric modeling using a basis of splines (Eilers & Marx, 1996)), $w(t)$ the water resonance (filtered either before quantification as explained in section 3.2.1, or during quantification as in (Sundin et al., 1999)) and $\epsilon(t)$ denotes white noise with standard deviation σ.

In order to assess quantification results, the Cramér-Rao lower bounds (CRLB) (Cavassila et al., 2001) are computed to provide an indication about the uncertainty and reliability of the estimated amplitudes (concentrations). Small CRLB values may (but not necessarily) indicate good parameter estimates and are proportional to the variance of the residue obtained from subtracting the fitted signal and the baseline from the original signal. Thus, acceptable CRLB should normally be below 40%.

3.2 Methods for quantification improvement

Although the quantification of *in vivo* MRS signals can often be reliably done using model (1) in AQSES, several issues appear when high field, short TE signals or multi-voxel MRSI data are being quantified. In this section, we present several quantification improvement methods implemented in AQSES (Croitor Sava, 2011; Osorio-Garcia, 2011). Whereas the filter of residual water is performed as a preprocessing step, the lineshape and baseline estimation methods are included inside the quantification method. Finally, a modified version of AQSES for MRSI data, which includes spatial knowledge is presented.

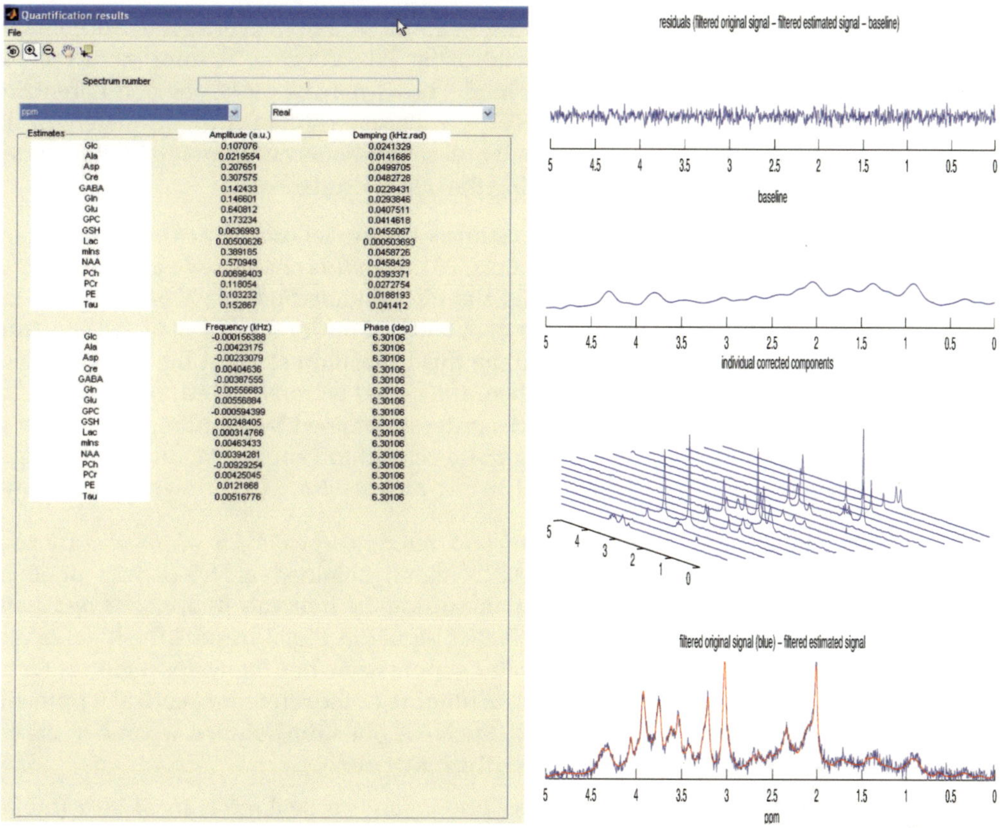

Fig. 2. Quantification results window for AQSES in SPID (left side) of an *in vivo* ^{1}H MRS signal from mouse brain acquired with a 9.4 T Bruker Biospec small animal MR scanner (Bruker BioSpin MRI, Ettlingen, Germany) with acquisition parameters: PRESS sequence, TR=4 s, TE=12 ms, SW=4 KHz, NDP=2048 points and 256 averages, volume of interest (VOI)= $3 \times 1.75 \times 1.75\ mm^3$. The basis set of 16 metabolites used for quantification was measured *in vitro*. Right: plots of residue, splines baseline, estimated metabolites and original with estimated signal.

3.2.1 Filtering of residual water

As described in section 2.2, the water component ($w(t)$ from Eq.(1)) can be filtered using HLSVD, however, appropriate filtering of this resonance in the case of distorted signals is often inaccurate. When HLSVD with one component (*i.e.*, a model order $K = 1$) is used to fit one non-Lorentzian peak, the result obtained by subtracting that modeled peak from the original signal produces a non-flat residual. In an ideal case, only white noise should be left in the residual.

The state-of-the-art methods proposed for determination of an optimal model order K in order to provide a reliable water peak removal have been described and studied on simulated, noiseless or non-overlapping peaks (Cabanes et al., 2001; Hu et al., 2010; Lin et al., 1997; Papy et al., 2007; Van Huffel & Vandewalle, 1991). For instance, (Cabanes et al., 2001) presented a method for optimal residual water removal of *in vivo* ^{1}H MRS signals of human brain using HLSVD with a model order of 25 ($K = 25$). Nevertheless, suppression of unwanted resonances of *in vivo* MRS signal using HLSVD may require more than 25 components. In fact, it is certain that a higher model order may better fit one non-Lorentzian peak. In such cases, the model order in HLSVD can be overestimated to adequately fit the experimental signal with distorted shape. Finally, all components encountered in the selected filtering region are suppressed without affecting the other resonances.

Therefore, we present a heuristic approach to estimate the model order by overestimating the number of components in HLSVD (Osorio-Garcia, 2011). In this chapter, we use the Lanczos algorithm with partial reorthogonalization, HLSVD-PRO (Laudadio et al., 2004). First, the tail of the time domain signal is truncated in order to obtain by Fourier transformation a spectrum with lower, but still adequate, spectral resolution; this truncation starts at the point at which the FID completely decays into the noise. Then, the signal is transformed to the frequency domain and an estimated number for the model order is obtained by counting the number of spectral points larger in absolute value than a noise-related threshold. We illustrate in Fig. 3 to 6 good peak suppression results on short TE *in vivo* and *in vitro* ^{1}H MRS signals, as follows:

- **1.5 T signals**. Filtering of residual water and reference peaks for an *in vivo* (normal human brain) and an *in vitro* (NAA) MRS signal obtained at 1.5 T was done by suppressing all peaks in the frequency region outside the intervals [0 ppm, 4.3 ppm] and [1 ppm, 4.44 ppm], respectively. For the *in vivo* signal in Fig. 3, results for $K = 25$ and K overestimated ($K = 44$) show a good water suppression, but the water region is flatter when $K = 44$. Fig. 4 illustrates the incomplete filtering of the reference peaks at 0 ppm and 8.4 ppm corresponding to solvents added to the NAA phantom solution when $K = 25$, but this is not the case when K is overestimated, thus, $K = 309$.
- **9.4 T signals**. Filtering of residual water and reference peaks for an *in vivo* (mouse brain) and an *in vitro* (Glucose (Glc)) MRS signal obtained at 9.4 T was done by suppressing all peaks in the frequency region outside the intervals [0 ppm, 4.3 ppm] and [2.95 ppm, 4.44 ppm], respectively. A residual reference peak located at 2.8 ppm contained in the *in vitro* signal could only be suppressed when K was overestimated. Figures 5 and 6 show the results for both signals.

3.2.2 Lineshape estimation

The metabolite profiles used for quantification have ideally a Lorentzian shape, however, the lineshape of the metabolite resonances in an *in vivo* signal might be distorted. We aim to estimate the lineshape distortion from the *in vivo* signal and impose the same distortion to each individual metabolite to ensure the same lineshape in both the *in vivo* and the model spectra. Here, we present a method (AQSES Lineshape) to estimate a common lineshape which has been successfully used in simulated, *in vitro* and *in vivo* signals (Osorio-Garcia et al., 2011; Sima et al., 2009).

In the presence of magnetic field inhomogeneities due to field perturbations or tissue heterogeneities, the symmetry and linewidth of the lineshapes are disturbed. Therefore, the fitting of the MR signal using an ideal lineshape (*e.g.*, Lorentzian, Gaussian or Voigt) becomes unreliable. Although some preprocessing methods can correct lineshape distortions, the use of a separate reference acquisition signal or a well-separated reference peak may limit their applicability.

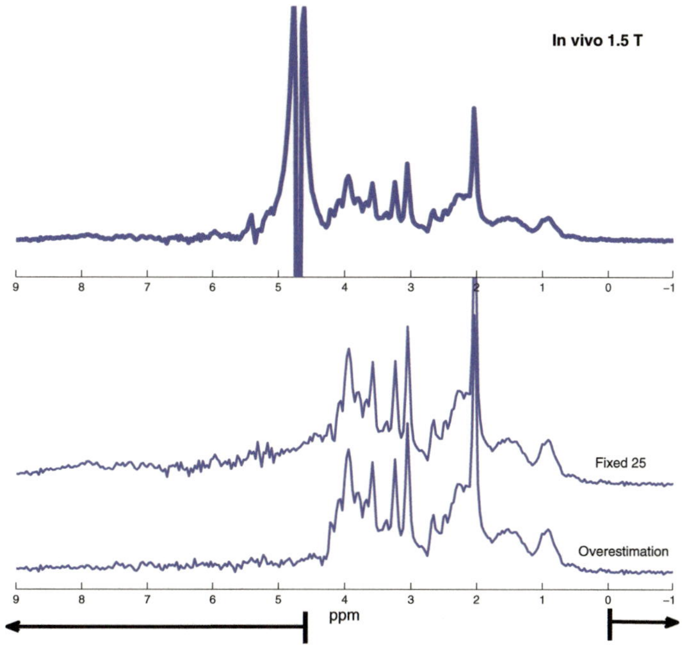

Fig. 3. Top: Real part of the spectrum of an *in vivo* MRS signal measured at 1.5 T with acquisition parameters: Philips scanner, PRESS sequence, TR=6 s, TE=23 ms, SW=1 KHz, NDP=512 points and 64 averages. Bottom: filtered signals using HLSVD-PRO with the model orders of $K = 25$ and overestimated as $K = 44$. All modeled peaks in the frequency region outside the interval [0 ppm, 4.3 ppm] were suppressed.

The lineshape of a peak in the frequency domain is determined by the decay function (damping) of the time domain signal. Self-deconvolution methods make use of the fact that within a measurement the most important factor that determines the decay rate is the local field heterogeneity, thus, all metabolites are distorted in the same way and therefore, a common lineshape can be estimated. Nevertheless, the computation of this lineshape produces a noisy function that needs to be converted into a smooth function. Methods in the literature differ in the approaches used for smoothing this noisy function. Here, we present a lineshape estimation method for correcting lineshape distortions during quantification with AQSES, where the exponential dampings $e^{(-d_k t)}$ in Eq.(1) are replaced by the common factor $g(t)$ of arbitrary shape:

$$y(t) = g(t) \sum_{k=1}^{K} a_k e^{(j\phi_k)} e^{(2\pi j f_k t)} v_k(t) + B(t) + \epsilon(t) \qquad (2)$$

The AQSES Lineshape algorithm for lineshape estimation is described below.

Step 1. Initial fitting. Quantification of the signal assuming a Lorentzian lineshape to extract the spectral parameters: amplitudes, frequencies, phases and dampings using the model in Eq. (1). Then, the signal is reconstructed from the estimated spectral parameters without considering the damping estimates.

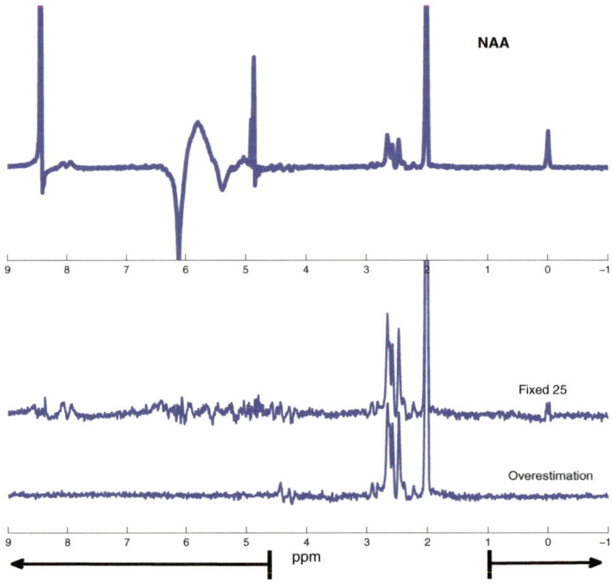

Fig. 4. Top: Real part of the spectrum of *in vitro* NAA measured at 1.5 T with acquisition parameters: Philips scanner, PRESS sequence, TR=6 s, TE=23 ms, SW=1 KHz, NDP=2048 points and 128 averages. Bottom: filtered signals using HLSVD-PRO with the model orders of $K = 25$ and overestimated as $K = 309$. All modeled peaks in the frequency region outside the interval [1 ppm, 4.44 ppm] were suppressed. Residual resonances are visible for $K = 25$ in the water and reference peak regions, *i.e.*, 4.7 ppm, 0 ppm and 8.44 ppm.

Step 2. Damping estimation. Computation of the damping function $g(t)$ as:

$$g(t) = \frac{y(t) - B(t)}{\sum_{k=1}^{K} a_k e^{(j\phi_k)} e^{(2\pi j f_k t)} v_k(t)} \tag{3}$$

where $y(t)$ is the experimental signal, $B(t)$ is the current baseline estimate, K is the number of metabolites, $v_k(t)$ the metabolite signal k in the basis set, and the amplitudes a_k, frequency shifts f_k and phase shift ϕ_k are estimated from a previous AQSES iteration from **Step 1** or **Step 4**.

Step 3. Smoothing. Outliers caused by numerical instability and division by small numbers are reduced using local regression (LOESS). This method assigns lower weight to outliers in the regression (Cleveland, 1979) and allows a robust smoothing. (See Fig. 7)

Step 4. Estimate. Spectral analysis is carried out again after point-wise multiplying the original metabolite basis set with the new smoothed function $g(t)$ from **Step 3**.

Steps 2-4 are repeated until a residual smaller than a chosen threshold is obtained or a convergence of amplitude estimates is reached.

Results of the lineshape estimation are shown below.

- **Simulated signals.** The simulated MRS signals were generated as a linear combination of 7 *in vitro* measured metabolites: Alanine (Ala), Creatine (Cr), Glutamine (Gln), Glutamate (Glu), Lactate (Lac), N-Acetyl-Aspartate (NAA), and Taurine (Tau). Then a distortion

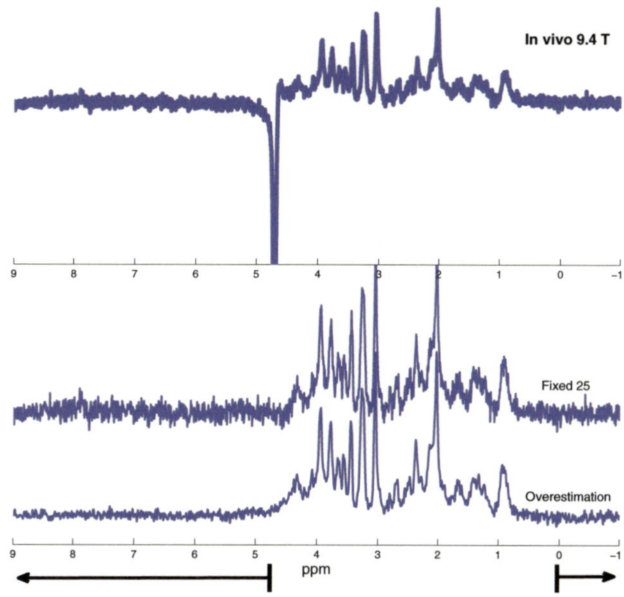

Fig. 5. Top: Real part of the spectrum of an *in vivo* MRS signal measured at 9.4 T with acquisition parameters: PRESS sequence with implemented pre-delay OVS as well as the water suppression method VAPOR, FASTMAP shimming correction, TR=4 s, TE=12 ms, SW=4 KHz, 2048 points and 256 averages. Bottom: Filtered signals with the model orders of $K = 25$ and overestimated as $K = 134$. All modeled peaks in the frequency region outside the interval [0 ppm,4.3 ppm] were suppressed.

was included to simulate a damping different from the ideal Lorentzian. Fig. 8 shows the quantification results obtained for a set of simulated signals with triangular and eddy current distortions having small and large dampings. The top row shows the fits with AQSES and AQSES Lineshape with the corresponding residuals when simulating the signals with a small (left) and a large (right) damping. The residual corresponding to AQSES contains some patterns corresponding to metabolite contributions that were not correctly quantified due to the Lorentzian lineshape model, whereas the residuals corresponding to AQSES Lineshape show a nearly flat line containing white noise that may be attributed to the estimated lineshape model. At the bottom of each plot, the amplitude estimates using AQSES and AQSES Lineshape are shown.

- ***In vitro* signals.** An *in vitro* signal containing Ala, Cr, Gln, Glu, Lac, NAA and Tau was acquired using the default shimming technique with linewidth=1.36 Hz and SNR=22. The magnetic field was afterwards intentionally distorted by mis-setting the shim current of the X coil in order to simulate lineshape distortions caused by incorrect shimming; two distorted signals were then acquired. Results of quantification of *in vitro* signals are shown in Fig. 9. The undistorted *in vitro* signal is fitted identically by AQSES and AQSES Lineshape, *i.e.*, AQSES Lineshape reports convergence after the first iteration (results not shown). For the distorted signals, the resonances of Cr at 3 ppm and 3.9 ppm and the one from NAA at 2 ppm are not very well fitted with AQSES, while AQSES Lineshape is able to fit these peaks. This is due to the fact that the lineshape distortions have a shape different from the typical Lorentzian type considered by AQSES.

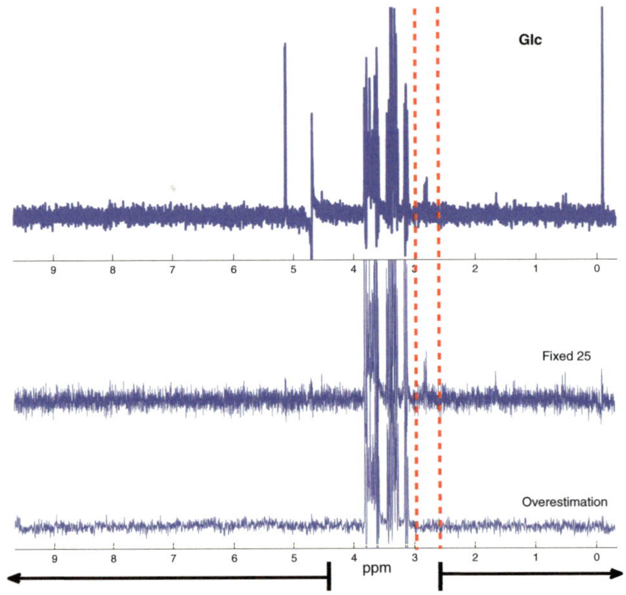

Fig. 6. Top: Real part of the spectrum of *in vitro* Glc measured at 9.4 T with acquisition parameters: PRESS sequence with implemented pre-delay OVS as well as the water suppression method VAPOR, FASTMAP shimming correction, TR=4 s, TE=12 ms, SW=4 KHz, 6144 points and 64 averages. Bottom: filtered signal with the model orders of $K = 25$ and overestimated as $K = 126$. All modeled peaks in the frequency region outside the interval [2.95 ppm,4.44 ppm] were suppressed. Residual resonances are visible at the region around 2.8 ppm (between the two vertical dashed lines).

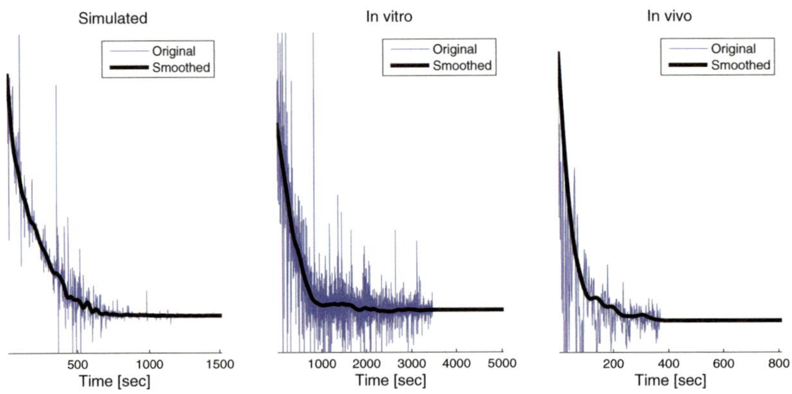

Fig. 7. Time domain signal of the resulting lineshape for simulated (left), *in vitro* (middle) and *in vivo* (right) signals. The signal labeled as 'Original' corresponds to the $g(t)$ function calculated with the ratio formula in Eq.(3) and the smoothed signal is its final denoised version after convergence.

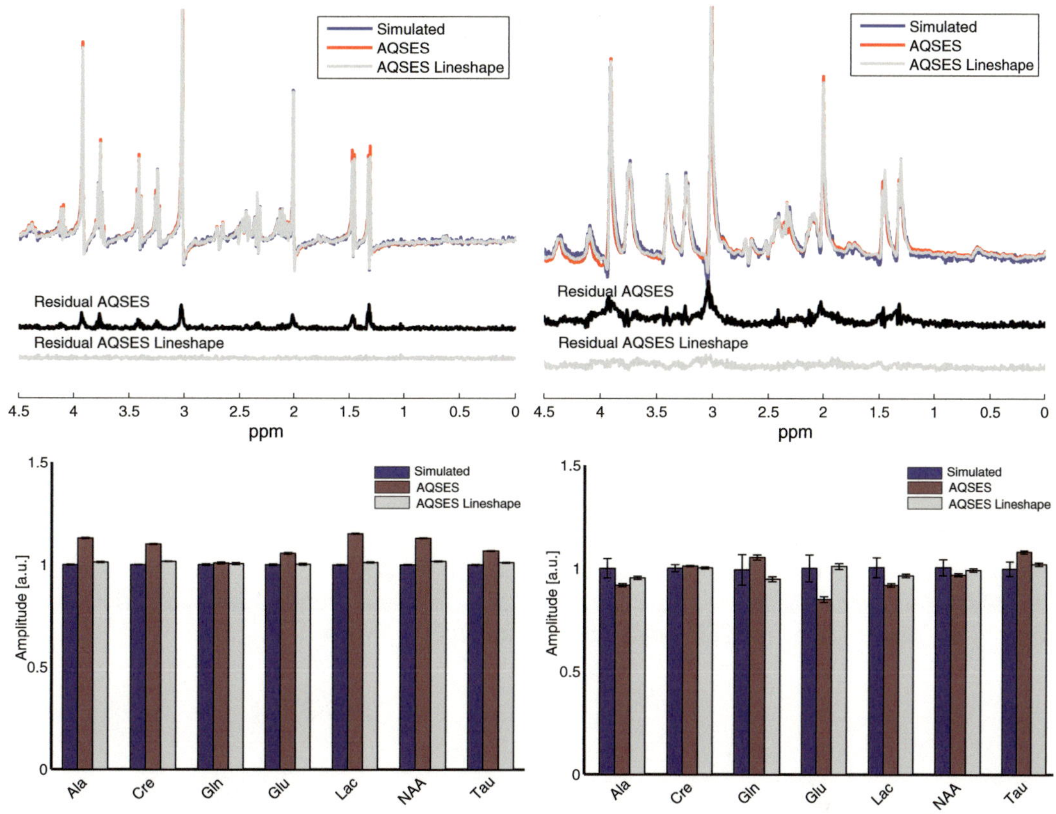

Fig. 8. Simulated MRS signals with lineshape distortions and the corresponding quantification results. These signals were obtained as the linear combination of 7 metabolites (Ala, Cr, Gln, Glu, Lac, NAA, and Tau) measured *in vitro* at 9.4 T with acquisition parameters: PRESS sequence, TR=8 s, TE=20 ms, SW=4 KHz and NDP=2048 points and 64 averages. Top left: small damping (to simulate *in vitro* signals). Top right: large damping (to simulate *in vivo* signals). The bottom plots represent the amplitude estimates for the corresponding simulated signals using AQSES and AQSES Lineshape.

- ***In vivo* signals.** An *in vivo* signal was acquired using the default shimming technique. Then, after modifying the first and second order shim coils X and Z^2, two mis-shimmed signals were also acquired. The undistorted *in vivo* signal was fitted similarly by AQSES and AQSES Lineshape, *i.e.*, AQSES Lineshape reports convergence after the first iteration (results not shown). Results of quantification for the two distorted *in vivo* signals are shown in Fig. 10.

3.2.3 Baseline estimation

The contribution from macromolecules and lipids may vary depending on the anatomical region or due to disease (tumor or metabolic disease), providing potentially useful diagnostic information, but also creating a sort of baseline in the spectra. As a consequence, some of these macromolecule/lipid resonances also overlap with metabolite peaks and it is necessary to account for these contributions during the quantification. Therefore, several baseline methods

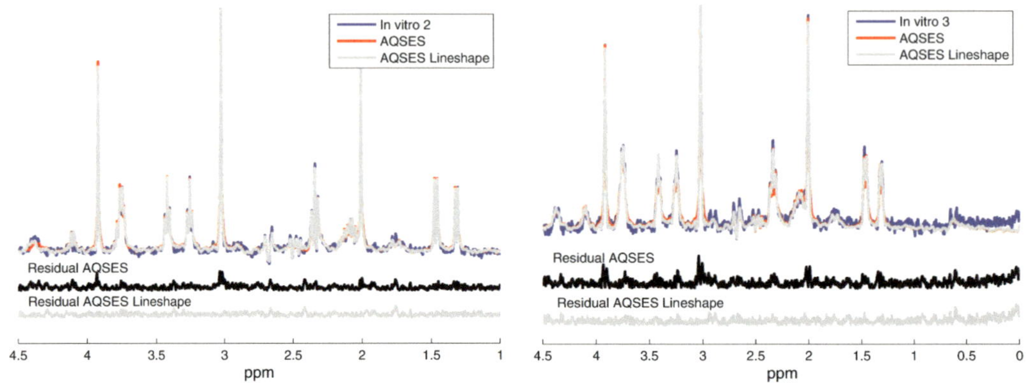

Fig. 9. Spectra of *in vitro* MRS signals measured with a Bruker scanner at 9.4 T containing 7 metabolites: Ala, Cr, Gln, Glu, Lac, NAA, and Tau. Acquisition parameters: PRESS sequence, TR=8 s, TE=20 ms, SW=4 KHz and NDP=2048 points and 128 averages. Two distorted signals were acquired by mis-setting the shim current of the X coil, Left: 'in vitro 2' with linewidth=3.92 Hz and SNR=20. Right: 'in vitro 3' with linewidth=6.52 Hz and SNR=18. Both were quantified by AQSES and AQSES Lineshape.

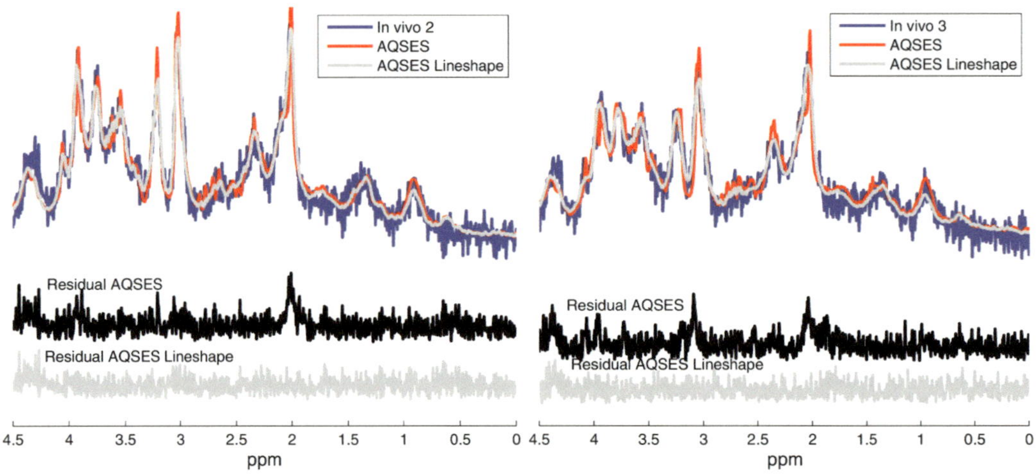

Fig. 10. Rat brain *in vivo* spectra from the right hemisphere of the thalamus measured with a Bruker scanner at 9.4 T with acquisition parameters: PRESS sequence, TR=8 s, TE=20 ms, SW=4 KHz, NDP=2048 points and 128 averages. 'In vivo 2' and 'in vivo 3' were acquired by mis-setting the shimming parameters of the first and second order shim coils X and Z^2. The linewidth for these signals was 27.8 Hz and 39.69 Hz, respectively with SNR=20. Both were quantified by AQSES and AQSES Lineshape.

have been developed based on advanced acquisition techniques using inversion recovery (*i.e.*, metabolite-nulled spectrum) (Cudalbu et al., 2009; Kunz et al., 2010; Mlynárik et al., 2008; Pfeuffer et al., 1999), parametric (Bartha et al., 1999; Seeger et al., 2003) and non-parametric estimation methods (Poullet et al., 2007; Provencher, 2001; Ratiney et al., 2004). Fig. 11 shows an *in vivo* MRS signal from a mouse brain obtained at 9.4 T and the macromolecule/lipid baseline obtained via inversion recovery.

Here, we present a method that extracts characteristic information from a set of inversion recovery MM signals. Thus, individual macromolecule/lipid components are computed and included in the metabolite basis set used in the AQSES quantification method.

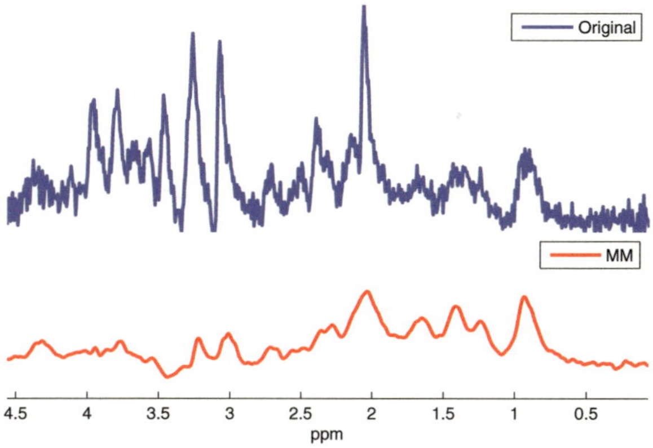

Fig. 11. Real part of the spectrum of an *in vivo* MRS signal and an MM signal obtained from a mouse brain. 'Original' acquisition parameters: Bruker 9.4 T scanner, PRESS sequence, TR=4 s, TE=12 ms, SW=4 KHz and 256 averages. 'MM' acquisition parameters: Bruker 9.4 T scanner, TI=800 ms, TR=3 s, NDP=2048 points and 1024 averages.

Characterization of the macromolecular baseline was addressed by modeling m previously identified profiles shown in Fig. 12 left. Thus, a set of 10 inversion recovery signals was first measured and m individual lipid and macromolecular peaks were identified as *prior knowledge*. These resonances were observed at frequency locations around: 0.89 (MM1), 1.20 (MM2), 1.36 (MM3), 1.63 (MM4), 2.02 (MM5), 2.29 (MM6), 2.65 (MM7), 3.03 (MM8), 3.21 (MM9), 3.75 (MM10), and 4.31 ppm (MM11). The spectral fitting method AMARES (Vanhamme et al., 1997) in jMRUI (Stefan et al., 2009) was used to quantify the set of inversion recovery signals as a sum of 11 damped sinusoids and the mean of amplitudes, frequency locations and linewidths were used to create the individual MM resonances shown in Fig. 12 right. The final MM components are included in the basis set of AQSES subject to small parameter variations.

When lineshape and baseline estimations are considered in the quantification, the model in Eq. (3) changes and $g(t)$ is estimated as:

$$g(t) = \frac{y(t) - B(t)}{\sum_{k=1}^{K} a_k e^{(j\phi_k)} e^{(2\pi j f_k t)} v_k(t) + \sum_{i=1}^{m} \tilde{a}_i e^{(j\tilde{\phi}_i)} e^{(2\pi j \tilde{f}_i t)} MM_i(t)} \quad (4)$$

where $y(t)$ is the experimental signal, $B(t)$ is the non-parametric (spline) baseline from the previous iteration, $MM_i(t)$ is the set of modeled profiles, K is the number of metabolites, $v_k(t)$

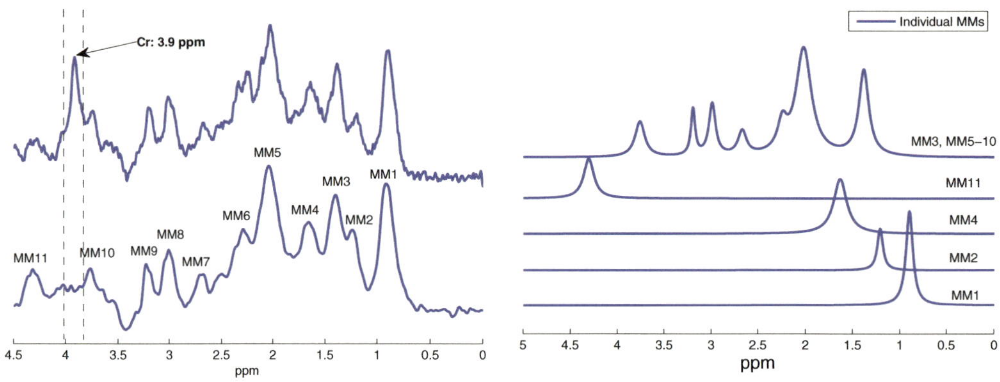

Fig. 12. **Left:** Real part of an *in vivo* metabolite-nulled MM spectrum acquired with a Bruker scanner at 9.4 T with acquisition parameters: TI=800 ms, TR=3 s, NDP=2048 points and 1024 averages. Spectra were post-processed with a 15 Hz Lorentzian line broadening. Due to a shorter T_1, the marked (Cr + PCr) resonance at 3.9 ppm was not completely minimized, therefore this peak was filtered out using HLSVD-PRO (top curve). Macromolecular resonances are labeled as MM from 1 until 11 at the following central frequencies: 0.89, 1.20, 1.36, 1.63, 2.02, 2.29, 2.65, 3.03, 3.21, 3.75, 4.31 ppm; the mean of 10 filtered MM signals is shown in the bottom curve. **Right:** Real part of the MM spectrum obtained with AMARES using *prior knowledge* from the measured inversion recovery signals. This plot shows the individual MMs computed based on the mean of the AMARES estimates of all measured MMs. Small variations are expected for different signals which are then corrected by AQSES.

the metabolite signal k in the basis set, and the amplitudes a_k, $\tilde{a}_i$, frequency shifts f_k, $\tilde{f}_i$ and phase shift ϕ_k, $\tilde{\phi}_i$ are estimated from the previous iteration of the AQSES Lineshape algorithm.

To avoid mis-quantification due to overlapping of MM resonances with metabolites, we combined MM3 with MM5-MM11 to obtain a single profile of seven resonances located in the region between 2 ppm - 4.1 ppm where all important metabolites are resonating. Fig. 13 shows the results of fitting using the mean of inversion recovery measured baselines and the mean of individual MMs obtained with AMARES (*i.e.*, five MM profiles).

3.2.4 Inclusion of spatial constraints in MRSI quantification

Magnetic Resonance Spectroscopic Imaging (MRSI) provides MR spectra from multiple adjacent voxels within a body volume represented as a 2 or 3 dimensional matrix, allowing measurement of the distribution of metabolites over this volume. Commonly, for estimating the metabolite concentrations, the signals within an MRSI grid are analyzed on a single voxel basis by quantifying each signal individually. To this aim, methods such as QUEST (Ratiney et al., 2005), AQSES (Poullet et al., 2007) or AMARES (Vanhamme et al., 1999) may be considered (the list can be extended, see the methods listed at the beginning of section 3). Compared with *in vitro*, *ex vivo* and single voxel *in vivo* MRS signals, *in vivo* MRSI data have a lower quality due to the spatial/spectral trade-off. Moreover, the magnetic field inhomogeneities, relatively low signal-to-noise ratio (SNR) and physiological motion that might appear during an MRSI acquisition compromise the spectral resolution and lead to strongly overlapping metabolite peaks. Therefore, quantifying metabolites within MRSI

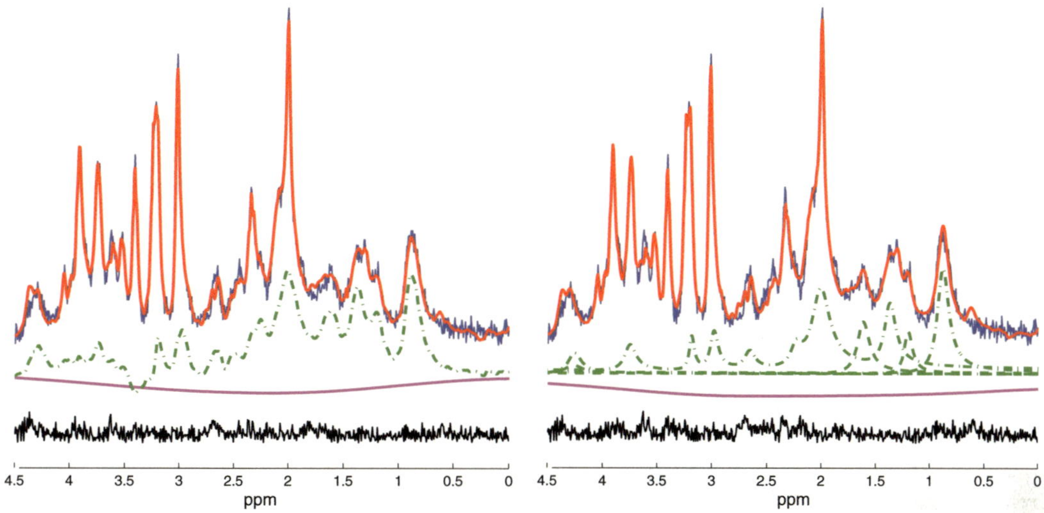

Fig. 13. AQSES fit for the mean spectra of short TE ^{1}H MRS *in vivo* from mouse brains. Real part of the *in vivo* spectrum (noisy signal) together with the fit using AQSES (bold line on top of the signal), MM (dash-dotted curve below the signal), spline baseline (smooth curve below the MM signal) and the residual (noisy line beneath). Quantification was made accounting for the baseline in two ways: (i) considering a metabolite-nulled signal computed as the mean of all measured signals (left) and (ii) considering 5 MM profiles obtained via AMARES (right). Additionally, a very smooth splines function was used to fit any broadening of the baseline.

data on a voxel-by-voxel basis can suffer from accuracy limitations that are inherent to maximum likelihood estimation, and, moreover, it can be prone to faulty convergence to local minima. Since MRSI provides spatial knowledge, in order to improve quantification results, and thus, metabolite estimates in MRSI data, a new metabolite quantification method, in which the available spatial information is exploited, has been proposed. The method, called AQSES-MRSI, is a modified version of AQSES for MRSI data (Croitor Sava et al., 2011).

AQSES-MRSI starts by individually fitting each signal in the grid using nonlinear least squares (Poullet et al., 2007; Sima & Van Huffel, 2007) to extract the spectral parameters, frequencies and dampings, from each voxel which will be further used as *prior knowledge*. Then, for the quantification of each voxel c within the MRSI grid, spatial information is taken into account in more steps. Moreover, several sweeps are performed through the grid and at each run some hyper-parameters may be tuned. Firstly, the starting values for the nonlinear parameters, θ_c (vector containing damping corrections and frequency shifts for voxel c) are optimized by setting them to the median of the parameter values from the considered neighbors $\theta_s (s = 1, \ldots, S$, where S is the total number of voxels in the considered neighborhood). Secondly, optimized bounds on the parameters' variability are computed so that the parameters of the neighboring voxels do not present a high variability. Thirdly, a penalty term that promotes a spatially smooth spectral parameter map for the frequency shifts and damping corrections are imposed, while allowing complete freedom to the metabolite amplitudes. The weight on the smoothness of individual parameters is adjustable:

$$\min_{\theta_c} \frac{1}{N} \sum_{t=t_0}^{t_{N-1}} \left| y_c(t) - \hat{y}_c(t,\theta_c) \right|^2 + \sigma^2 \sum_{\theta_c \neq \theta_s} \varepsilon_s \beta_{cs} \left\| W(\theta_c - \theta_s) \right\|_2^2 \tag{5}$$

where the signal $y_c(t)$ corresponds to voxel c in the grid and the model $\hat{y}_c(t,\theta_c)$ is considered as a weighted sum of metabolite signals with nonlinear corrections θ_c, similarly to the model in Eq. (1). The second term, called penalty term, encourages a smooth solution for the problem. ε_s accounts for the trade-off between an optimal fitting of the current signal and the penalty, σ^2 is an estimate of the noise variance computed from the tail of the signal in time domain in voxel c, β_{cs} is a weighting scalar which gives the influence of the parameters θ_s on the parameters θ_c (as described below), W is a diagonal weighting matrix, with $W \in R^{Km \times Km}$, which accounts for the scale differences between parameters, where K is the number of metabolite profiles and m is the number of parameters per metabolite.

AQSES-MRSI's performance on simulated MRSI data with several types of disturbances and on short echo time *in vivo* proton MRSI data showed improved metabolites estimates compared to quantification of each voxel signal individually, see Fig. 14 and 15. With

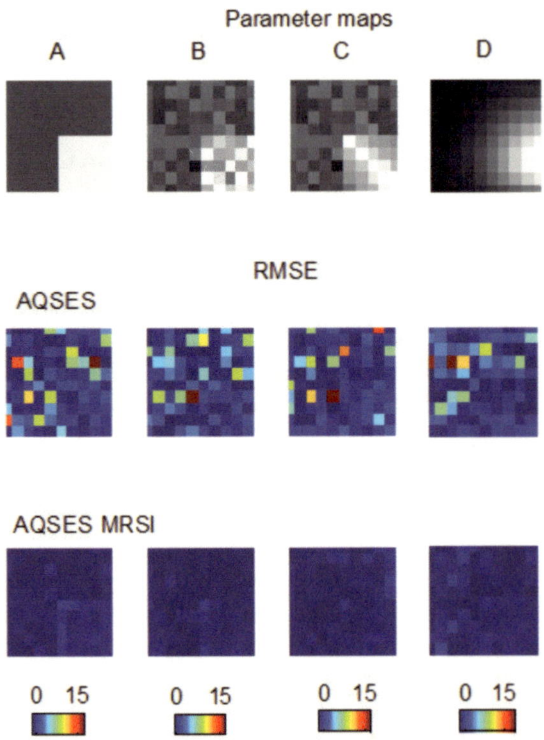

Fig. 14. First row: simulated MRSI grids with different parameter maps: A-D. 2nd and 3rd row illustrate color maps with the values of the error in estimating the metabolite concentrations, computed as a root mean square error (RMSE computed as in (Croitor Sava et al., 2011)), for each voxel for AQSES and AQSES-MRSI, respectively.

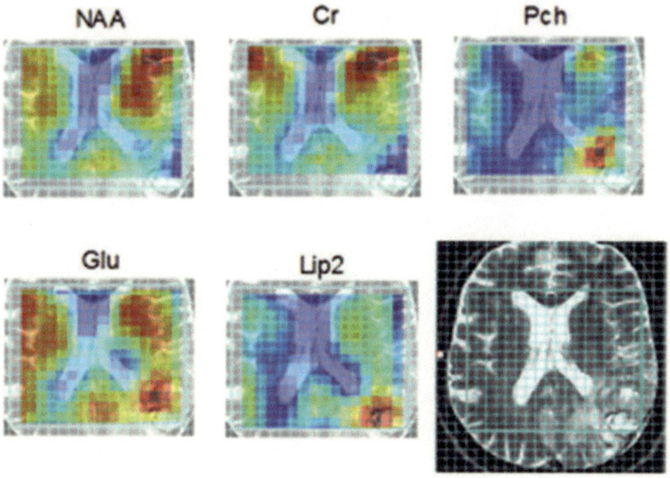

Fig. 15. Metabolic maps obtained after applying AQSES-MRSI. The color scheme is relative to each metabolite. The patient is diagnosed to have glioblastoma tumor (lower right corner of the MRI image).

AQSES-MRSI, overlapping peaks or peaks of compounds present at low concentration can be better resolved than in single-voxel approaches.

Fig. 14 presents four simulated MRSI data sets of 10×10 voxels generated with different levels of inhomogeneities within the parameter maps. 75% of each simulated MRSI grid contains a region with normal-tissue-like spectra and 25% of the grid presents tumor-tissue-like spectra (damping, frequency and amplitude values were set to values corresponding to the signals measured in normal brain and tumor region, respectively). The simulated MRSI signals were obtained as a linear combination of 11 metabolite profiles: NAA, myo-inositol (Myo), Cr, Phosphocholine (PCh), Glu, Lac, Ala, Glc, Tau plus two simulated lipids profiles located at 1.3 ppm (Lip1) and 0.9 ppm (Lip2). These profiles were selected from a measured database acquired with a 1.5 T Philips NT Gyroscan using a PRESS sequence with TE=23 ms, and a PRESS box of $2 \times 2 \times 2$ cm^3. The results illustrated in Fig. 14 show that regardless of the degree of inhomogeneity, AQSES-MRSI outperforms the single voxel approach, AQSES.

Results on an *in vivo* MRSI case (see Fig. 15) show that AQSES-MRSI method provides a much less noisy spatial metabolite distribution compared to single voxel approaches (Croitor Sava et al., 2011). Well-contoured metabolic maps are obtained for all illustrated metabolites. Even metabolites that are difficult to quantify with conventional approaches (see Glu) are well estimated with AQSES-MRSI.

4. Discussion and conclusions

When using HLSVD for filtering the water and unwanted resonances in *in vitro* and *in vivo* MRS(I) signals, the model order plays an important role. Compared to other methods, the overestimation approach is able to suppress distorted lineshape peaks in the presence of low or high SNR. Although we focused on ^{1}H MRS signals, potential implementation with other nuclei is also feasible. Thus, in MRS signals a good peak suppression is essential to achieve accurate quantification results and is therefore important for a correct usage of the signals.

Even though increasing importance has been given to the lineshape of MR signals, many *in vivo* studies seem to still ignore this problem. For not heavily distorted MRS signals, the Lorentzian lineshape is a good approximation to the shape of the experimental data. However, it is advantageous to rely on a method that takes any shape into account. Therefore, AQSES Lineshape works iteratively and evaluates the performance of tuning a more flexible lineshape starting with the Lorentzian model. As a result, quantification of distorted signals with lineshape estimation showed good quantification results for simulated, *in vitro* and *in vivo* distorted signals.

Although the MM signal acquired by inversion recovery is known to provide a good approximation of the macromolecular contamination, it is also true that it requires a long acquisition time and is not reproducible when the conditions of the region of interest are affected by acquisition problems and various diseases. Moreover, it also contains some unsuppressed metabolites. Nevertheless, the baseline information acquired with this method is a good approximation to the expected MM contributions. Therefore, the presented approach includes *prior knowledge* about the frequency locations, amplitudes and linewidths of individual MM profiles, which are beneficial for the quantification method.

Exploiting spatial *prior knowledge* when analyzing MRSI data has been tackled previously (Bao & Maudsley, 2007; Kelm, 2007; Pels, 2005). In all these approaches a common quantification solution is formulated for the whole MRSI grid. Still, due to the heterogeneity of the tissue that characterizes brain tumors, and to the variations induced by magnetic field inhomogeneities, a common optimization over the whole MRSI array may not always provide satisfactory results. With AQSES-MRSI the bounds on the relevant values of the parameters are iteratively adapted, and/or the parameters of the model function take at each iteration new starting values for each voxel. Such a dynamic approach shows improved quantification results and demonstrates that considering spatial information can improve the estimation of metabolite levels.

5. Acknowledgments

Research supported by: GOA MaNet, CoE EF/05/006 Optimization in Engineering (OPTEC), PFV/10/002 (OPTEC), FWO postdoc grants, IBBT, IUAP P6/04 (DYSCO, 'Dynamical systems, control and optimization', 2007-2011), FAST (FP6-MC-RTN-035801), K.U. Leuven Center of Excellence 'MoSAIC'.

6. References

Antoine, J.-P., Coron, A. & Dereppe, J.-M. (2000). Water peak suppression: Time-frequency vs time-scale approach, *Journal of Magnetic Resonance* 144(2): 189 – 194.

Bao, Y. & Maudsley, A. (2007). Improved reconstruction for MR Spectroscopic Imaging, *IEEE Transactions on Medical Imaging* 26(5): 686 –695.

Barkhuijsen, H., de Beer, R. & van Ormondt, D. (1987). Improved algorithm for noniterative time-domain model fitting to exponentially damped magnetic resonance signals, *Journal of Magnetic Resonance* 73(3): 553 – 557.

Bartha, R., Drost, D. J. & Williamson, P. C. (1999). Factors affecting the quantification of short echo *in vivo* ^{1}H MR spectra: prior knowledge, peak elimination, and filtering, *NMR in Biomedicine* 12(4): 205–216.

Bartha, R., Drost, D., Menon, R. & Williamson, P. (2000). Spectroscopic lineshape correction by QUECC: Combined QUALITY deconvolution and eddy current correction, *Magnetic Resonance in Medicine* 44(4): 641–645.

Behar, K. L. & Ogino, T. (1993). Characterization of macromolecule resonances in the ^{1}H NMR spectrum of rat brain, *Magnetic Resonance in Medicine* 30(1): 38–44.

Belkić, D. & Belkić, K. (2006). *In vivo* Magnetic Resonance Spectroscopy by the fast Padé transform, *Physics in Medicine and Biology* 51(5): 1049.

Bhat, H., Sajja, B. R. & Narayana, P. A. (2006). Fast quantification of proton Magnetic Resonance Spectroscopic Imaging with artificial neural networks, *Journal of Magnetic Resonance* 183(1): 110 – 122.

Blamire, A. M., Rothman, D. L. & Nixon, T. (1996). Dynamic shim updating: A new approach towards optimized whole brain shimming, *Magnetic Resonance in Medicine* 36(1): 159–165.

Cabanes, E., Confort-Gouny, S., Fur, Y. L., Simond, G. & Cozzone, P. J. (2001). Optimization of residual water signal removal by HLSVD on simulated short echo time proton MR spectra of the human brain, *Journal of Magnetic Resonance* 150(2): 116 – 125.

Cavassila, S., Deval, S., Huegen, C., van Ormondt, D. & Graveron-Demilly, D. (1999). The beneficial influence of prior knowledge on the quantitation of *In vivo* Magnetic Resonance Spectroscopy signals, *Investigative Radiology* 34: 242–246.

Cavassila, S., Deval, S., Huegen, C., van Ormondt, D. & Graveron-Demilly, D. (2001). Cramér-Rao bounds: an evaluation tool for quantitation, *NMR in Biomedicine* 14(4): 278–283.

Chang, D., Banack, C. D. & Shah, S. L. (2007). Robust baseline correction algorithm for signal dense NMR spectra, *Journal of Magnetic Resonance* 187(2): 288 – 292.

Chen, H., Van Huffel, S., van Ormondt, D. & de Beer, R. (1996). Parameter estimation with *Prior Knowledge* of known signal poles for the quantification of NMR spectroscopy data in the time domain, *Journal of Magnetic Resonance, Series A* 119(2): 225 – 234.

Chen, J.-H., Sambol, E. B., Kennealey, P. T., O'Connor, R. B., DeCarolis, P. L., Cory, D. G. & Singer, S. (2004). Water suppression without signal loss in HR-MAS ^{1}H NMR of cells and tissues, *Journal of Magnetic Resonance* 171(1): 143 – 150.

Chen, L., Weng, Z., Goh, L. & Garland, M. (2002). An efficient algorithm for automatic phase correction of NMR spectra based on entropy minimization -ACME, *Journal of Magnetic Resonance* 158(1-2): 164 – 168.

Chu, W. C. W., Chik, K., Chan, Y., Yeung, D. K. W., Roebuck, D. J., Howard, R. G., Li, C. & Metreweli, C. (2003). White matter and cerebral metabolite changes in children undergoing treatment for acute lymphoblastic leukemia: Longitudinal study with MR imaging and ^{1}H MR spectroscopy, *Radiology* 229(3): 659–669.

Cleveland, W. S. (1979). Robust locally weighted regression and smoothing scatterplots, *Journal of the American Statistical Association* 74(368): pp. 829–836.

Cobas, J. C., Bernstein, M. A., Martín-Pastor, M. & Tahoces, P. G. (2006). A new general-purpose fully automatic baseline-correction procedure for 1D and 2D NMR data, *Journal of Magnetic Resonance* 183(1): 145 – 151.

Cobas, J. C. & Sardina, F. J. (2003). Nuclear Magnetic Resonance data processing. MestRe-C: A software package for desktop computers, *Concepts in Magnetic Resonance Part A* 19A(2): 80–96.

Croitor Sava, A. R., Sima, D. M., Poullet, J.-B., Wright, A. J., Heerschap, A. & Van Huffel, S. (2011). Exploiting spatial information to estimate metabolite levels in two-dimensional MRSI of heterogeneous brain lesions, *NMR in Biomedicine* 24(7): 824–835.

Croitor Sava, A. R. (2011). *Signal processing and classification for Magnetic Resonance Spectroscopy with clinical applications*, PhD thesis.

Cudalbu, C., Mlynárik, V., Xin, L. & Gruetter, R. (2009). Quantification of *in vivo* short echo-time proton magnetic resonance spectra at 14.1 T using two different approaches of modelling the macromolecule spectrum, *Measurement Science and Technology* 20(10): 104034 (7pp).

de Graaf, A. A., van Dijk, J. E. & BoéE, W. M. M. J. (1990). Quality: quantification improvement by converting lineshapes to the Lorentzian type, *Magnetic Resonance in Medicine* 13(3): 343–357.

de Graaf, R. (1998). *In vivo NMR Spectroscopy – Principles and Techniques*, Wiley: Chichester.

De Neuter, B., Luts, J., L., V., Lemmerling, P. & Van Huffel, S. (2007). Java-based framework for processing and displaying short-echo-time Magnetic Resonance Spectroscopy signals, *Computer Methods and Programs in Biomedicine* 85: 129–137.

Devos, A., Lukas, L., Suykens, J., Vanhamme, L., Tate, A., Howe, F., Majós, C., Moreno-Torres, A., van der Graaf, M., Arús, C. & Huffel, S. V. (2004). Classification of brain tumours using short echo time ^{1}H MR spectra, *Journal of Magnetic Resonance* 170(1): 164 – 175.

Dologlou, I., Van Huffel, S. & Van Ormondt, D. (1998). Frequency-selective MRS data quantification with frequency *Prior Knowledge*, *Journal of Magnetic Resonance* 130(2): 238 – 243.

Dong, Z., Dreher, W. & Leibfritz, D. (2006). Toward quantitative short-echo-time *in vivo* proton MR spectroscopy without water suppression, *Magnetic Resonance in Medicine* 55(6): 1441–1446.

Eilers, P. H. C. & Marx, B. D. (1996). Flexible smoothing with B-splines and penalties, *Statistical Science* 11: 89–121.

Elster, C., Schubert, F., Link, A., Walzel, M., Seifert, F. & Rinneberg, H. (2005). Quantitative Magnetic Resonance Spectroscopy: Semi-parametric modeling and determination of uncertainties, *Magnetic Resonance in Medicine* 53(6): 1288–1296.

Gabr, R. E., Ouwerkerk, R. & Bottomley, P. A. (2006). Quantifying *in vivo* MR spectra with circles, *Journal of Magnetic Resonance* 179(1): 152 – 163.

Giskeødegård, G. F., Bloemberg, T. G., Postma, G., Sitter, B., Tessem, M.-B., Gribbestad, I. S., Bathen, T. F. & Buydens, L. M. (2010). Alignment of high resolution magic angle spinning magnetic resonance spectra using warping methods, *Analytica Chimica Acta* 683(1): 1 – 11.

Gruetter, R. (1993). Automatic localized *in vivo* adjustment of all first- and second- order shim coils, *Magnetic Resonance in Medicine* 29(6): 804–811.

Guo, Y., Ruan, S., Landré, J. & Constans, J. M. (2010). A sparse representation method for Magnetic Resonance Spectroscopy quantification, *IEEE Transactions on Biomedical Engineering* 57(7): 1620 –1627.

Hao, J., Zou, X., Wilson, M. P., Davies, N. P., Sun, Y., Peet, A. C. & Arvanitis, T. N. (2009). A comparative study of feature extraction and blind source separation of independent component analysis (ICA) on childhood brain tumour ^{1}H magnetic resonance spectra, *NMR in Biomedicine* 22(8): 809–818.

Hiltunen, Y., Kaartinen, J., Pulkkinen, J., Häkkinen, A.-M., Lundbom, N. & Kauppinen, R. A. (2002). Quantification of human brain metabolites from *in vivo* ^{1}H NMR magnitude spectra using automated artificial neural network analysis, *Journal of Magnetic Resonance* 154(1): 1 – 5.

Hofmann, L., Slotboom, J., Boesch, C. & Kreis, R. (2001). Characterization of the macromolecule baseline in localized ^{1}H-MR spectra of human brain, *Magnetic Resonance in Medicine* 46(5): 855–863.

Hu, S.-L. J., Bao, X. & Li, H. (2010). Model order determination and noise removal for modal parameter estimation, *Mechanical Systems and Signal Processing* 24(6): 1605 – 1620.

Huang, W., Alexander, G. E., Chang, L., Shetty, H. U., Krasuski, J. S., Rapoport, S. I. & Schapiro, M. B. (2001). Brain metabolite concentration and dementia severity in Alzheimer's disease, *Neurology* 57(4): 626–632.

Jiru, F. (2008). Introduction to post-processing techniques, *European journal of radiology* 67(2): 202–217.

Juchem, C., Nixon, T. W., McIntyre, S., Rothman, D. L. & de Graaf, R. A. (2010). Magnetic field homogenization of the human prefrontal cortex with a set of localized electrical coils, *Magnetic Resonance in Medicine* 63(1): 171–180.

Kelm, B. (2007). *Evaluation of Vector-Valued Clinical Image Data Using Probabilistic Graphical Models: Quantification and Pattern Recognition*, PhD thesis.

Klose, U. (1990). *In vivo* proton spectroscopy in presence of eddy currents, *Magnetic Resonance in Medicine* 14(1): 26 – 30.

Knight-Scott, J. (1999). Application of multiple inversion recovery for suppression of macromolecule resonances in short echo time ^{1}H NMR spectroscopy of human brain, *Journal of Magnetic Resonance* 140(1): 228 – 234.

Kunz, N., Cudalbu, C., Mlynárik, V., Hüppi, P. S., Sizonenko, S. V. & Gruetter, R. (2010). Diffusion-weighted spectroscopy: A novel approach to determine macromolecule resonances in short-echo time ^{1}H-MRS, *Magnetic Resonance in Medicine* 64(4): 939–946.

Laudadio, T., Mastronardi, N., Vanhamme, L., Hecke, P. V. & Huffel, S. V. (2002). Improved Lanczos algorithms for blackbox MRS data quantitation, *Journal of Magnetic Resonance* 157(2): 292 – 297.

Laudadio, T., Selén, Y., Vanhamme, L., Stoica, P., Hecke, P. V. & Huffel, S. V. (2004). Subspace-based MRS data quantitation of multiplets using *prior knowledge*, *Journal of Magnetic Resonance* 168(1): 53 – 65.

Lazariev, A., Allouche, A.-R., Aubert-Frécon, M., Fauvelle, F., Elbayed, K., Piotto, M., Namer, I. J., van Ormondt, D. & Graveron-Demilly, D. (2011). Optimization of metabolite basis-sets prior to quantitation: a quantum mechanics approach, *Proc. of the 19th International Society of Magnetic Resonance in Medicine - ISMRM 2011*.

Lin, Y.-Y., Hodgkinson, P., Ernst, M. & Pines, A. (1997). A novel detection-estimation scheme for noisy NMR signals: Applications to delayed acquisition data, *Journal of Magnetic Resonance* 128(1): 30 – 41.

Maudsley, A. A. (1995). Spectral lineshape determination by self-deconvolution, *Journal of Magnetic Resonance, series B* 106(1): 47 – 57.

Metz, K. R., Lam, M. M. & Webb, A. G. (2000). Reference deconvolution: A simple and effective method for resolution enhancement in Nuclear Magnetic Resonance Spectroscopy, *Concepts in Magnetic Resonance* 12(1): 21–42.

Metzger, G. J., Patel, M. & Hu, X. (1996). Application of genetic algorithms to spectral quantification, *Journal of Magnetic Resonance, Series B* 110(3): 316 – 320.

Mierisová, S. & Ala-Korpela, M. (2001). MR Spectroscopy quantitation: a review of frequency domain methods, *NMR in Biomedicine* 14(4): 247–259.

Mlynárik, V., Cudalbu, C., Xin, L. & Gruetter, R. (2008). ^{1}H NMR Spectroscopy of rat brain *in vivo* at 14.1 Tesla: Improvements in quantification of the neurochemical profile, *Journal of Magnetic Resonance* 194(2): 163 – 168.

Osorio-Garcia, M. (2011). *Advanced signal processing for Magnetic Resonance Spectroscopy*, PhD thesis.

Osorio-Garcia, M. I., Sima, D. M., Nielsen, F. U., Himmelreich, U. & Van Huffel, S. (2011). Quantification of Magnetic Resonance Spectroscopy signals with lineshape estimation, *Journal of Chemometrics* 25(4): 183–192.

Papy, J.-M., De Lathauwer, L. & Van Huffel, S. (2007). A shift invariance-based order-selection technique for exponential data modelling, *IEEE Signal Processing Letters* 14(7).

Pels, P. (2005). *Analysis and Improvement of Quantification Algorithms for Magnetic Resonance Spectroscopy*, PhD thesis.

Pfeuffer, J., Tkáč, I., Provencher, S. & Gruetter, R. (1999). Toward an *in vivo* neurochemical profile: Quantification of 18 metabolites in short-echo-time ^{1}H NMR spectra of the rat brain, *Journal of Magnetic Resonance* 141(1): 104 – 120.

Pijnappel, W. W. F., van den Boogaart, A., de Beer, R. & van Ormondt, D. (1992). SVD-based quantification of Magnetic Resonance signals, *Journal of Magnetic Resonance (1969)* 97(1): 122 – 134.

Popa, E., Karras, D., Mertzios, B., Sima, D., de Beer, R., van Ormondt, D. & Graveron-Demilly, D. (2011). Semi-parametric estimation without searching in function space. Application to *in vivo* metabolite quantitation, *Measurement Science and Technology* (Epub) ahead of print, 2011.

Poullet, J.-B. (2008). Spid: Simulation Package based on *in vitro* databases.
URL: *http://homes.esat.kuleuven.be/ biomed/software.php*

Poullet, J.-B., Sima, D. M., Simonetti, A. W., De Neuter, B., Vanhamme, L., Lemmerling, P. & Van Huffel, S. (2007). An automated quantitation of short echo time MRS spectra in an open source software environment: AQSES, *NMR in Biomedicine* 20(5): 493–504.

Poullet, J.-B., Sima, D. M. & Van Huffel, S. (2008). MRS signal quantitation: A review of time- and frequency-domain methods, *Journal of Magnetic Resonance* 195(2): 134 – 144.

Provencher, S. W. (1993). Estimation of metabolite concentrations from localized *in vivo* proton NMR spectra, *Magnetic Resonance in Medicine* 30(6): 672–679.

Provencher, S. W. (2001). Automatic quantitation of localized *in vivo* ^{1}H spectra with LCModel, *NMR Biomed.* 14(4): 260–264.

Ratiney, H., Coenradie, Y., Cavassila, S., van Ormondt, D. & Graveron-Demilly, D. (2004). Time-domain quantitation of ^{1}H short echo-time signals: background accommodation, *Magnetic Resonance Materials in Physics, Biology and Medicine* 16: 284–296.

Ratiney, H., Sdika, M., Coenradie, Y., Cavassila, S., Ormondt, D. v. & Graveron-Demilly, D. (2005). Time-domain semi-parametric estimation based on a metabolite basis set, *NMR in Biomedicine* 18(1): 1–13.

Reynolds, G., Wilson, M., Peet, A. & Arvanitis, T. N. (2006). An algorithm for the automated quantitation of metabolites in *in vitro* NMR signals, *Magnetic Resonance in Medicine* 56(6): 1211–1219.

Romano, R., Motta, A., Camassa, S., Pagano, C., Santini, M. T. & Indovina, P. L. (2002). A new time-domain frequency-selective quantification algorithm, *Journal of Magnetic Resonance* 155(2): 226 – 235.

Ruiz-Pena, J. L., Pinero, P., Sellers, G., Argente, J., Casado, A., Foronda, J., Ucles, A. & Izquierdo, G. (2004). Magnetic resonance spectroscopy of normal appearing white matter in early relapsing-remitting multiple sclerosis: correlations between disability and spectroscopy, *BMC Neurology* 4(1): 8.

Seeger, U., Klose, U., Mader, I., Grodd, W. & Nägele, T. (2003). Parameterized evaluation of macromolecules and lipids in proton MR Spectroscopy of brain diseases, *Magnetic Resonance in Medicine* 49(1): 19–28.

Sima, D. M., Osorio-Garcia, M. I., Poullet, J.-B., Suvichakorn, A., Antoine, J.-P., Huffel, S. V. & van Ormondt, D. (2009). Lineshape estimation for Magnetic Resonance Spectroscopy (MRS) signals: self-deconvolution revisited, *Measurement Science and Technology* 20(10): 104031.

Sima, D. M. & Van Huffel, S. (2007). Separable nonlinear least squares fitting with linear bound constraints and its application in magnetic resonance spectroscopy data quantification, *Journal of Computational and Applied Mathematics* 203: 264–278.

Slotboom, J., Boesch, C. & Kreis, R. (1998). Versatile frequency domain fitting using time domain models and *prior knowledge*, *Magnetic Resonance in Medicine* 39(6): 899–911.

Soher, B. J., Young, K., Govindaraju, V. & Maudsley, A. A. (1998). Automated spectral analysis III: Application to *in vivo* proton MR spectroscopy and spectroscopic imaging, *Magnetic Resonance in Medicine* 40(6): 822–831.

Stefan, D., Di Cesare, F., Andrasescu, A., Popa, E., Lazariev, A., Vescovo, E., Strbak, O., Williams, S., Starčuk, Z., Cabanas, M., van Ormondt, D. & Graveron-Demilly, D. (2009). Quantitation of Magnetic Resonance Spectroscopy signals: the jMRUI software package, *Measurement Science and Technology* 20(10): 104035.

Stoyanova, R. & Brown, T. R. (2001). NMR spectral quantitation by Principal Component Analysis, *NMR in Biomedicine* 14(4): 271–277.

Sundin, T., Vanhamme, L., Van Hecke, P., Dologlou, I. & Van Huffel, S. (1999). Accurate quantification of ^{1}H spectra: From finite impulse response filter design for solvent suppression to parameter estimation, *Journal of Magnetic Resonance* 139(2): 189 – 204.

van den Boogaart, A. (1997). Quantitative data analysis of *in vivo* MRS data sets, *Magnetic Resonance in Chemistry* 35(13): 146–152.

van der Veen, J. W., de Beer, R., Luyten, P. R. & van Ormondt, D. (1988). Accurate quantification of *in vivo* ^{31}P NMR signals using the variable projection method and *prior knowledge*, *Magnetic Resonance in Medicine* 6(1): 92–98.

Van Huffel, S. & Vandewalle, J. (1991). *The Total Least Squares Problem: Computational Aspects and Analysis*, SIAM.

Vanhamme, L., Huffel, S. V., Hecke, P. V. & van Ormondt, D. (1999). Time-domain quantification of series of biomedical magnetic resonance spectroscopy signals, *Journal of Magnetic Resonance* 140(1): 120 – 130.

Vanhamme, L., Sundin, T., Van Hecke, P. & Van Huffel, S. (2001). MR spectroscopy quantitation: a review of time-domain methods, *NMR in Biomedicine* 14(4): 233–246.

Vanhamme, L., van den Boogaart, A. & Van Huffel, S. (1997). Improved method for accurate and efficient quantification of MRS data with use of *Prior Knowledge*, *Journal of Magnetic Resonance* 129(1): 35 – 43.

Vermathen, P., Laxer, K. D., Schuff, N., Matson, G. B. & Weiner, M. W. (2003). Evidence of neuronal injury outside the medial temporal lobe in temporal lobe epilepsy: N-Acetylaspartate concentration reductions detected with multisection Proton MR Spectroscopic Imaging - Initial experience, *Radiology* 226(1): 195–202.

Veselkov, K. A., Lindon, J. C., Ebbels, T. M. D., Crockford, D., Volynkin, V. V., Holmes, E., Davies, D. B. & Nicholson, J. K. (2009). Recursive segment-wise peak alignment of biological ^{1}H NMR spectra for improved metabolic biomarker recovery, *Analytical Chemistry* 81(1): 56–66.

Wilson, M., Reynolds, G., Kauppinen, R. A., Arvanitis, T. N. & Peet, A. C. (2011). A constrained least-squares approach to the automated quantitation of *in vivo* ^{1}H Magnetic Resonance Spectroscopy data, *Magnetic Resonance in Medicine* 65(1): 1–12.

Xi, Y. & Rocke, D. (2008). Baseline correction for NMR spectroscopic metabolomics data analysis, *BMC Bioinformatics* 9(1): 324.

Young, K., Govindaraju, V., Soher, B. J. & Maudsley, A. A. (1998). Automated spectral analysis I: Formation of *a priori* information by spectral simulation, *Magnetic Resonance in Medicine* 40(6): 812–815.

2

^{13}C Magnetic Resonance Spectroscopy in Neurobiology - Its Use in Monitoring Brain Energy Metabolism and in Identifying Novel Metabolic Substrates and Metabolic Pathways

Bjørnar Hassel
Department of Neurohabilitation, Oslo University Hospital-Ullevål, Oslo
Norwegian Defense Research Establishment, Kjeller
Norway

1. Introduction

A wealth of information on brain metabolism has been gathered from studies in which ^{13}C-labeled metabolic substrates (often glucose) have been administered to human subjects or experimental animals. ^{13}C Magnetic resonance spectroscopy (MRS[1]) of the brain (or extracts of brain) has shown to what degree the ^{13}C-labeled compound has been metabolized, and, to some extent, along which metabolic pathways. The latter interpretation derives from the fact that ^{13}C MRS shows the ^{13}C labeling not of individual compounds, e.g. amino acids, but of individual carbon positions in those different compounds (Fig. 1). Because some enzymes of amino acid metabolism have a cell-specific expression, it is possible to study the metabolic activity of individual cell types or the transfer of amino acids between them. Finally, ^{13}C MRS allows studies of a host of substrates to examine their potential as metabolic substrates for the brain. An extensive review, which included an overview of technical aspects of ^{13}C MRS in studies of brain and cultured brain cells, appeared recently (Rodrigues et al., 2009).

2. ^{13}C MRS for the visualization of brain energy metabolism

Glucose is considered the physiologic energy substrate of the brain and is used by all brain cells, neurons and glial cells alike. Glucose consumption is tightly coupled to the need for energy (ATP), which in the brain largely reflects neuronal activity, or more specifically, depolarization of neuronal cell membranes. The membrane potential derives from the ionic gradients created by ion pumps that transport sodium and potassium against their concentration gradients across cell membranes, an activity that is fuelled by ATP (Attwell and Laughlin, 2001). Therefore, alterations in neuronal activity will be reflected in changes in glucose consumption, and, conversely, constraints in the availability of glucose and oxygen will limit neuronal activity. ^{13}C MRS after administration of ^{13}C-labeled glucose to

[1] Abbreviations:ATP: adenosine triphosphate, CoA: coenzyme A, GABA: γ-aminobutyrate, i.v. intravenously, MRS: magnetic resonance spectroscopy, PET; positron emission tomography, TCA cycle: tricarboxylic acid cycle.

human volunteers or to experimental animals is well suited to investigate the relationship between neuronal activity, energy requirements, and glucose metabolism, because several of the downstream metabolites of glucose (lactate, alanine, glutamate, glutamine GABA, aspartate – see Fig. 1) can be detected by ^{13}C MRS.

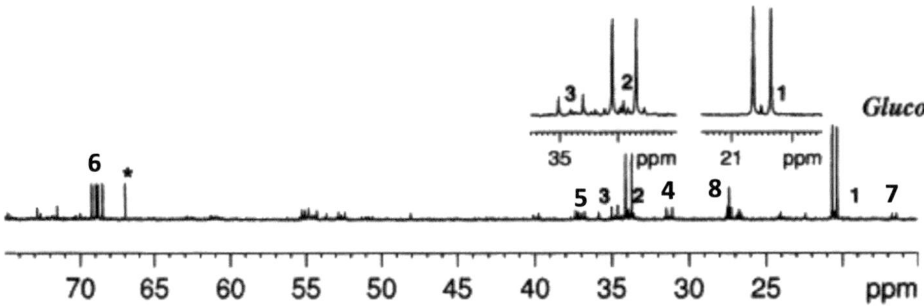

Fig. 1. ^{13}C MR spectrum of a brain extract from a mouse that received 150 μmol [U- ^{13}C] glucose intravenously in the awake state and was sacrificed after 5 minutes. Peak numbers: 1, lactate C3; 2, glutamate C4; 3, GABA C2; 4, glutamine C4, 5, aspartate C3, 6: lactate C2; 7, alanine C3, 8: glutamate C3, which is labeled after a full turn of the TCA cycle. *Internal standard (dioxane). Note the strong ^{13}C labeling of glutamate C4 and lactate C3 from [U-^{13}C]glucose. Reprinted from Nguyen et al., 2003, with permission from the publisher.

Administration of ^{13}C-labeled glucose intravenously (i.v.) or intraperitoneally leads to predominant labeling of glutamate in the brain (Figs. 1 and 2). This is so, because glutamate is present in concentrations that allow detection by ^{13}C MRS, and because virtually all glucose that enters the brain is metabolized through glutamate: glutamate equilibrates with α-ketoglutarate of the tricarboxylic acid (TCA) cycle, through which glucose is metabolized oxidatively. Briefly, ^{13}C-glucose is metabolized to ^{13}C-acetyl-CoA, which reacts with oxaloacetate to form citrate. Acetyl-CoA gives rise to the 1st and 2nd carbons of citrate, which correspond to the 5th and 4th carbon positions in α-ketoglutarate and glutamate (Fig. 2). Logically, these two positions are the first to be labeled from glucose, provided that uniformly labeled glucose, [U-^{13}C]glucose is being used. If [1-^{13}C]glucose is used, which is often the case, the 2nd position of acetyl-CoA becomes labeled, and hence the 4th position of glutamate (e.g. Fitzpatrick et al., 1990; Shank et al., 1993; Mason et al., 1999; see Figs. 1 and 2).

However, when α-ketoglutarate is metabolized further through the TCA cycle, succinate is formed. Succinate has four carbon atoms and is symmetrical, so the label is now scrambled between the 1st + 2nd positions and the 3rd + 4th positions (or the 2nd and 3rd positions if [1-^{13}C]glucose is being used). From succinate fumarate, malate, and oxaloacetate are formed before another molecule of acetyl-CoA enters the TCA cycle to form citrate. The labeling of the 2nd and 3rd positions in succinate, fumarate, malate, and oxaloacetate correspond to the 2nd and 3rd positions in glutamate. Labeling of these positions in glutamate reflects passage of ^{13}C through the TCA cycle (Fig. 1 and 2). From the labeling of the 2nd and 3rd vs. the 4th positions in glutamate from [1-^{13}C]glucose an impression of the TCA cycle rate may be gained, or the rate may even be calculated (Hassel et al., 1995a; 1997; Mason et al., 1999; Hyder et al., 2003).

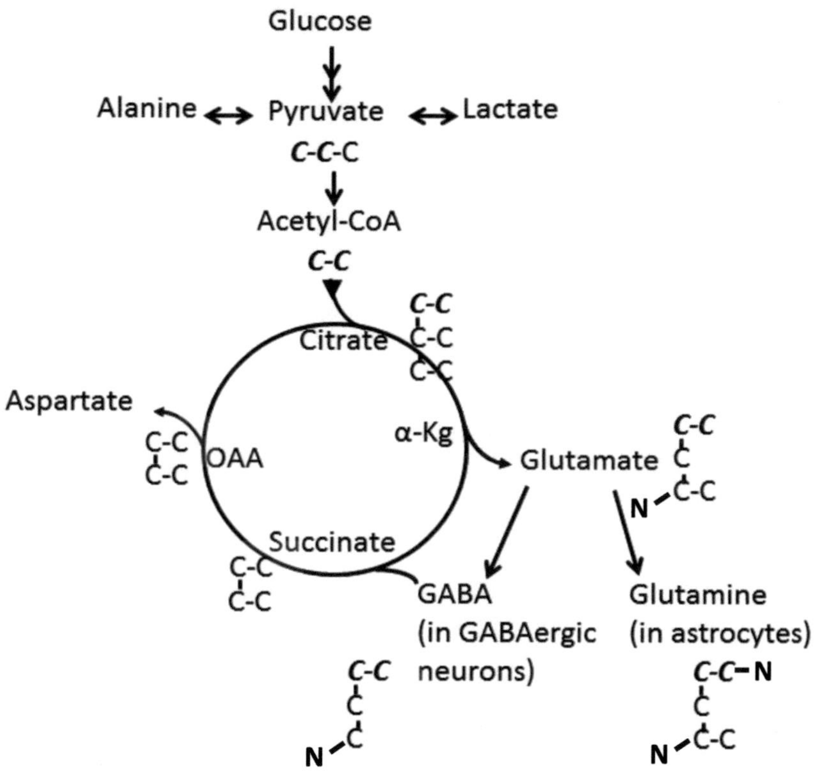

Fig. 2. Simplified scheme of glycolysis and the TCA cycle. Glucose is metabolized glycolytically to pyruvate, which may undergo decarboxylation in the pyruvate dehydrogenase reaction to become acetyl-CoA. Acetyl-CoA enters the TCA cycle to condense with oxaloacetate (OAA) and form citrate. The two carbons from acetyl-CoA that contribute to citrate (and hence α-ketoglutarate, glutamate, glutamine and GABA) are shown in italics. Due to the symmetry of succinate these two carbons are distributed evenly between the C1+C2 positions and the C3+C4 positions in succinate and in fumarate, malate and oxaloacetate, which are formed downstream of succinate. Pyruvate may also become aminated to alanine or reduced to lactate.

Oxaloacetate equilibrates with aspartate, and whereas oxaloacetate at a tissue concentration of ~10 nmol/g brain tissue (Siesjö, 1978) defies detection by ^{13}C MRS, aspartate is readily detected, especially its 2nd and 3rd carbon positions, the labeling of which reflects the passage of ^{13}C through the TCA cycle (Figs. 1 and 2). It has been shown with various techniques that aspartate is concentrated in GABAergic neurons (Ottersen and Storm-Mathisen, 1985; Hassel et al., 1992; 1995b). With ^{13}C MRS this has been verified by blocking the TCA cycle of GABAergic neurons specifically; this leads to a marked reduction in the ^{13}C labeling of aspartate from [1-^{13}C]glucose (Hassel and Sonnewald, 1995a; Johannessen et al., 2001).

Inhibition of TCA cycle activity by drugs or toxins may reduce the ^{13}C labeling of glutamate, GABA, or glutamine from [^{13}C]glucose (e.g. Hassel and Sonnewald, 1995a). But because TCA cycle activity is closely coupled to neuronal activity, any influence that reduces brain activity (e.g. anesthetics, antiepileptic drugs) will reduce glucose metabolism in the brain and hence ^{13}C labeling of glucose metabolites. Therefore, a reduction in the labeling of cerebral metabolites from [^{13}C]glucose must be interpreted with some caution. Such a reduction does not necessarily imply a direct effect, e.g. of a drug, on TCA cycle activity, for instance through enzyme inhibition.

Conversely, any influence that leads to increased activation of the brain may increase glucose metabolism and increase ^{13}C labeling from [^{13}C]glucose. Such effects have been seen in human subjects and in rats (Hyder et al., 1996; Patel et al., 2004). However, it should be noted that although previous studies on a variety of experimentally induced conditions, including epileptic seizures and stroke, have shown increased uptake of the glucose analogue deoxyglucose by positron emission tomography (PET) or autoradiographic methods, data obtained with ^{13}C MRS seem to indicate that the oxidative metabolism of glucose may be only little affected or even reduced (Petroff et al., 2002; Eloqayli et al., 2004; Nguyen et al., 2007a; Pan et al., 2008; Håberg et al., 2009). The same is true for other conditions that would be expected to entail an increased energy demand, e.g. traumatic brain injury (Bartnik et al., 2007; Scafidi et al., 2009). Deoxyglucose is a substrate for the glucose transporter in the blood-brain barrier and in neurons, as well as for the first enzyme of glucose metabolism, hexokinase, which phopsphorylates glucose and deoxyglucose to their 6-phospho- derivatives. But once phophorylated deoxyglucose is not metabolized further and accumulates intracellularly; this allows its detection by PET or autoradiography. It follows that the deoxyglucose-based methods strictly detect the transport and initial phosphorylation of deoxyglucose, whereas ^{13}C MRS detection of glutamate labeling from [^{13}C]glucose reflects both glycolytic and oxidative metabolic activity in the brain.

The possibility of visualizing brain energy metabolism appeared to pave the way for studies in which brain activity, including sensory activation and thought processes, could be monitored by ^{13}C MRS. It soon became clear, however, that the increase in glucose metabolism caused by various forms of physiological activation, was quite small, and not always readily detectable on the background of a high basal metabolic rate in the un-anesthetized brain (Shulman et al., 2004).

3. Visualization of the metabolic interplay between astrocytes and neurons

The cellular complexity of the brain makes it difficult to assess the metabolic activity of individual cell types separately. However, because some metabolic pathways are unique to certain cells, and because some metabolic substrates are metabolized selectively by certain cell types, some degree of metabolic dissection of the brain is made possible. First we consider the transfer of glutamine from astrocytes to neurons as a precursor for glutamate and GABA in neurons. Thereafter we discuss the transfer of glutamate from neurons to astrocytes during glutamatergic neurotransmission.

In the brain, acetate is metabolized oxidatively by astrocytes and not by neurons. Because astrocytes express glutamine synthetase (Martinez-Hernandez et al., 1977), isotopically labeled acetate (given i.v. or intracerebrally) leads to preferential labeling of glutamine (van den Berg et al., 1969; Hassel et al., 1997; Lebon et al., 2002; Deelchand et al., 2009). Glutamine is exported from astrocytes to the extracellular fluid, from where it is taken up by neurons, both glutamatergic and GABAergic. Inside neurons glutamine becomes deamidated to glutamate by phosphate-activated glutaminase (Kvamme et al., 2001), a mitochondrial enzyme, which in the brain appears to be expressed only by neurons. In GABAergic neurons the glutamine-derived glutamate becomes decarboxylated to GABA by glutamic acid decarboxylase (GAD), an enzyme that in the brain is expressed in inhibitory GABAergic neurons (Fonnum et al., 1970). Therefore, when administration of ^{13}C-labeled acetate to experimental animals leads to ^{13}C labeling of GABA, this labeling illustrates a series of metabolic and transport-related events (Fig. 3) that highlights the role of (astrocytic) glutamine as a precursor of (neuronal) glutamate and GABA (Hassel et al., 1997).

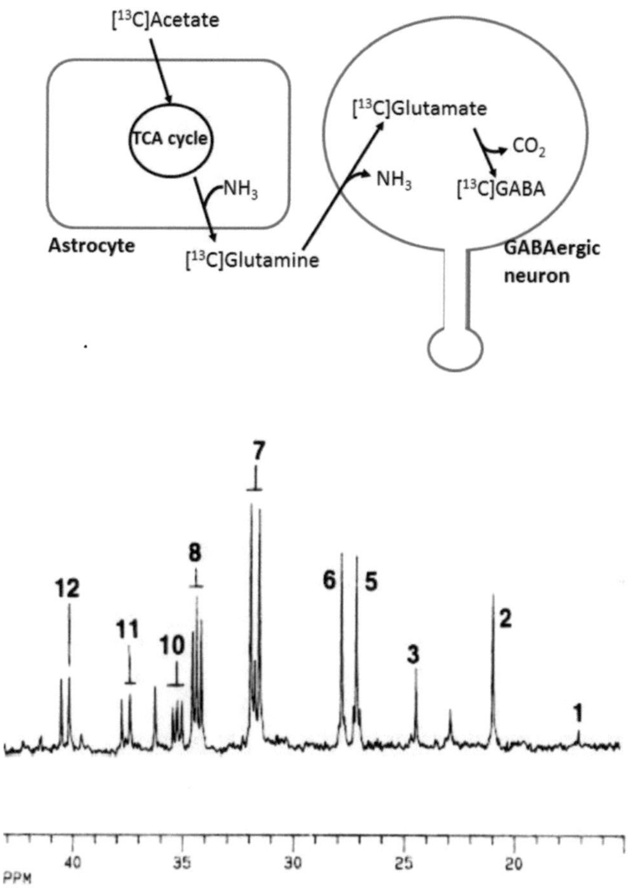

Fig. 3. Metabolism of [^{13}C]acetate in astrocytes with formation of [^{13}C]glutamine, which is transferred to neurons, where it is deamidated to [^{13}C]glutamate. In GABAergic neurons [^{13}C]glutamate is decarboxylated to [^{13}C]GABA. The spectrum is from a brain extract from a mouse that received [1,2-^{13}C]acetate, 150 µmol i.v. and was sacrificed after 15 minutes. Peaks are: 1, alanine C-3; 2, lactate C-3; 3, GABA C-3; 5, glutamine C-3; 6, glutamate C-3; 7, glutamine C-4; 8, glutamate C-4; 10, GABA C-2; 11, aspartate C-3; 12, GABA C-4. Note the strong labeling of glutamine compared to results with [^{13}C]glucose (Fig. 1) (From Hassel et al., 1997, with permission from the publisher). Thus, formation of [^{13}C]GABA from [^{13}C]acetate illustrates astrocytic uptake and oxidative metabolism of [^{13}C]acetate, glutamine synthetase activity, the activity of glutamine transporters at the astrocytic and neuronal cell membranes, neuronal glutaminase activity, and glutamate decarboxylase activity.

An enigma of brain metabolism is why acetate is oxidized only by astrocytes and not by neurons. Waniewski and Martin (1998) provided evidence that acetate is taken up across the cell membrane only in astrocytes. This finding was unexpected, since acetate is a small monocarboxylate, for which neurons are richly equipped with transporters (Bergersen, 2007). Nguyen et al (2007b) later found that neurons take up propionate (which is closely related to acetate), which suggested that even acetate is taken up (but not metabolized) by neurons. Later it was found that administration of propionate to mice leads to an increase in brain GABA levels, suggesting an inhibitory action of propionate on the GABA-degrading enzyme GABA transaminase (Hassel et al., unpublished). GABA transaminase is an intramitochondrial enzyme in GABAergic neurons (Schousboe et al., 1974), and its inhibition by a small monocarboxylate such as propionate suggests that propionate (and acetate) is taken up by neurons and neuronal mitochondria, but that the latter are deficient in the enzyme that converts acetate and propionate into their mitochondrial CoA derivatives.

Because glutamate is readily labeled from ^{13}C-labeled precursors, there has been considerable interest in identifying transmitter glutamate with ^{13}C MRS. Glutamate is the main excitatory neurotransmitter in the central nervous system. While glutamate serves many functions in the brain, it has been estimated that 2-20% of the total amount of brain glutamate serves a neurotransmitter function (Hassel and Dingledine, 2006). After release from synaptic nerve endings glutamate is largely taken up by astrocytes that surround the synaptic cleft, and converted into glutamine (Danbolt, 2001). This process may be illustrated with ^{13}C MRS. Administration of ^{13}C-labeled glucose to experimental animals leads to rapid ^{13}C labeling of glutamate and, after a delay, of glutamine. This labeling of glutamine to a large extent reflects uptake of (neuronal) transmitter glutamate into astrocytes. This was shown in an experiment in which mice had their astrocytic TCA cycle inhibited by the glia-specific metabolic inhibitor fluoroacetate (Hassel et al., 1997). The mice could not form glutamate or glutamine through their TCA cycle activity, but they still produced ^{13}C-glutamine from ^{13}C-glucose. Formation of glutamine from ^{13}C-glucose was interpreted to reflect formation of ^{13}C-glutamate from ^{13}C-glucose in neurons, release of ^{13}C-labeled transmitter glutamate from neurons, uptake into astrocytes of the released ^{13}C-labeled transmitter glutamate and subsequent amidation by glutamine synthetase (Fig. 4).

The exchange between neurons and astrocytes of glutamate and glutamine has been the subject of many studies, in both human subjects and experimental animals (Shen et al., 1999; see Rothman et al., 1999; 2003, for review). Interpretation of ^{13}C MRS after infusion of ^{13}C-labeled glucose into awake humans indicated that the flux of glutamate from neurons to astrocytes was close to 50% of the cerebral metabolism of glucose. This would suggest a massive transfer of glutamate from neurons to astrocytes. However, if this is true, it is still not known whether all this glutamate is transmitter glutamate in the sense that it originates from presynaptic vesicles.

In ^{13}C MRS studies of the brain, acetate is used as a glial substrate, and glucose is used as an energy substrate for all brain cells, but with a dominant contribution from (glutamatergic) neurons. As will become evident below ('Identification of alternative substrates for brain energy metabolism'), lactate and pyruvate have become regarded as more purely neuronal substrates that are used by glutamatergic and GABAergic neurons alike, whereas glycerol appears to be a substrate specifically used by GABAergic neurons (Nguyen et al., 2003). Thus, some degree of metabolic dissection of the brain is made possible by combining the administration of an appropriate ^{13}C-labeled energy substrate with ^{13}C MRS.

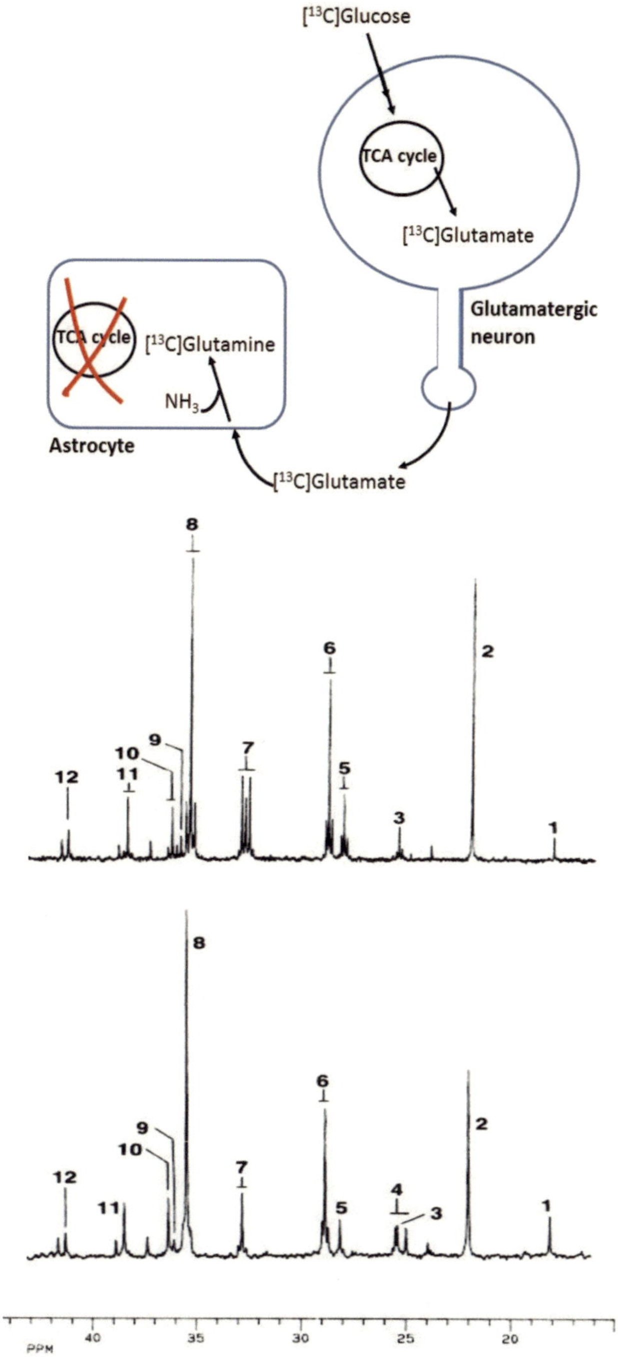

Fig. 4. Uptake of transmitter glutamate by astrocytes. In this experiment mice received the glia-specific metabolic inhibitor fluoroacetate, which blocks the astrocytic TCA cycle at the level of aconitase. Thus, the ability of astrocytes to form glutamate and hence glutamine from α-ketoglutarate from their own TCA cycle was blocked. Even so, glutamine was

formed from [^{13}C]glucose, presumably because ^{13}C-labeled transmitter glutamate was still being released from neurons and taken up by astrocytes with subsequent formation of [^{13}C]glutamine. The upper spectrum is from the brain of a mouse that received [1,2-^{13}C]acetate and [1-^{13}C]glucose. The doubly labeled acetate gives rise to the double peaks in glutamine C4 (peak 7). The lower spectrum is from a mouse, whose astrocytic TCA ycle was blocked by fluoroacetate; here only glutamine labeled from [1-^{13}C]glucose (single peak 7) can be seen (From Hassel et al., 1997, with permission from the publisher).

4. Identification of alternative substrates for brain energy metabolism

Serum glucose is considered the physiological energy substrate of the brain. Even so, a number of substrates may feed into the glycolytic pathway or the TCA cycle of brain cells. For example, lactate, which was shown by ^{13}C MRS to be a substrate for brain metabolism in mice (Hassel and Bråthe, 2000), was recently shown by ^{13}C MRS to contribute importantly to energy metabolism in the human brain under physiological conditions (Gallagher et al., 2009; Boumezbeur et al., 2010). The ability of a substrate to function as a metabolic substrate for brain cells depends on its ability to cross the blood-brain barrier, i.e. on the presence of specific transporter proteins in the barrier. Further, brain cells must have the necessary transporters to take the substrates up from the extracellular fluid as well as the enzymes necessary for their metabolism. A substrate that is not metabolized in the brain after i.v. injection may prove to be metabolized after intracerebral injection, a finding that points to transport limitations at the blood-brain barrier; this holds true for dicarboxylates like fumarate and malate (Hassel et al., 2002); if injected directly into the brain parenchyma, these substrates are taken up into astrocytes and rapidly metabolized through the TCA cycle to glutamine, indicating the presence of the plasma membrane dicarboxylate transporter predominantly in astrocytes. A similar situation exists for the monosaccharide fructose (Hassel et al., submitted), which hardly crosses the blood-brain barrier at all. This can be shown by giving mice [^{13}C]fructose i.v.; in contrast to liver, the brain does not accumulate the injected [^{13}C]fructose, as can be shown by ^{13}C MRS of brain and liver extracts. However, if fructose is injected into the brain parenchyma, it becomes metabolized. The oxidation of fructose by brain tissue would explain the ability of fructose to support energy-requiring processes, such a axonal activity, in vitro (Meakin et al., 2007).

Even though a substrate crosses the blood-brain barrier, the enzymatic machinery required for its metabolism may not be present in the brain. An example is propionate, which readily crosses the blood-brain barrier, but hardly becomes metabolized in the brain (Nguyen et al., 2007b; Morland et al., in prep). The enzymes required for the initial metabolism of propionate, propionyl-CoA synthetase is expressed at low levels, making it difficult to detect propionate metabolites by ^{13}C MRS after i.v. administration of [^{13}C]propionate to experimental animals. Cerebral metabolism of propionate may be detected with radiolabeled propionate, however, owing to the higher sensitivity of radiodetective methods (scintillation counting) than of ^{13}C MRS (Nguyen et al., 2007b).

With the use of ^{13}C MRS β-hydroxybutyrate (Künnecke et al., 1993; Pan et al., 2002; Andrews et al., 2009), lactate (Hassel and Bråthe, 2000; Tyson et al., 2003; Boumezbeur et al., 2010), and pyruvate (Gonzalez et al., 2005) have been shown to be energy substrates for the brain after i.v. injection, pointing to the existence of the appropriate monocarboxylate transporters at the blood-brain barrier. The predominant labeling of glutamate (over glutamine) points to a predominantly neuronal metabolism of these subtrates (Fig. 5). Even octanoate has been shown to be metabolized by the brain (Ebert et al., 2003), suggesting a certain capacity for fatty acid metabolism in the brain; the preferential labeling of glutamine pointed to astrocytes as the main metabolic compartment.

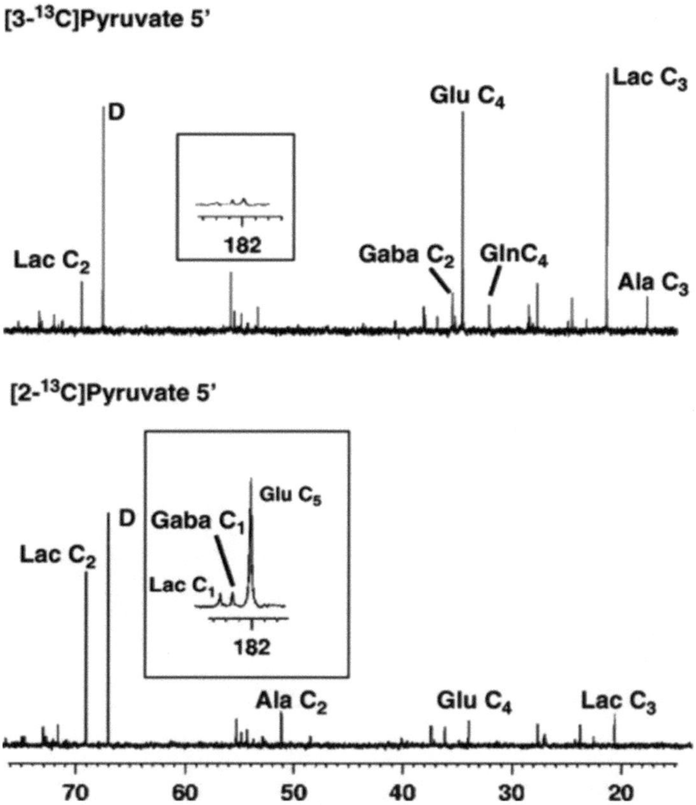

Fig. 5. ^{13}C MR spectra of brain extracts of mice that received [3-^{13}C]pyruvate or [2-^{13}C]pyruvate i.v. The (labeling of) individual carbon positions in certain metabolites is indicated. Wake mice received 9 mmoles/kg [3-^{13}C]pyruvate (upper panel) or [2-^{13}C]pyruvate (lower panel) i.v. Survival time was 5 min. [3-^{13}C]Pyruvate labels the C3 of lactate (Lac) and alanine (Ala), the C4 of glutamate (Glu) and glutamine (Gln), and GABA C2 (but not glutamate C5 or the C1 of GABA or lactate; insert). [2-^{13}C]Pyruvate labels lactate and alanine C2, and glutamate C5, GABA C1 and lactate C1 (insert). D is dioxane (internal standard). The peak corresponding to Glu C4 in lower spectrum represents naturally abundant ^{13}C-glutamate. Reprinted from Gonzalez et al., 2005, with permission from the publisher.

^{13}C-Labeled acetate also yields good labeling of cerebral amino acids, predominantly glutamine, after i.v. injection, a finding that points to their metabolism in astrocytes (see above, 3. Visualization of the metabolic interplay between astrocytes and neurons). The labeling of amino acids in the brain from [^{13}C]acetate is on a level similar to that achieved with [^{13}C]glucose (Hassel et al., 1995a;1997), which suggests that acetate could support brain energy metabolism; this has been shown in hypoglycemic mice (Urion et al., 1979).

An interesting example of the power of ^{13}C MRS in elucidating cell-specific metabolism in the CNS is the avid labeling of GABA from [^{13}C]glycerol (Nguyen et al., 2003); this labeling greatly exceeded that of glutamate and glutamine (Fig. 6), pointing to GABAergic neurons as the predominant cell compartment for glycerol metabolism. A later ^{13}C MRS study showed that glycerol is being produced from glucose by both neurons and astrocytes and that this production increases during hypoxia or epileptic seizures (Nguyen et al., 2007c). The two findings put together (formation of glycerol in both neurons and astrocytes and its metabolism by GABAergic neurons) could point to a 'glycerol cycle' in the brain.

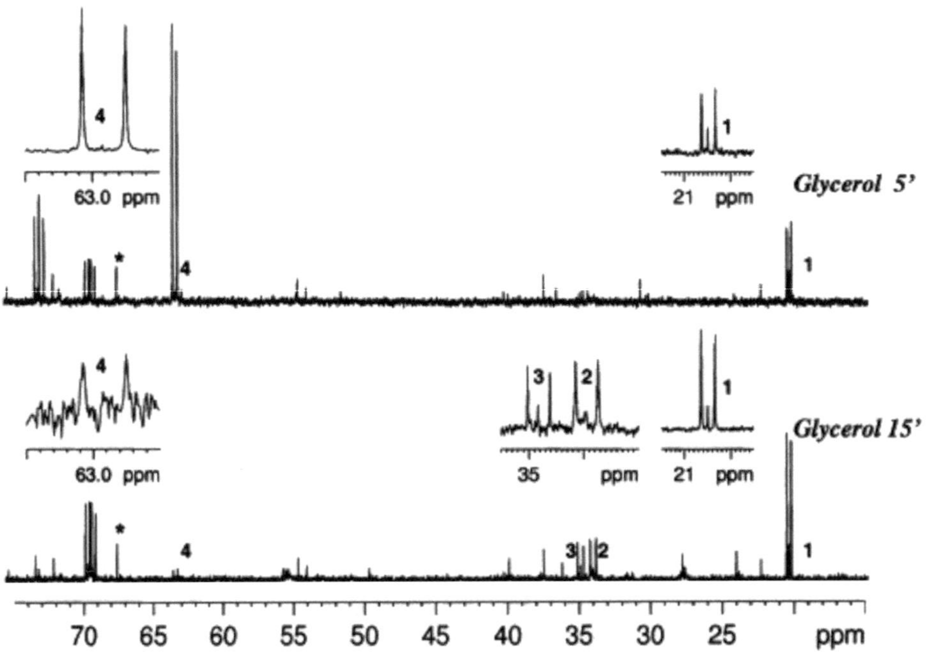

Fig. 6. ^{13}C MR spectra of brain extracts from mice that received [U- ^{13}C]glycerol i.v. Wake mice received 150 µmol [U-^{13}C]glycerol and were killed at 5 or 15 min. Peak numbers: 1, lactate C3; 2, glutamate C4; 3, GABA C2; 4, glycerol C1 + C3. *Internal standard (dioxane). Note the strong labeling of GABA C2 relative to glutamate C4 at 15 min after injection of [U-^{13}C]glycerol in comparison with the much higher labeling of glutamate from ^{13}C-labeled glucose or pyruvate (Figs. 1 and 5). Reprinted from Nguyen et al., 2003, with permission from the publisher.

5. Identification of metabolic pathways from the ^{13}C labeling of specific carbon positions in glutamate and glutamine

In the second paragraph of this paper ('^{13}C MRS for the visualization of brain energy metabolism') the ^{13}C labeling of glutamate from [^{13}C]glucose through TCA cycle activity is described. In fact, any ^{13}C-labeled substrate that gives rise to ^{13}C-labeled acetyl-CoA will label glutamate and glutamine in positions that reflect the entry of label into the TCA cycle and its subsequent turning in the cycle. This applies to ^{13}C-labeled lactate, pyruvate, alanine, beta-hydroxybutyrate, acetate, butyrate, glycerol, and others. However, substrates that give rise to ^{13}C-labeled pyruvate in the brain (glucose, pyruvate, lactate, alanine, glycerol) may enter the TCA cycle through two different enzymatic routes. The first, which gives rise to acetyl-CoA, is pyruvate dehydrogenase, which removes a carboxylic group from pyruvate in the form of CO_2. The second route involves the addition of a carboxylic group (from CO_2 or HCO_3^-) to pyruvate to produce oxaloacetate or its immediate precursor malate (See upper part of Fig. 7); these reactions are known as pyruvate carboxylation. In astrocytes, the reaction is catalyzed by pyruvate carboxylase, in neurons, it may be catalyzed by malic enzyme. These reactions are 'anaplerotic', meaning that they function to 'fill up' the TCA cycle with intermediates. They are thought to compensate for the loss of α-ketoglutarate inherent in export of glutamine from astrocytes and for the similar loss of α-ketoglutarate inherent in glutamatergic and GABAergic neurotransmission when (See below) astrocytes take up glutamate or GABA from the synaptic cleft.

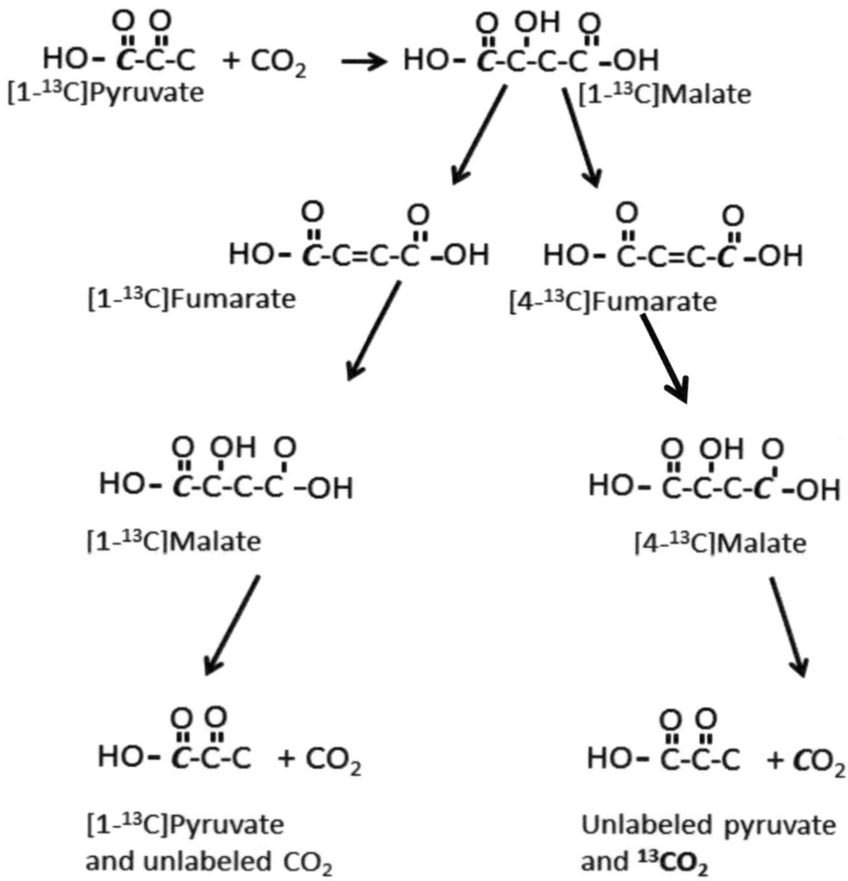

Fig. 7. Reversible pyruvate carboxylation and equilibration of malate with fumarate, which explains rapid formation of $^{13}CO_2$ from [1-^{13}C]pyruvate. [1-^{13}C]Pyruvate undergoes carboxylation to [1-^{13}C]malate, presumably by malic enzyme. [1-^{13}C]Malate equilibrates with the symmetrical fumarate, so that both [1-^{13}C]malate and [4-^{13}C]malate are formed. Decarboxylation of these malates produces $^{13}CO_2$ as well as unlabeled CO_2. The ^{13}C is represented in italics.

When pyruvate is ^{13}C-labeled these reactions lead to the formation of ^{13}C-labeled malate and oxaloacetate. Pyruvate labeled in the 3rd carbon (which originates from glucose labeled in the 1st position, [1-^{13}C]glucose) leads to formation of malate or oxaloacetate labeled in the 3rd carbon. This carbon position corresponds to the 2nd carbon in glutamate and glutamine. In several studies the greater labeling of the 2nd than the 3rd carbon in glutamine has been taken as evidence of pyruvate carboxylase activity in astrocytes (Shank et al., 1993; Hassel et al., 1995a; Serres et al., 2008). A similar preferential labeling of the 2nd over the 3rd carbon in glutamate has not been consistently found, apparently pointing to the absence of pyruvate carboxylation in neurons. However, oxaloacetate and malate tend to equilibrate with the symmetrical fumarate, leading to scrambling of label between the two carbon position. ^{13}C MRS evidence of such scrambling in neurons has been reported in both cultured neurons (Merle et al., 1996) and in vivo (Hassel et al., 2000; Gonzalez et al., 2005). Another way to study pyruvate carboxylation is to use glucose labeled in the 2nd position. Glucose labeled in this position ([2-^{13}C]glucose) does not label acetyl-CoA, but it may label the 2nd and 3rd positions in glutamate and glutamine through pyruvate carboxylation. Mason et al (2007) showed in awake human subjects the flux through pyruvate carboxylation to be approximately 6% of that through pyruvate dehydrogenase (the activity of which was studied with [1-^{13}C]glucose). This value was in good agreement with previous ^{13}C MRS studies in rats (Shank et al., 1993) and with previous estimates based on radiolabeling studies (Van den Berg, 1973).

Formation of pyruvate from TCA cycle intermediates malate or oxaloacetate (through the decarboxylating activities of malic enzyme and phosphoenolpyruvate carboxykinase, respectively) is termed pyruvate recycling. This process takes place in the brain (Cerdan et al., 1990; Hassel and Sonnewald, 1995b; Cruz et al., 1998) as it does in liver. In one study this process was identified in brain by ^{13}C MRS of brain extracts from rats that had received [^{13}C]acetate, which labeled lactate (Hassel and Sonnewald, 1995b). Such labeling can only occur through formation of pyruvate from TCA cycle intermediates. When pyruvate thus formed (and labeled) enters the TCA cycle through pyruvate dehydrogenase a distinct labeling pattern may be seen in glutamate (Cerdan et al., 1990; Håberg et al., 1998). Valid criticism of the interpretation of previous studies has come from Serres et al. (2008) who pointed out that hepatic gluconeogenesis with ^{13}C labeling of serum glucose from [^{13}C]acetate may influence findings in the brain. However, pyruvate recycling also occurs in cultured brain cells (astrocytes), in which hepatic gluconeogenesis is not an issue (Sonnewald et al., 1996).

With the use of ^{13}C MRS Gruetter and colleagues were able to determine the concentration and turnover of glycogen in the intact brain (van Heeswijk et al., 2010), and they also described the formation of N-acetyl-aspartate, which is present in the brain at high concentrations, from [^{13}C]glucose, and they determined the turnover rate of this presumed 'inert' compound (Choi et al., 2004).

6. The use of hyperpolarization of ^{13}C to increase MRS sensitivity

A problem with ^{13}C MRS is the low sensitivity of the method. This weakness implies that ^{13}C-labeled metabolic substrates have to be given in large amounts to achieve detection of their metabolites. In contrast, radiolabeling studies are done with minute quantities of substrate. In an attempt to improve ^{13}C MRS sensitivity, hyperpolarization of ^{13}C-labeled substrates has been done prior to i.v. injection. The MRS signal may thus be enhanced more than 10,000 times (Ardenkjaer-Larsen et al., 2003). In some studies pyruvate, which is labeled in the carboxylic position, [1-^{13}C]pyruvate, has been used (Hurd et al., 2010; Marjańska et al., 2010; Mayer et al., 2011). The [^{13}C]pyruvate is hyperpolarized immediately before i.v. injection. The hyperpolarization is lost within some seconds, however, and the detection of metabolism of pyruvate is restricted to ^{13}C-labeled lactate, alanine, and CO_2 (see Fig. 2). Formation of $^{13}CO_2$ has been interpreted to reflect pyruvate dehydrogenase activity, i.e. the formation of acetyl-CoA, which may enter the TCA cycle to form citrate. But in the brain the activity of pyruvate dehydrogenase is quite low (Morland et al., 2007), and formation of TCA cycle intermediates and related amino acids takes several minutes (Gonzalez et al., 2005), so a more likely explanation for the formation of $^{13}CO_2$ within a few seconds is reversible pyruvate carboxylation (Fig. 3): [^{13}C]pyruvate is carboxylated to [^{13}C]malate, which equilibrates with (the symmetrical) fumarate, so that ^{13}C is distributed evenly between the two carboxylic groups of fumarate. [^{13}C]Fumarate equilibrates with malate, which may become decarboxylated to pyruvate and CO_2. Some of this CO_2 will then be ^{13}C-labeled. This series of reactions has been described in the brain with the use of [2-^{13}C]pyruvate and [3-^{13}C]pyruvate (Gonzalez et al., 2005), and they occur much more rapidly than the pyruvate dehydrogenase reaction. Another issue in studies that use hyperpolarized substrates is the use of anesthesia, which reduces brain metabolism of ^{13}C-labeled substrates markedly (Shank et al., 1993).

Hyperpolarized [^{13}C]pyruvate may prove useful in the diagnostic workup of malignant tumors, including brain tumors, which show a greater tendency to convert [^{13}C]pyruvate into [^{13}C]lactate than the normal surrounding tissue. Some recent studies even suggest the possibility of monitoring tumor response to therapy from the reduced conversion of pyruvate into lactate within a day's time after irradiation or chemotherapy (Day et al., 2007; 2011; Park et al., 2011).

7. References

Andrews MT, Russeth KP, Drewes LR, Henry PG. (2009) Adaptive mechanisms regulate preferred utilization of ketones in the heart and brain of a hibernating mammal during arousal from torpor. Am. J. Physiol. Regul. Integr. Comp. Physiol. 296:R383-393.

Ardenkjaer-Larsen JH, Fridlund B, Gram A, Hansson G, Hansson L, Lerche MH, Servin R, Thaning M, Golman K. (2003) Increase in signal-to-noise ratio of > 10,000 times in liquid-state NMR. Proc. Natl. Acad. Sci. U. S. A. 100:10158-10163.

Attwell D, Laughlin SB. (2001) An energy budget for signaling in the grey matter of the brain. J. Cereb. Blood Flow Metab. 21:1133-1145.

Bartnik BL, Lee SM, Hovda DA, Sutton RL. (2007) The fate of glucose during the period of decreased metabolism after fluid percussion injury: a 13C NMR study. J. Neurotrauma. 24:1079-1092.

Bergersen LH. (2007) Is lactate food for neurons? Comparison of monocarboxylate transporter subtypes in brain and muscle. Neuroscience 145:11-19.

Boumezbeur F, Petersen KF, Cline GW, Mason GF, Behar KL, Shulman GI, Rothman DL. (2010) The contribution of blood lactate to brain energy metabolism in humans measured by dynamic ^{13}C nuclear magnetic resonance spectroscopy. J. Neurosci. 30:13983-13991.

Cerdan S, Künnecke B, Seelig J. (1990) Cerebral metabolism of [1,2-$^{13}C_2$]acetate as detected by in vivo and in vitro ^{13}C NMR. J. Biol. Chem. 265:12916-12926.

Choi IY, Gruetter R. (2004) Dynamic or inert metabolism? Turnover of N-acetyl aspartate and glutathione from D-[1-^{13}C]glucose in the rat brain in vivo. J. Neurochem. 91:778-787.

Cruz F, Scott SR, Barroso I, Santisteban P, Cerdán S. (1998) Ontogeny and cellular localization of the pyruvate recycling system in rat brain. J. Neurochem. 70:2613-2619.

Danbolt NC. (2001) Glutamate uptake. Prog. Neurobiol. 65:1-105.

Day SE, Kettunen MI, Gallagher FA, Hu DE, Lerche M, Wolber J, Golman K, Ardenkjaer-Larsen JH, Brindle KM. (2007) Detecting tumor response to treatment using hyperpolarized ^{13}C magnetic resonance imaging and spectroscopy. Nat. Med. 13:1382-1387.

Day SE, Kettunen MI, Cherukuri MK, Mitchell JB, Lizak MJ, Morris HD, Matsumoto S, Koretsky AP, Brindle KM. (2011) Detecting response of rat C6 glioma tumors to radiotherapy using hyperpolarized [1- ^{13}C]pyruvate and ^{13}C magnetic resonance spectroscopic imaging. Magn. Reson. Med. 65:557-563.

Deelchand DK, Shestov AA, Koski DM, Uğurbil K, Henry PG. (2009) Acetate transport and utilization in the rat brain. J. Neurochem. 109 Suppl 1:46-54.

Ebert D, Haller RG, Walton ME. (2003) Energy contribution of octanoate to intact rat brain metabolism measured by ^{13}C nuclear magnetic resonance spectroscopy. J. Neurosci. 23:5928-5935.

Eloqayli H, Dahl CB, Götestam KG, Unsgård G, Sonnewald U. (2004) Changes of glial-neuronal interaction and metabolism after a subconvulsive dose of pentylenetetrazole. Neurochem. Int. 45:739-745.

Fitzpatrick SM, Hetherington HP, Behar KL, Shulman RG. (1990) The flux from glucose to glutamate in the rat brain in vivo as determined by ^{1}H-observed, ^{13}C-edited NMR spectroscopy. J. Cereb. Blood Flow Metab. 10:170-179.

Fonnum F, Storm-Mathisen J, Walberg F. (1970) Glutamate decarboxylase in inhibitory neurons. A study of the enzyme in Purkinje cell axons and boutons in the cat. Brain Res. 20:259-275.

Gallagher CN, Carpenter KL, Grice P, Howe DJ, Mason A, Timofeev I, Menon DK, Kirkpatrick PJ, Pickard JD, Sutherland GR, Hutchinson PJ. (2009) The human brain utilizes lactate via the tricarboxylic acid cycle: a ^{13}C-labelled microdialysis and high-resolution nuclear magnetic resonance study. Brain 132:2839-2849.

Gonzalez SV, Nguyen NH, Rise F, Hassel B. (2005) Brain metabolism of exogenous pyruvate. J. Neurochem. 95:284-293.

Hassel B, Paulsen RE, Johnsen A, Fonnum F. (1992) Selective inhibition of glial cell metabolism in vivo by fluorocitrate. Brain Res. 576:120-124.

Hassel B, Sonnewald U, Fonnum F. (1995a) Glial-neuronal interactions as studied by cerebral metabolism of [2-^{13}C]acetate and [1-^{13}C]glucose: an ex vivo ^{13}C NMR spectroscopic study. J. Neurochem. 64:2773-2782.

Hassel B, Westergaard N, Schousboe A, Fonnum F. (1995b) Metabolic differences between primary cultures of astrocytes and neurons from cerebellum and cerebral cortex. Effects of fluorocitrate. Neurochem. Res. 20:413-420.

Hassel B, Sonnewald U. (1995a) Selective inhibition of the tricarboxylic acid cycle of GABAergic neurons with 3-nitropropionic acid in vivo. J. Neurochem. 65:1184-1191.

Hassel B, Sonnewald U. (1995b) Glial formation of pyruvate and lactate from TCA cycle intermediates: implications for the inactivation of transmitter amino acids? J. Neurochem. 65:2227-2234.

Hassel B, Bachelard H, Jones P, Fonnum F, Sonnewald U. (1997) Trafficking of amino acids between neurons and glia in vivo. Effects of inhibition of glial metabolism by fluoroacetate. J. Cereb. Blood Flow Metab. 17:1230-1238.

Hassel B, Bråthe A. (2000) Cerebral metabolism of lactate in vivo: evidence for neuronal pyruvate carboxylation. J. Cereb. Blood Flow Metab. 20:327-336.

Hassel B, Dingledine R. (2006) Glutamate. In GJ Siegel (ed) *Basic Neurochemistry*. Elsevier, pp. 267-290.

Hurd RE, Yen YF, Mayer D, Chen A, Wilson D, Kohler S, Bok R, Vigneron D, Kurhanewicz J, Tropp J, Spielman D, Pfefferbaum A. (2010) Metabolic imaging in the anesthetized rat brain using hyperpolarized [1-^{13}C] pyruvate and [1-^{13}C] ethyl pyruvate. Magn. Reson. Med. 63:1137-1143.

Hyder F, Chase JR, Behar KL, Mason GF, Siddeek M, Rothman DL, Shulman RG. (1996) Increased tricarboxylic acid cycle flux in rat brain during forepaw stimulation detected with ^{1}H[^{13}C]NMR. Proc. Natl. Acad. Sci. U. S. A. 93:7612-7617.

Hyder F, Brown P, Nixon TW, Behar KL. (2003) Mapping cerebral glutamate ^{13}C turnover and oxygen consumption by in vivo NMR. Adv. Exp. Med. Biol. 530:29-39.

Håberg A, Qu H, Bakken IJ, Sande LM, White LR, Haraldseth O, Unsgård G, Aasly J, Sonnewald U. (1998) In vitro and ex vivo ^{13}C-NMR spectroscopy studies of pyruvate recycling in brain. Dev. Neurosci. 20:389-398.

Håberg AK, Qu H, Sonnewald U. (2009) Acute changes in intermediary metabolism in cerebellum and contralateral hemisphere following middle cerebral artery occlusion in rat. J. Neurochem. 109 Suppl 1:174-181.

Johannessen CU, Qu H, Sonnewald U, Hassel B, Fonnum F. (2001) Estimation of aspartate synthesis in GABAergic neurons in mice by 13 C NMR spectroscopy. Neuroreport 12:3729-3732.

Künnecke B, Cerdan S, Seelig J. (1993) Cerebral metabolism of [1,2-$^{13}C_2$]glucose and [U-$^{13}C_4$]3-hydroxybutyrate in rat brain as detected by ^{13}C NMR spectroscopy. NMR Biomed. 6:264-277.

Kvamme E, Torgner IA, Roberg B. (2001) Kinetics and localization of brain phosphate activated glutaminase. J. Neurosci. Res. 66:951-958.

Lebon V, Petersen KF, Cline GW, Shen J, Mason GF, Dufour S, Behar KL, Shulman GI, Rothman DL. (2002) Astroglial contribution to brain energy metabolism in humans revealed by ^{13}C nuclear magnetic resonance spectroscopy: elucidation of the dominant pathway for neurotransmitter glutamate repletion and measurement of astrocytic oxidative metabolism. J. Neurosci. 22:1523-1531.

Marjańska M, Iltis I, Shestov AA, Deelchand DK, Nelson C, Uğurbil K, Henry PG. (2010) In vivo ^{13}C spectroscopy in the rat brain using hyperpolarized [1-^{13}C]pyruvate and [2-^{13}C]pyruvate. J. Magn. Reson. 206:210-218.

Martinez-Hernandez A, Bell KP, Norenberg MD. (1977) Glutamine synthetase: glial localization in brain. Science 195:1356-1358.

Mason GF, Pan JW, Chu WJ, Newcomer BR, Zhang Y, Orr R, Hetherington HP. (1999) Measurement of the tricarboxylic acid cycle rate in human grey and white matter in vivo by ^{1}H-[^{13}C] magnetic resonance spectroscopy at 4.1T. J. Cereb. Blood Flow Metab. 19:1179-1188.

Mason GF, Petersen KF, de Graaf RA, Shulman GI, Rothman DL. (2007) Measurements of the anaplerotic rate in the human cerebral cortex using ^{13}C magnetic resonance spectroscopy and [1-^{13}C] and [2-^{13}C] glucose. J. Neurochem. 100:73-86.

Mason GF, Petersen KF, Lebon V, Rothman DL, Shulman GI. (2006) Increased brain monocarboxylic acid transport and utilization in type 1 diabetes. Diabetes 55:929-934.

Mayer D, Yen YF, Takahashi A, Josan S, Tropp J, Rutt BK, Hurd RE, Spielman DM, Pfefferbaum A. (2011) Dynamic and high-resolution metabolic imaging of hyperpolarized [1-^{13}C]-pyruvate in the rat brain using a high-performance gradient insert. Magn. Reson. Med. 65:1228-1233.

Merle M, Martin M, Villégier A, Canioni P. (1996) [1-^{13}C]glucose metabolism in brain cells: isotopomer analysis of glutamine from cerebellar astrocytes and glutamate from granule cells. Dev. Neurosci. 18:460-468.

Morland C, Henjum S, Iversen EG, Skrede KK, Hassel B. (2007) Evidence for a higher glycolytic than oxidative metabolic activity in white matter of rat brain. Neurochem. Int. 50:703-709.

Nguyen NH, Bråthe A, Hassel B. (2003) Neuronal uptake and metabolism of glycerol and the neuronal expression of mitochondrial glycerol-3-phosphate dehydrogenase. J. Neurochem. 85:831-842.

Nguyen N, Gonzalez SV, Rise F, Hassel B. (2007a) Cerebral metabolism of glucose and pyruvate in soman poisoning. A ^{13}C nuclear magnetic resonance spectroscopic study. Neurotoxicology 28:13-18.

Nguyen NH, Morland C, Gonzalez SV, Rise F, Storm-Mathisen J, Gundersen V, Hassel B. (2007b) Propionate increases neuronal histone acetylation, but is metabolized oxidatively by glia. Relevance for propionic acidemia. J. Neurochem. 101:806-814.

Nguyen NH, Gonzalez SV, Hassel B. (2007c) Formation of glycerol from glucose in rat brain and cultured brain cells. Augmentation with kainate or ischemia. J. Neurochem. 101:1694-1700.

Ottersen OP, Storm-Mathisen J. (1985) Different neuronal localization of aspartate-like and glutamate-like immunoreactivities in the hippocampus of rat, guinea-pig and Senegalese baboon (Papio papio), with a note on the distribution of gamma-aminobutyrate. Neuroscience 16:589-606.

Pan JW, Williamson A, Cavus I, Hetherington HP, Zaveri H, Petroff OA, Spencer DD. (2008) Neurometabolism in human epilepsy. Epilepsia. 49 Suppl 3:31-41.

Pan JW, de Graaf RA, Petersen KF, Shulman GI, Hetherington HP, Rothman DL. (2002) [2,4-$^{13}C_2$]-beta-Hydroxybutyrate metabolism in human brain. J. Cereb. Blood Flow Metab. 22:890-898.

Park I, Bok R, Ozawa T, Phillips JJ, James CD, Vigneron DB, Ronen SM, Nelson SJ. (2011) Detection of early response to temozolomide treatment in brain tumors using hyperpolarized ^{13}C MR metabolic imaging. J. Magn. Reson. Imaging 33:1284-1290.

Patel AB, de Graaf RA, Mason GF, Kanamatsu T, Rothman DL, Shulman RG, Behar KL. (2004) Glutamatergic neurotransmission and neuronal glucose oxidation are coupled during intense neuronal activation. J. Cereb. Blood Flow Metab. 24:972-985.

Petroff OA, Errante LD, Rothman DL, Kim JH, Spencer DD. (2002) Glutamate-glutamine cycling in the epileptic human hippocampus. Epilepsia 43:703-710.

Rodrigues TB, Fonseca CP, Castro MM, Cerdán S, Geraldes CF. (2009) ^{13}C NMR tracers in neurochemistry: implications for molecular imaging. Q. J. Nucl. Med. Mol. Imaging 53:631-645.

Rothman DL, Sibson NR, Hyder F, Shen J, Behar KL, Shulman RG. (1999) In vivo nuclear magnetic resonance spectroscopy studies of the relationship between the glutamate-glutamine neurotransmitter cycle and functional neuroenergetics. Philos. Trans. R. Soc. Lond. B Biol. Sci. 354:1165-1177.

Rothman DL, Behar KL, Hyder F, Shulman RG. (2003) In vivo NMR studies of the glutamate neurotransmitter flux and neuroenergetics: implications for brain function. Annu. Rev. Physiol. 65:401-27.

Scafidi S, O'Brien J, Hopkins I, Robertson C, Fiskum G, McKenna M. (2009) Delayed cerebral oxidative glucose metabolism after traumatic brain injury in young rats. J. Neurochem. 109 Suppl 1:189-197.

Serres S, Bezancon E, Franconi JM, Merle M. (2007) Brain pyruvate recycling and peripheral metabolism: an NMR analysis ex vivo of acetate and glucose metabolism in the rat. J. Neurochem. 101:1428-1240.

Serres S, Raffard G, Franconi JM, Merle M. (2008) Close coupling between astrocytic and neuronal metabolisms to fulfill anaplerotic and energy needs in the rat brain. J. Cereb. Blood Flow Metab. 28:712-724.

Shank RP, Leo GC, Zielke HR. (1993) Cerebral metabolic compartmentation as revealed by nuclear magnetic resonance analysis of D-[1-^{13}C]glucose metabolism. J. Neurochem. 61:315-323.

Shen J, Petersen KF, Behar KL, Brown P, Nixon TW, Mason GF, Petroff OA, Shulman GI, Shulman RG, Rothman DL. (1999) Determination of the rate of the glutamate/glutamine cycle in the human brain by in vivo ^{13}C NMR. Proc. Natl. Acad. Sci. U. S. A. 96:8235-8240.

Shulman RG, Rothman DL, Behar KL, Hyder F. (2004) Energetic basis of brain activity: implications for neuroimaging. Trends Neurosci. 27:489-495.

Siesjö BK. (1978) *Brain Energy Metabolism*, New York.

Sonnewald U, Westergaard N, Jones P, Taylor A, Bachelard HS, Schousboe A. (1996) Metabolism of [U-$^{13}C_5$] glutamine in cultured astrocytes studied by NMR spectroscopy: first evidence of astrocytic pyruvate recycling. J. Neurochem. 67:2566-2572.

Tyson RL, Gallagher C, Sutherland GR. (2003) ^{13}C-Labeled substrates and the cerebral metabolic compartmentalization of acetate and lactate. Brain Res. 992:43-52.

Urion D, Vreman HJ, Weiner MW. (1979) Effect of acetate on hypoglycemic seizures in mice. Diabetes 28:1022-1026.

Van den Berg, C. J. (1973) *Metabolic compartmentation in the brain* (Balázs R and Cremer JE, eds), Macmillan, London, pp. 137–166.

van Heeswijk RB, Morgenthaler FD, Xin L, Gruetter R. (2010) Quantification of brain glycogen concentration and turnover through localized ^{13}C NMR of both the C1 and C6 resonances. NMR Biomed. 23:270-276.

Waniewski RA, Martin DL. (1998) Preferential utilization of acetate by astrocytes is attributable to transport. J. Neurosci. 18:5225-5233.

3

MR Spectroscopy in Multiple Sclerosis - A New Piece of the Puzzle or Just a New Puzzle

Fahmy Aboul-Enein
SMZ-Ost Donauspital, Department of Neurology
Austria

Systems do not exist in Nature but only in man's minds.[1]

1. Introduction

In the late '80s magnetic resonance imaging (MRI) and magnetic resonance spectroscopy (MRS) revolutionized the care and monitoring of patients with multiple sclerosis (MS). For the first time detailed, high resolution images of the brain, spinal cord and lesions could be made by MRI *in vivo*, and followed over time. However, the changes detectable on T1- or T2-weighted magnetic resonance images are non-specific for the underlying pathology, especially in MS patients, and slow down the enthusiasm. They may reflect edema, demyelination, axonal loss, inflammation, gliosis, remyelination, or Wallerian degeneration in MS.

Similar it is with MRS. Early on it was suggested that metabolites within the tissue may reflect certain cellular compartments and tissue conditions in health and disease. First reports about *in vivo* detection of brain metabolites in humans were published in 1989 (Bruhn et al., 1989; Frahm et al., 1989a; 1989b). Combined with conventional MRI technique spatial anatomical and chemical information about the analysed tissue may be achieved. MRS was approved by the FDA in 1996. However, only few metabolites are detectable (table 1), limiting the main applications of MRS yet to (1) brain tumors (low grade vs. high grade gliomas, metastasis, lymphoma, meningeoma), (2) follow-up of tumors (under chemotherapy and radiotherapy), (2) infectious, mostly focal CNS processes such as pyogenic abscesses, toxoplasmosis, tuberculosis, cryptococcosis, and (3) hepatic encephalopathy, other metabolic disorders, inborn errors of metabolism or hypoxic encephalopathy. In some selected MS cases MRS might be useful to differentiate tumor-like MS brain lesions or Balo-like MS lesions from tumor lesions (table 1) or confluent MS lesions from leucodystrophies or leucoencephalopathies.

Well characterized peaks obtained at long echo times (more than TE 135ms, highlighted in grey) are: (1) at 2.0 ppm ('NAA-peak'; N-acetyl-aspartate (NAA)), (2) at 3.0 ppm ('Cr-peak'; creatine (Cr)), (3) at 3.2 ppm ('Cho-peak'; choline (cho)), (4) at 1.3 ppm ('Lac-peak'; lactate (Lac)), (5) at 1.48ppm ('Alanine Peak'; alanine (Ala)),

---

[1] **Claude Bernard** (French physiologist, 1813 – 1878)

marker (metabolite)	ppm	[mM]	indicates	possible to find in...
lipids	0.9-1.2	-	tissue necrosis (highly specific)	brain tumors, abscesses, tissue necrosis
cytosolic amino acids (valine, leucine, and iso-leucine)	0.9	-	products of proteolysis (neutrophil cells)	abscesses, neurocysticerkosis (but not in neoplasms!)
lactate (Lac)	1.2	-	anaerobic glycolysis; inverted double peak (TE136ms)	Balo like MS lesions, malignant tumors, infarcts, abscesses, mitochondrial disorders
alanine (Ala)	1.48	-	inverted double peak (TE 136ms)	meningeomas brain abscesses
acetate	1.5	-	product of propionic acid fermentation and mixed acid fermentation (anaerobic bacteria)	abscesses, neurocysticercosis
N-acetylaspartate (NAA)	2.0	7-17	neurons, axons	decreased in tumors, and any process with tissue destruction
glutamate and glutamine (glx)	2.2-2.7	6-12 and 3-12	excitatory neurotransmitter	increased in stroke, lymphoma, hepatic encephalopathy, metabolic disorders
succinate	2.4	-	product of propionic acid fermentation and mixed acid fermentation	abscesses, neurocysticercosis
Creatine (Cr)	3.0	4.5-10.5	cell energy/ metabolism	mostly stable, used as reference peak
Choline (Cho)	3.2	0.5-3.0	cell membranes (cell turnover, cell destruction)	tumors, lymphomas, stroke, infectious processes, MS
myo-Inositol (mIns)	3.5	4.0-9.0	glucose metabolism mainly in astrocytes	gliosis, hepatic encephalopathy, pontine myelinolysis, MS

Table 1. Brain metabolites

And at short echo times (less than TE 30ms) are : (6) at 3.5 ppm ('mIns-Peak'; myo-inositol, (mIns)), (7) at 0.9-1.2 ppm ('free lipids peak').

Normal peak levels are given in [mM].

Brain metabolites were suggested as markers for (1) neurons (NAA), (2) energy metabolism (Cr), (3) cell membranes or cell membrane turnover (Cho), (4) anaerobic glykolysis, i.e. tissue necrosis (Lac, lipids, cytosolic amino acids, Ala, acetate, succinate), (5) astrogliosis (mIns), and (6) myelin break down (lipids, cytosolic amino acids). Abnormally strong or weak peaks or certain patterns of several peaks may be indicative for various pathological processes, and may help to interpret changes found by conventional MRI.

For instance, lac is normally only detectable if the lac concentration in the CNS parenchyma has reached at least the lac concentration in the cerebrospinal fluid (CSF). Lac is the end product of anaerobic glycolysis and may occur in severe tissue necrosis or abscesses (table 1).

The most discussed MRS peaks (or brain metabolites) yet are, NAA, Cho, Crea and mIns.

1.1.1 N-acetyl-aspartate (NAA), at 2.0 ppm

In normal CNS tissue the highest peak in the proton spectrum is found at 2.0 ppm, resembling the sharp resonance signal from NAA, largely composed of NAA itself, and to a lesser proportion out of N-acetyl-aspartate-glutamate. NAA is an amino-acid derivative synthesized from L-aspartate and acetyl-CoA. NAA was found to be mainly expressed in the mitochondria of neurons, their cell bodies, dendrites and axons, and thus was suggested to indicate either the structural or functional integrity of neurons or axons. However, its function remains unknown. In principal three scenarios, where a reduction of the NAA peak might occur, are discussed: (1) if neurons or axons are damaged irreversible, and degenerate, (2) if their density is reduced relatively in the tissue due to oedema, or (3) if their function is impaired, only.

1.1.2 Choline (Cho), at 3.2 ppm

Cho and Cho-containing phospholipids hardly resonate under normal conditions because they are mainly insoluble and immobile as they constitute all cell membranes and myelin. In tumors, inflammation, infarcts, leucoencephalopathy, leucodystrophies or in certain MS lesions, high cell membrane turnover due to cellular mitosis and cell death, or myelin break down may lead to higher concentration of soluble, freely mobile Cho, which may be detected at 3.2 ppm on the frequency scale. If freely mobile Cho molecules are abundant and resonate, an increased 'Cho-peak' may be found.

Note that severe tissue destruction, i.e. necrosis, where cell membranes are heavily damaged, torn asunder and single cell membrane compounds released into the necrosis, may produce other resonances or peaks (such as free lipids, lac, acetate, succinate).

1.1.3 Creatine (Cr), at 3.0 ppm

The 'Cr-peak' is composed of Cr and phosphor-creatine, and lies at 3.0 ppm on the frequency scale, representing a marker for cellular energy metabolism. As the Cr concentration was found relatively stable throughout the CNS, **and** found relatively resistant to change, Cr is often used as internal standard, and thus the signals strength of the other metabolites are expressed as ratio to Cr. However, under certain conditions such as higher age, tumors, infarcts or trauma Cr is found decreased. (Sometimes Cr was also found increased in the NAWM of MS patients, see below).

1.1.4 Myo-Inositol (mINS), at 3.5 ppm

The 'mIns-peak' is believed to resemble an 'activated' state of higher cell metabolism or proliferation of astrocytes. mIns is a sugar-like molecule which may be crucial for the osmotic regulation in the CNS parenchyma. An elevated 'mIns-peak' may be interpreted as higher astroglial activity and proliferation or gliosis.

But MRS allows a limited view only. From a scientific point of view, it is hardly conceivable that a few metabolites really allow the complete representation of complex biological processes of individual cells within the spectroscopied CNS tissue. Note that the function of the metabolites and that their (resonance) characteristics under certain conditions are still largely unknown.

One of the most important and controversially discussed hypotheses today is that 'early axonal damage already exists in very early stages of (all) MS patients'. This view may open the way for 'an (very) early treatment' of MS patients, also if clinical symptoms are minor or even absent (Miller et al., 2008; Gilmore et al., 2010). This hypothesis comes mainly from MRI and MRS findings reporting reduced NAA levels in the normal appearing white matter (NAWM). NAA levels are suggested as marker for neuronal integrity and function and should reflect the burden of disease in MS patients (figure 1).

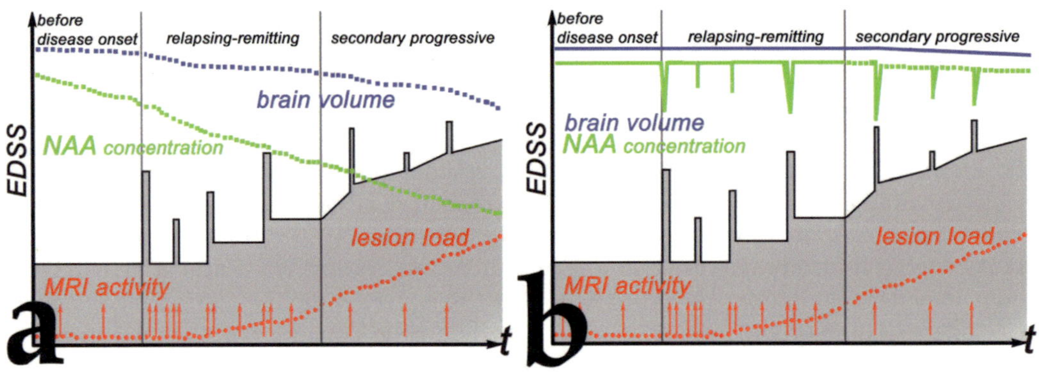

Fig. 1. A hypothesis, nothing else. **a,** It remains unclear, simply hypothetically, whether progressive, i.e. steadily ongoing 'silent', axonal damage exists in all MS patients, or not and if so, whether it can be reliable detected and monitored over time. It was suggested that NAA levels in the NAWM decline in some MS patients continuously. This NAA decline would be expected more than naturally occurring declines by age. **b,** Objective and neutral interpretation of the data allows also a second scenario, where brain volume (and NAA concentration?) only slightly decreases with age, or secondary progression. And during relapses temporarily a decrease of NAA can be found, that may recover fully.

However, due to the most often relapsing-remitting course of MS patients, with remission over years and sometimes over decades, early treatment per se must be carefully considered and risks and benefits carefully weighed.

In biological sciences, the role of a method is even more important than in other sciences, because of the immense complexity of the phenomena and the countless sources of error, which complexity brings into experimentation.[2]

1.2 Recently the pivotal role of advanced MR technique was emphasized

1.2.1 'Differential diagnosis of suspected multiple sclerosis: A consensus approach'

Miller DH, Weinshenker BG, Filippi M, Banwell BL, Cohen JA, Freedman MS, Galetta SL, Hutchinson M, Johnson RT, Kappos L, Kira J, Lublin FD, McFarland HF, Montalban X, Panitch H, Richert JR, Reingold SC, Polman CH.

Multiple Sclerosis, Vol. 14, No. 9, pp. 1157-1174.

P 1164, [...] *Although symptoms and signs of a monophasic illness have been an essential prerequisite for diagnosis of CIS, there is an exceptional scenario that the Panel feels warrants inclusion as CIS Type 5 (Table 2): patients who have no symptoms or only non-specific symptoms (e.g., headache, dizziness), but have MRI evidence for multifocal abnormalities typical for demyelination. Such patients are increasingly identified using MRI for incidental indications (e.g., headache) especially with high-field strength magnets with greater sensitivity for such lesions [17]. Current criteria preclude a diagnosis of MS without objective clinical evidence for CNS abnormality and the ability to establish a confident diagnosis of MS in such individuals and their natural history should be addressed through prospective studies* [18]. [...]

P 1172, [...] *Disease biomarkers will aid enormously in differential diagnosis. Accurate and sensitive disease markers – imaging or laboratory based – may provide non-invasive aids to differential diagnosis. The discovery of NMO-IgG that helps to distinguish NMO from MS is a good example. Relevant imaging advances may include non-conventional MR techniques to quantitate change in normal appearing white matter that may be relatively specific for MS, and high-field MRI to better visualize Dawson's fingers [17] or cortical lesions that may be specific to MS.* [...]

Interestingly, the reference No. 17 (title 'Cerebral Cortical Lesions in Multiple Sclerosis Detected by MR Imaging at 8 Tesla') is a case report where the *post mortem/ex vivo* findings of a single patient, a male aged 42 years, were described (Kangarlu et al., 2007). Coronal slices of the patient's formalin fixed brain were examined using MRI at 8T. Details about the disease course, or how the diagnosis 'MS' were made was not specified, p262, [...]

'Cerebral cortical lesions in multiple sclerosis detected by MR imaging at 8 Tesla.' Kangarlu A, Bourekas EC, Ray-Chaudhury A, Rammohan KW.

AJNR American Journal of Neuroradiology, Vol. 28, No. 2, pp. 262-266.

A 42-year-old man with severe disabilities secondary to MS died of aspiration pneumonia. In the year before his death, he had been seen at our medical center on 2 occasions, mostly for palliative care. He was bed-bound and very dependent for all activities of daily living. He was paraplegic with additional severe weakness of the upper extremities, which were also severely ataxic. The ataxia also affected his trunk and prevented him from sitting unassisted in a standard wheelchair. He had complete bilateral internuclear ophthalmoplegia, vertical nystagmus, and severe

[2] **Claude Bernard** (French physiologist, 1813 – 1878)

titubation of his head. His ability to communicate was intact, though his speech was barely intelligible. His mentation seemed intact; he remained completely oriented and participated in all decisions of his care, including his desire to have his brain evaluated for scientific endeavors after death. He needed to be fed through a percutaneous gastrostomy tube. Cognitive status could not be formally evaluated because of the severity of his disabilities. The duration of his disease was estimated to be approximately 12 years. At the time of his demise, he was considered to be in the advanced stages of the secondary-progressive form of MS. His general health was otherwise excellent, and he had no known cardiovascular, cerebrovascular, hypertensive, or diabetes-related disabilities. [...].

[...]

For reference No. 18 see, Lebrun at al., 2008 and the comment by Chattaway, 2008.

[...]

As critical readers we are aware that we must read more than the headlines and abstracts of the papers and that the hypothesis that 'early axonal damage already exists in very early stages of (all) MS patients' has yet to be proven (Figure 1), and that the very controversial discussion is still ongoing (e.g. Chattaway, 2008 and 2010; Gilmore et al., 2010; Lebrun et al., 2008; Miller et al., 2008). In any case, we must keep in mind that direct scientific evidence is still lacking.

I consider the hospital as the antechamber of medicine.
It is the first place where the physician makes his observations.
But the laboratory is the temple of the science of medicine.[3]

2. Multiple sclerosis

Multiple sclerosis (MS) is a chronic idiopathic disease of the central nervous system (CNS). Inflammation, demyelination and axonal injury are most typical pathological features, but their underlying pathogenetic mechanisms are still unclear (Barnett et al., 2009; Hibberd, 1994; Lassmann et al., 2007). They are probably complex and heterogeneous, and may be triggered outside the CNS or conversely, may be triggered within the CNS. And they may initiate focally and further disperse, or they may affect the whole CNS diffusely at once. In either case, blood brain barrier (BBB) alterations are conceivable, focally or diffusely, visible or invisible (Figure 2). But at least the primary cause of MS, and whether BBB alterations are the initial detectable pathological event in the evolution of the MS lesions, or why and whatever, the MS lesions are caused by, remains unknown (Aboul-Enein & Lassmann, 2006; Allen & McKeown, 1979; Allen et al., 1989; Barnes et al., 1991; Barnett et al., 2004; Barnett & Prineas, 2009; Henderson et al., 2009; Höftberger et al., 2004; Lassmann et al., 2007).

If an idea presents itself to us, we must not reject it simply,
because it does not agree with the logical deductions of a reigning theory.[4]
It is what we know already that often prevents us from learning.[5]

[3] **Claude Bernard** (French physiologist, 1813 – 1878)
[4] **Claude Bernard** (French physiologist, 1813 – 1878)
[5] **Claude Bernard** (French physiologist, 1813 – 1878)

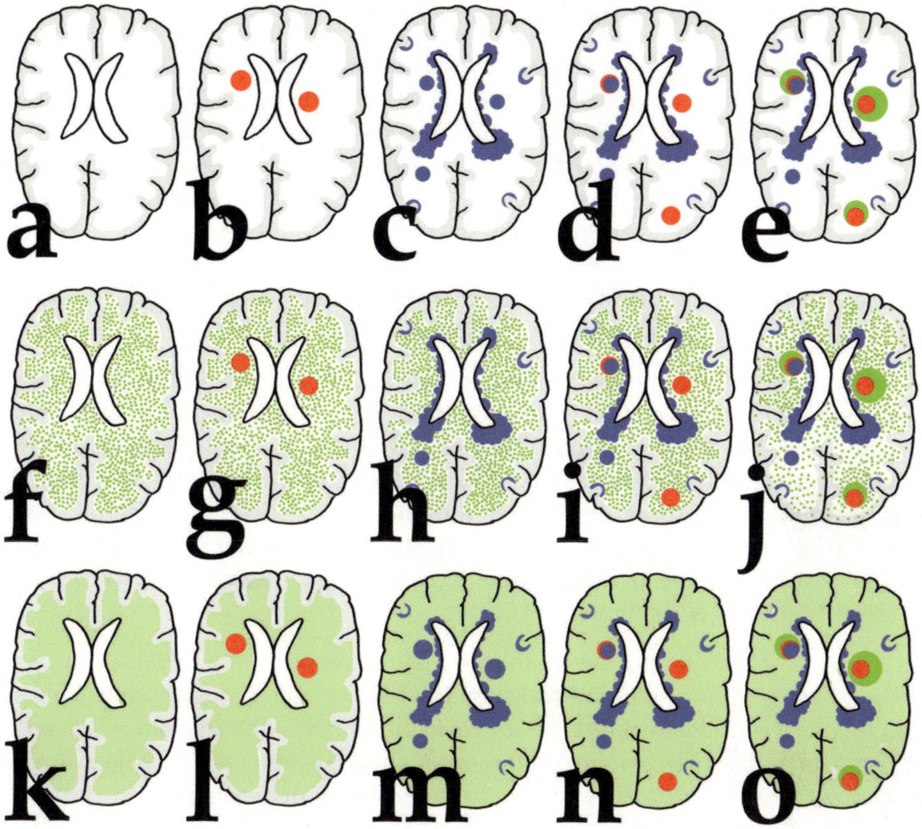

Fig. 2. 'The chicken or the egg causality dilemma' in MS lesion evolution.
Red, enhancing (active) MR lesions; **blue,** old(er), at least not enhancing lesions; **green,** in MR invisible inflammation or an underlying, yet not determined, pathogenetic mechanism around focal MS lesions; **lime,** hypothesized invisible, yet not determined, compartmentalized focal or diffuse inflammation or yet not determined pathogenetic process. **a-e, the disease might be triggered from outside the CNS. a,** normal brain without any lesion or invisible disease activity; **b,** the naïve brain with two enhancing lesions (red) only; **c,** brain with typical periventricular and subcortical old (not enhancing) white matter (WM) lesions only; **d,** same scenario as in c, but with new enhancing lesions (red). **e,** older non enhancing WM lesions (blue) of which one enhances in its right anterior margin (red margin) with ongoing (invisible) activity (green) beyond the in MR visible lesion border and two new enhancing (red) with invisible activity in the left hemisphere. **f-o, the disease might be already compartmentalized within the CNS from the very beginning, but invisible with MRI (lime): f-j,** focally, but widely dispersed; **k-o,** diffusely within the CNS. **f-o,** show the same enhancing (red) and old/er (blue) in MRI detectable lesions as presented in *a-d*. In both scenarios, the in MRI detectable lesions may resemble only the 'tip of the iceberg', leading to over time and space disseminated focal lesions with BBB alterations. In other words, the hypothesized underlying, invisible disease activity may lead from inside out to focal 'eruptions' with BBB alterations and influx of inflammation, or might attract inflammatory cells which lead to the BBB breakdown. The infiltrating inflammatory cells might be primarily harmful to the CNS, or otherwise, they might be primarily beneficial but may cause substantial bystander tissue damage, or both.

2.1 Diagnostic criteria and the disease course of MS

The diagnosis 'MS' is a clinical one, if stringent diagnostic criteria are fulfilled and if there is no better explanation for the clinical presentation (Mc Donald et al., 2001; Polman et al. 2005, 2010; Poser et al., 1983; Schuhmacher et al., 1965). The diagnosis 'MS' is based on the clinical evidence for typical disseminated CNS lesions, and may be supported by cerebrospinal fluid (CSF) analysis, magnetic resonance imaging (MRI), and evoked potentials. However, all findings are non-specific by themselves, but overall, they might be typical for the diagnosis 'MS'. Up till now, a reliable specific para-clinical marker neither for the diagnosis nor for monitoring disease activity of MS could yet be established (e.g. Aboul-Enein et al., 2010; Gilmore et al., 2010; Kuhle et al., 2007; Serbecic et al., 2010, 2011).

In most of the cases MS starts between the age of 20 to 40 years and follows a relapsing-remitting course with clear defined relapses with no apparent clinical deterioration between the relapses. Each MS patient follows his/her individual disease course (Gilmore et al., 2010). It is unclear why MS sometimes follows a benign disease course with clinical remission over decades, or changes after an uncertain period of time into secondary progression with or without superimposed relapses (SPMS, secondary progressive MS), or follows rarely a progressive disease course right from the disease onset (PPMS, primary progressive MS) (Lublin & Reingold, 1996).

To sum up, no clinical or paraclinical parameter could yet be found, which allows a reliable prognosis of the 'relapse-free intervals', the relapses, the sequelae and the possible 'conversion into secondary progression'. In particular, neither the frequency nor severity of relapses nor disability in the first years after onset nor the lesion load in magnetic resonance images (MRI) correlates strictly with the disease activity or its impact on the individual clinical disease course (e.g. Brex et al., 2002; Fisniku et al., 2008; Gilmore et al., 2010; Weinshenker et al., 1989a, 1989b). And axonal alterations or axonal loss, which is yet suggested as main pathological substrate, unfortunately, provides only some explanation.

In teaching man, experimental science results in lessening his pride more and more by proving to him every day that primary causes, like the objective reality of things, will be hidden from him forever and that he can only know relations.[6]

2.2 The clinical-pathological paradox of MS

Pathologists and neurologists have known for a long time that a considerable amount of CNS lesions with demyelination, axonal changes, inflammation and gliosis might be found, although clinical signs and symptoms were absent or should have never occurred (Lumdsen, 1970). A plausible explanation could be that in such cases the lesions were small, or that they occurred in non-eloquent CNS areas, but in any way, it means that recovery of function is possible. Axonal loss of function may be caused either by structural damage such as demyelination and (secondary) axonal injury (McDonald and Sears, 1970) or may be caused without any detectable structural damage by certain immune mediators only, which might interfere with axonal conductance (Aboul-Enein et al., 2006; Smith & Lassmann, 2002). Block of conduction is in principal reversible as axons may be remyelinated and the axonal

[6] **Claude Bernard** (French physiologist, 1813 - 1878)

sodium channels may be restored, or the conduction block causing mediators may be removed (Smith, 2007). Of course, other mediators derived from any other tissue or incorporated from outside, and being not associated with the body's immune system might be worth considering. But neither remyelination nor gliosis, both can be extensive in autopsies, correlate to permanent functional loss, if at all, only the irreversible axonal loss was found to correlate. And pathologists have only a very limited point of view (as neurologists and radiologists, too!). They can merely try to reconstruct the *in vivo* situation in most of the cases after long disease courses with very specific markers which however, allow mostly no further statement about the in vivo integrity and function over the patients' lifetime.

2.3 The clinical-radiological paradox of MS

On a more philosophical - someone might argue - on a very 'realistic' level, we must remember that we merely know nothing about the disease's origin or the disease's specific processes. Direct scientific evidence is lacking for almost every little so far identified experimental, pathological, clinical, radiological or epidemiological fragment. We even do not know whether MS is one disease or a whole spectrum of disorders, or vice versa, whether the same pathogenetic mechanisms may have different effects in different individuals, or at different times in one individual MS patient. Otherwise not a specific primary cause itself, but the lack of specific resistant factor(s) or repair mechanisms might be responsible that some individuals become ill (and diagnosed), whereas all the others remain healthy. In other words, how many healthy people (Also you, dear readers!) could have a considerable lesion load or brain atrophy in MRI suggestive for MS, but without any further consequence as they feel healthy (and never see a doctor). Patients diagnosed with MS may be that ones with lesions mainly in eloquent areas. Thus they may resemble only a very small portion, the so called 'tip of the iceberg', but of course, they shape our view about MS.

However, by occasion some patients, who receive a MRI of their brain (because of a wide range of 'unspecific' symptoms, and because MRI is now widely available), show asymptomatic lesions suggestive for MS (Chataway, 2010). Recently, these 'patients' were classified as radiological isolated syndrome (RIS) or clinical isolated syndrome (CIS) type 5 (Miller et al., 2008). It is controversially discussed, whether these 'patients' should be followed closely, or even treated (Chataway, 2008, 2010; Gilmore et al., 2010; Lebrun et al., 2008; Miller et al., 2008; Sellner et al., 2010; Siva et al., 2009).

The link between disease onset and possible irreversible end-stage parameters such as glial scar tissue formation and brain and spinal cord atrophy is still missing. MRI and magnetic resonance spectroscopy (MRS) allows to visualize changes during individual disease courses in vivo, but they provide at least information from magnetic fields of certain molecules, mostly hydrogen nuclei (protons, or ^{1}H) of water molecules, nothing else.

A fact in itself is nothing.
It is valuable only for the idea attached to it,
or for the proof which it furnishes.[7]

[7] **Claude Bernard** (French physiologist, 1813 - 1878)

3. Of what we believe about MRI lesion evolution

3.1 Acute enhancing lesions

It is believed, that the alteration of the BBB may be the earliest event in formation of a focal MS lesion which may be visualized by gadolinium enhancement in T1-weighted MRI images with high sensitivity. Prerequisite for this is that gadolinium must be able to reach the specific region and that the BBB alterations are rather gross ('BBB leakage', in a strict sense). Gadolinium enhancement was suggested to be more sensitive in detecting disease activity than either clinical examination or T2 weighted MRI (Miller et al., 1993). Theoretically, all relapses should be accompanied by new, active enhancing MRI lesions (Figure 1b, d, e g, i, j, l, n o). But, enhancement is dependent on the dose and the technique used, and dependent on the lesion size and location. This must be borne in mind when different studies are compared.

Higher doses of gadolinium (triple dose, 0.3mmol/kg body weight), longer delay between injection and the MRI scan (30-60 minutes), and the combination with a magnetization transfer pulse which suppresses the normal brain tissue, but spares areas with enhancement, can increase the sensitivity of MRI, i.e. make an higher number of enhancing MS lesions visualized (Filippi et al., 1996; Miller et al., 1998). Caveat is the increase of false positive results. However it remains unclear, if all lesions, in particular, those with only subtle BBB alterations can be detected hereby (Barnes et al., 1991; Kwon & Prineas et al., 1994, Waubant, 2006). Very often neurological symptoms may occur without any (correlating) acute enhancing MRI lesions, especially in the spinal cord. And most confusing is that acute enhancing MRI lesions that are clinically silent, may be found between relapses, even though they are located in eloquent areas (Davie et al., 1994; Schubert et al., 2002).

Put off your imagination as you take off your overcoat,
when you enter the laboratory.[8]

In contrast to usual CNS immune surveillance with regular, always occurring transmigration of only few immune cells (Aboul-Enein et al., 2004), it is supposed that the lesion evolution starts with large numbers of immune cells that cross the BBB into the CNS parenchyma, and thus may lead to BBB leakage (Barnes et al., 1991; Hawkins et al., 1991). This is mainly supported by animal models of experimental autoimmune encephalomyelitis (EAE) that however, must not be uncritically translated to humans. In EAE huge masses of CNS antigen specific immune cells or antibodies, or both, are injected, and initiate an acute, but mostly monophasic inflammatory disease in the CNS (Flugel et al., 2001, 2007; Floris et al., 2004; Hawkins et al., 1991; Kawakami et al., 2005). The situation in humans with MS remains unclear. It is even unknown whether the inflammation is primary, whether the infiltrating immune cells themselves cause the tissue damage, or whether some other primary event within the CNS leads to the actual lesion formation and attracts the inflammatory cells into the CNS. The inflammation may be beneficial or conversely, may cause some bystander damage (Barnett & Prineas, 2004; Henderson et al., 2009; Hohlfeld et al., 2006). Anyway, corticosteroids may decrease or may completely suppress the enhancement of MS lesions for several weeks (Barkhof et al., 1991, 1994; Burnham et al., 1991). Conceivable are various mechanisms of action such as apoptosis of circulating

[8] **Claude Bernard** (French physiologist, 1813 - 1878)

immune cells, down-regulation of adhesion molecules on immune cells or endothelial cells, or both, or another yet not determined mechanism, that seals the BBB (Engelhardt, 2006; Gelati et al., 2002; Leussink et al., 2001; Prat et al., 2002).

3.2 Others than acute enhancing lesions

Most of the acute gadolinium enhancing MS lesions change their MR characteristics in further follow up. Some convert to mildly or severly hpointense T1 lesions which might reflect severe underlying tissue damage with marked axonal loss and correlating reduced NAA levels (e.g. van Walderveen et al., 1998), others convert to persistent T2 lesions after several months. The latter may appear hyperintense in T1 weighted images or become undectable in T1 weighted images. In persistent T2 lesions, no matter what behavior they had in T1, nearly all thinkable metabolite constellations were described (increase, decrease, no changes of NAA, Cr, Cho, mIns etc., e.g. Davie et al., 1997; van Walderveen et al., 1997.). Reduced NAA levels might reflect axonal injury, dysfunction or loss. They might be temporarily or permanently, within lesions or remote from lesions due to secondary axonal degeneration or Wallerian degeneration. (Increased NAA levels have yet been described in Canavan's disease only). Elevated Cr, mIns levels were suggested to reflect 'higher metabolism' in astrocytes, and increased Cho was suggested to reflect higher cell membrane turnover or proliferation of astrocytes within MS lesions or NAWM. Decreased levels might be due to decreased cell numbers or lower 'cellular energy state'. These divergent results may be explained by the very small and heterogeneous patient cohorts (e.g. 2 RRMS and 12 SPMS aged from 28 to 61 years, and 4 controls aged 33 to 48 years in van Walderveen et al., 1999), by the use of a 1.5 Tesla 1H-MRS and by the measurement of metabolite ratios instead of absolute metabolite concentrations.

Only single reports of histopathological correlations to *in vivo* MR data have been published (Bitsch et al., 1997) that are of most importance for our understanding, but must be interpreted very carefully. Biopsies are only very seldom performed in MS patients, mostly if tumor lesions must be ruled out or verified. Whether demyelinating tumor-like MS lesions have the same characteristics and behavior like common unspecific smaller MS lesions, is unclear. Moreover, it is still unknown, if MS is one disease or a syndrome of many disorders, or if the same trigger causes the same pathological changes in different MS patients or if the same trigger at different time points leads to different types of lesions in one individual MS patient. Therefore, any general interpretation must be done with caution.

Men who have excessive faith in their theories or ideas
are not only ill prepared for making discoveries.
They also make very poor observations.[9]

4. Of what we believe to see with MRT and MRS

MRI allows the detailed visualization of the anatomical and pathological structures based on different signals of freely mobile hydrogen protons between different tissues or anatomical compartments.

[9] **Claude Bernard** (French physiologist, 1813 - 1878)

The signals from freely mobile hydrogen protons are up to 1000 fold more than the resonances from other brain metabolites. The selective suppression of the signal from hydrogen protons 'unmasks' the spectra of various specific metabolites within the magnetic resonance frequency spectrum, and thus allows to detect and separate them, as each brain metabolite resonates at a characteristic position along the frequency scale expressed in parts per million (ppm). The sharpness and the amplitude of a specific peak along the frequency scale is determined by the specific metabolite itself, its concentration and most importantly, by its mobility. The brain metabolites must be freely mobile to produce well detectable peaks. In general, the more freely mobile specific metabolites in a specific volume of interest (VOI) resonate the higher their resulting peak is. If the specific peak is low, or even absent, this could mean that the protons in the examined VOI are either not occurring or not freely mobile or might require specific MR technique/parameters to be detected.

For instance, lipids are abundant within the brain, but under normal conditions immobile, as they constitute mainly highly compacted myelin. If myelin breaks down, they become mobile and may produce a 'free lipid peak' in the frequency spectrum at 0.9-1.2 ppm.

'NAA-peak' reduction or reduction of NAA absolute concentration in the spectroscopied tissue may occur due to axonal injury, damage or even loss, and might be irreversible or reversible. Infarcts, tumors, traumatic injury may lead to severe tissue destruction, heavy axonal damage and loss of axons, and thus may lead to irreversible NAA reduction. In the case of temporarily NAA reduction, various scenarios are conceivable: firstly, the NAA reduction correlates with structural axonal damage, i.e. axonal loss that in principle may be restored by remyelination and regain more or less the same NAA concentrations as before. Secondly, NAA reduction might reflect mitochondrial dysfunction in neurons or axons, whatever the underlying cause might be (e.g. inflammatory mediators, or any other molecule which might interfere with mitochondrial function), and might be restored when the interfering stimulus or agent is removed. The numbers of axons can be unchanged, or can be markedly reduced but have the same NAA levels, i.e. more 'active mitochondria' per axon or neuron. In other words, the loss of axons might be compensated with increase of numbers of mitochondria or increase of the NAA content in axonal mitochondria. (It was suggested that NAA might play a crucial role in the mitochondrial function).

A tumor or tumor-like brain lesion may either show profound reduction of NAA and relative high Cr concentrations in a first baseline scan. Several weeks later the NAA levels might be found still reduced or restored. In the first case, a tumor must be considered, whereas in the latter case a demyelinating tumor-like lesion with subsequent remyelination seems conceivable. (Tumors do not recover spontaneously).

A discovery is generally an unforeseen relation not included in theory,
for otherwise it would be foreseen.[10]

5. Of what could be found with MRS in early stages of RRMS or even in CIS

Medline Database Research using following search term/key words {"multiple sclerosis" AND (NAWM OR "normal appearing white matter") AND ("N-acetyl-aspartate" OR NAA) and ("spectroscopy") and "absolute concentration"} yielded 67 results (until March 2011).

[10] **Claude Bernard** (French physiologist, 1813 - 1878)

Only **38** original articles providing MRS data (NAA/Cr ratios and/or NAA absolute concentrations) of RRMS or CIS patients could be further analysed. Other search results had to be excluded because they included MRS studies on SPMS or PPMS patients only (Leary et al., 1999; Cucurella et al., 2000; Sastre-Garriga et al., 2005), or did not compare the NAWM of matched controls (Hiehle et al., 1994), or were reviews, post mortem studies, MRS studies on patients with neuromyelitis optica, systemic lupus erythematodes or relatives of MS patients who were not afflicted with MS.

A meta-analysis of the remaining 38 identified MRS studies could not be performed as they differ from study design (inclusion criteria and technical parameters), and do not provide all necessary data such as detailed demographic data and individual values for metabolite ratios and concentrations. However, following characteristics of the NAWM of CIS and RRMS patients could be identified (table 2, references are listed chronologically by publication date).

		TESLA		controls			CIS			RRMS			SPMS			PPMS			abs.		NAA	Cho	mIns	Cr
	Reference	1,5	3,0	n	m	f	n	m	f	n	m	f	n	m	f	n	m	f	con	rati				
1	Davie et al., 1994	■		8						8										■	↓	↓*		
2	Husted et al., 1994									13										■	↓	=	↑	
4	Peters et al., 1995	■		3	1	2				4	2	2	5	4	1	2	1	1		■	↓	=		
5	Fu et al., 1998	■		12						11			17							■	↓*			
6	Schiepers et al., 1997	■		9	4	5				3			6			4				■	↓	=		
7	Davie et al., 1997	■		9			9			9			10			8				■	=	=		
8	Sarchielli et al., 1999	■		6						10										■	=	=	=	=
9	Foong J et al., 1999	■		38	18	20				25	10	15								■	↓*	=		
10	Sarchielli et al., 1999	■		12						27			13						■	■	↓*	=		=
11	Brex et al., 1999	■					20	10	10										■		=	=	=	=
12	van Walderveen et al., 1999	■		4	0	4				2			12							■	↓*	=		↑*
13	Suhy et al., 2000	■		20	13	7				13	7	6				15	10	5		■	↓*	=		↑*
14	de Stefano et al., 2001	■		17	?	?				55	23	32	33	17	16					■	↓*	=		
15	Tedeschi et al., 2001	■		50	25	25				19	7	12	5	3	2					■	↓	↓		
16	Kapeller et al., 2001	■		12	9	3				16	7	9							■		↓*	=	↑*	=
17	Chard et al., 2002	■		28	15	13				25	6	19							■		↓*	=	↑*	=
18	de Stefano et al., 2002	■		21	8					60	19	41								■	↓*	=		
19	Kapeller et al., 2002	■		21	15	6	9	2	7	32	12	20								■	=	=		=
20	Casanova et al. 2003,	■		4	2	2				21	3	10								■	↓*	=		
21	Inglese et al., 2004	■		9	2	7				11	3	8							■		↓	=		=
22	Adalsteinsson et al., 2004	■		9	1	8				5	0	5	5	1	4				■		↓	=		=
23	Fernando et al., 2004	■		44	22	22	96	63	33										■		=	=	↑	=
24	Ruiz-Pena et al., 2004	■		10	5	5				31	9	22							■	■	=	=		=
25	He et al., 2005	■		9	2	7				9	3	6							■		↓	↑	↑	
26	Vrenken et al., 2005	■		25	14	11				42	13	29	20	9	11	14	8	6	■	■	=	=	↑*	↑*
27	Mathiesen et al., 2005	■								14	4	10								■	=	=		=
28	Srinivasan et al., 2005		■	16	8	8				16			4			7			■		=	↑*	↑*	=
29	Staffen et al., 2005	■		21						21										■	↓			
30	Khan et al., 2005	■								22										■	↑	=		=
31	Tiberio et al., 2006	■								20	4	16							■		↓*			
32	Sijens et al., 2006	■		6						7			4			4			■		↓*	=	=	=
33	Pascual et al., 2007	■		10	3	7				43	18	25								■	↓*	↑*		=
34	Wattjes et al., 2008		■	20			25	8	17										■	■	↓	=	=	=
35	Wattjes et al., 2008		■	20			31	9	22										■	■	↓	=	=	=
36	Khan et al., 2008	■								22										■	↑	=		=
37	Bellmann-Strobl et al., 2009	■								17	7	10								■	=	=		=
38	Aboul-Enein et al., 2010		■	8	1	7				27	4	23	10	3	7				■	■	=*	=		=

Table 2. Synopsis of literature research.

5.1 Reported NAA changes

5.1.1 Decreased NAA ratios or NAA concentrations

Twenty-four MRS studies were published with decreased ratios of NAA to Cr or Cho, or decreased NAA absolute concentrations in the NAWM in a total of **56 CIS** or **418 RRMS** patients (Davie et al., 1994; Husted et al., 1994; Peters et al., 1995; Fu et al., 1998; Schiepers et al., 1997; Foong J et al., 1999; Sarchielli et al., 1999; van Walderveen et al., 1999; Suhy et al., 2000; de Stefano et al., 2001; Tedeschi et al., 2001; Kapeller et al., 2001; Chard et al., 2002; de Stefano et al., 2002; Casanova et al. 2003; Inglese et al., 2004; Adalsteinsson et al., 2004; He et al., 2005; Staffen et al., 2005; Tiberio et al., 2006; Sijens et al., 2006; Pascual et al., 2007; Wattjes et al., 2008; Wattjes et al., 2008).

5.1.2 No significant changes of NAA ratios or NAA concentrations

Fourteen MRS studies were published with no significant NAA changes in the NAWM in a total of **184 CIS** or **263 RRMS** patients (Davie et al., 1997; Sarchielli et al., 1998; Brex et al., 1999; Kapeller et al., 2002; Fernando et al., 2004; Ruiz-Pena et al., 2004; Vrenken et al., 2005; Mathiesen et al., 2005; Srinivasan et al., 2005; Khan et al., 2005; Khan et al., 2008; Kirov et al., 2008; Bellmann-Strobl et al., 2009; Aboul-Enein et al., 2010).

5.2 Reported Cho changes

5.2.1 No significant changes of Cho ratios or Cho concentrations

Twenty-nine MRS studies were published with no significant Cho changes in the NAWM in a total of **190 CIS** or **513 RRMS** patients (Husted et al., 1994; Peters et al., 1995; Schiepers et al., 1997;Davie et al., 1997; Sarchielli et al., 1999; Foong J et al., 1999; Sarchielli et al., 1999; Brex et al., 1999; van Walderveen et al., 1999; Suhy et al., 2000; de Stefano et al., 2001; Kapeller et al., 2001; Chard et al., 2002; de Stefano et al., 2002; Kapeller et al., 2002; Casanova et al. 2003; Inglese et al., 2004; Adalsteinsson et al., 2004; Fernando et al., 2004; Ruiz-Pena et al., 2004; Vrenken et al., 2005; Mathiesen et al., 2005; Khan et al., 2005; Sijens et al., 2006; Wattjes et al., 2008; Wattjes et al., 2008; Khan et al., 2008; Bellmann-Strobl et al., 2009; Aboul-Enein et al., 2010).

5.2.2 Significant changes of Cho ratios or Cho concentrations

In **two MRS studies** (**8** and **19 RRMS** patients) Cho was found decreased (Davie et al., 1994; Tedeschi et al., 2001) and in **4 MRS studies** (**9, 16, 43** and **21 RRMS** patients) Cho levels were found increased (He et al., 2005; Srinivasan et al., 2005; Pascual et al., 2007; Kirov et al., 2008).

5.3 Reported mIns changes

5.3.1 No significant changes of mIns ratios or mIns concentrations

Five out of 12 MRS studies reported no significant mINS changes in the NAWM of in a total of **76 CIS** or **17 RRMS** patients (Brex et al., 1999; Sarchielli et al., 1998; Sijens et al., 2006; Wattjes et al., 2008a; Wattjes et al., 2008b).

5.3.2 Significant changes of mIns ratios or mIns concentrations

Seven out of 12 MRS studies reported **increased** levels of mIns in the NAWM of in a total of **96 CIS** or **116 RRMS** patients (Kapeller et al., 2001; Chard et al., 2002; Fernando et al., 2004; He et al., 2005; Vrenken et al., 2005; Srinivasan et al., 2005; Kirov et al., 2008).

Keep in mind, that in most of the cases statistical characteristics of groups of MS patients were reported. Only very rarely the presentation of the data allow the readers their own interpretation because data are summarized in tables (with means, standard errors or standard deviations, range) and bar charts, instead of tables and scatter plots presenting all data for each individual patients. That groups of patients differ significantly, does not necessarily mean that all patients differ significantly from age and sex matched normal controls. They even may lie within normal range. For instance, the NAA levels of RRMS patients and even a proportion of SPMS patients were found within the range of NAA absolute concentrations that were found in healthy controls (Aboul-Enein et al., 2010; fig.3 squares, RRMS patients (n=27); circles, SPMS patients (n=10); triangles, controls (n=8); bars, means). However the mean NAA levels of SPMS patients were found significantly decreased compared to controls and RRMS patients.

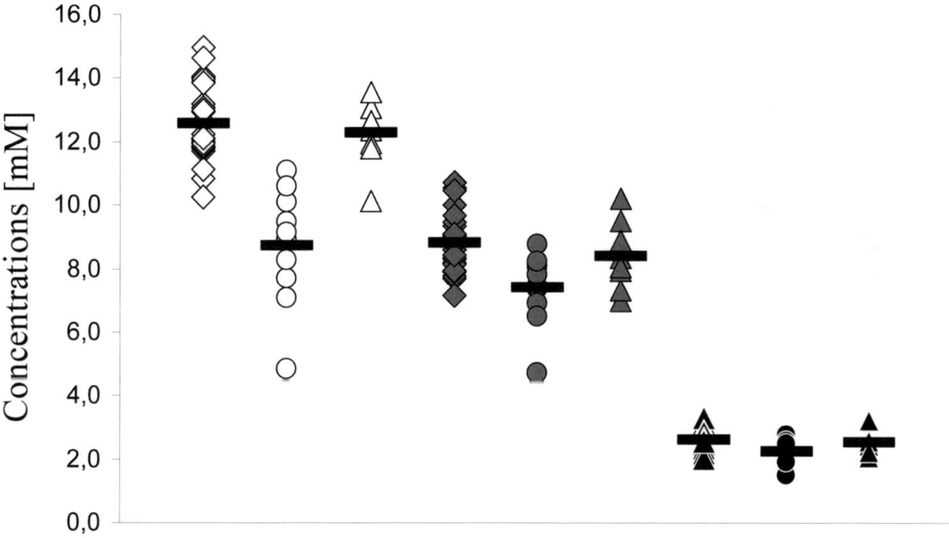

Fig. 3. MRS absolute concentrations of brain metabolites in the NAWM of MS patients and controls (from Aboul-Enein F et al., 2010). White, NAA [mM]; grey, Cr [mM]; black, Cho [mM].

6. Conclusion

Currently the potpourri of data allows no reliable general information or even evidence about metabolite changes in the NAWM that were hypothesized to occur in all CIS or RRMS patients. Sophisticated meta-analysis is yet not possible as different MR methods were used, and individual data such as age, sex, disease duration, disease activity, lesion load, therapy, and metabolites concentrations cannot be extracted. Moreover, it remains unclear, what the specific metabolites reflect in the tissue of individual MS patients. In any case, we must be aware that the magnetic resonances of freely mobile hydrogen protons or certain other freely mobile metabolites are converted to images, and thus 'are made visible for the human's eye'.

7. Acknowledgment

The author is thankful to Atbin for substantial help. In love, dedicated to my little daughter and my wife.

8. References

Aboul-Enein F, Krssák M, Höftberger R, Prayer D, Kristoferitsch W. (2010). Reduced NAA-levels in the NAWM of patients with MS is a feature of progression. A study with quantitative magnetic resonance spectroscopy at 3 Tesla. *PLoS One,* Vol. 5, No. 7, (July 2010), e11625, ISSN 1932-6203.

Aboul-Enein F, Bauer J, Klein M, Schubart A, Flügel A, Ritter T, Kawakami N, Siedler F, Linington C, Wekerle H, Lassmann H, Bradl M. (2004). Selective and antigen-dependent effects of myelin degeneration on central nervous system inflammation. *J Neuropathol Exp Neurol,* Vol. 63, No. 12, (December 2004), pp. 1284-1296, ISSN 0022-3069.

Aboul-Enein F, Lassmann H. (2005). Mitochondrial damage and histotoxic hypoxia: a pathway of tissue injury in inflammatory brain disease? *Acta Neuropathol,* Vol. 109, No. 1, (January 2005), pp. 49-55, ISSN 0001-6322.

Aboul-Enein F, Weiser P, Höftberger R, Lassmann H, Bradl M. (2006). Transient axonal injury in the absence of demyelination: a correlate of clinical disease in acute experimental autoimmune encephalomyelitis. *Acta Neuropathol,* Vol. 111, No. 6, (June 2006), pp. 539-547, ISSN 0001-6322.

Aboul-Enein F, Krssák M, Höftberger R, Prayer D, Kristoferitsch W. (2010). Diffuse white matter damage is absent in neuromyelitis optica. *AJNR Am J Neuroradiol,* Vol. 31, No. 1, (January 2010), pp. 76-79, ISSN 0195-6108.

Adalsteinsson E, Langer-Gould A, Homer RJ, Rao A, Sullivan EV, Lima CA, Pfefferbaum A, Atlas SW. (2003). Gray matter N-acetyl aspartate deficits in secondary progressive but not relapsing-remitting multiple sclerosis. *AJNR Am J Neuroradiol,* Vol. 24, No. 10, (November 2003), pp. 1941-1945, ISSN 0195-6108.

Allen IV, McKeown SR. (1979). A histological, histochemical and biochemical study of the macroscopically normal white matter in multiple sclerosis. *J Neurol Sci,* Vol. 41, No. 1. (March 1979), pp. 81-91, ISSN 1300-1817.

Allen IV, Glover G, Anderson R. (1981). Abnormalities in the macroscopically normal white matter in cases of mild or spinal multiple sclerosis (MS). *Acta Neuropathol,* Vol. 7, No. Supplement, (1981), pp. 176-178, ISSN 0001-6322.

Arnold DL, Matthews PM, Francis G, Antel J. (1990). Proton magnetic resonance spectroscopy of human brain in vivo in the evaluation of multiple sclerosis: assessment of the load of disease. *Magn Reson Med,* Vol. 14 , No 1., (April 1990), pp. 154-159, ISSN 1522-2594.

Arnold DL, Riess GT, Matthews PM, Francis GS, Collins DL, Wolfson C, Antel JP. (1994). Use of proton magnetic resonance spectroscopy for monitoring disease progression in multiple sclerosis. *Ann Neurol,* Vol. 36, No. 1, (July 1994), pp. 76-82, ISSN 0364-5134.

Barkhof F, Hommes OR, Scheltens P, Valk J. (1991). Quantitative MRI changes in gadolinium-DTPA enhancement after high-dose intravenous methylprednisolone in multiple sclerosis. *Neurology,* Vol. 41, No. 8, (August 1991), pp. 1219-1222, ISSN 0028-3878.

Barkhof F, Tas MW, Frequin ST, Scheltens P, Hommes OR, Nauta JJ, Valk J. (1994). Limited duration of the effect of methylprednisolone on changes on MRI in multiple sclerosis. *Neuroradiology,* Vol. 36, No. 5, (July 1994), pp. 382-387, ISSN 0028-3940.

Barnes D, Munro PM, Youl BD, Prineas JW, McDonald WI. (1991) The longstanding MS lesion. A quantitative MRI and electron microscopic study. *Brain,* Vol. 114, No. 3, (June 1991), pp. 1271-1280; ISSN 0006-8950.

Barnett MH, Prineas JW. (2004). Relapsing and remitting multiple sclerosis: pathology of the newly forming lesion. *Ann Neurol,* Vol. 55, No. 4, (April 2004), pp. 458-468, ISSN 0364-5134.

Barnett MH, Parratt JD, Pollard JD, Prineas JW. (2009). MS: is it one disease? *Int MS J,* Vol. 16, No. 2, (June 2009), pp. 57-65, ISSN 1352-8963.

Benedetti B, Rovaris M, Rocca MA, Caputo D, Zaffaroni M, Capra R, Bertolotto A, Martinelli V, Comi G, Filippi M. (2009). In-vivo evidence for stable neuroaxonal damage in the brain of patients with benign multiple sclerosis. *Mult Scler,* Vol. 15, No. 7, (July 2009), pp. 789-794, ISSN 1352-4585.

Bitsch A, Bruhn H, Vougioukas V, Stringaris A, Lassmann H, Frahm J, Brück W. (1999). Inflammatory CNS demyelination: histopathologic correlation with in vivo quantitative proton MR spectroscopy. *AJNR Am J Neuroradiol,* Vol. 20, No. 9, (October 1999), pp. 1619-1627, ISSN 0195-6108.

Brex PA, Gomez-Anson B, Parker GJ, Molyneux PD, Miszkiel KA, Barker GJ, MacManus DG, Davie CA, Plant GT, Miller DH. (1999). Proton MR spectroscopy in clinically isolated syndromes suggestive of multiple sclerosis. *J Neurol Sci,* Vol. 166, No. 1, (June 1999), pp. 16-22, ISSN 1300-1817.

Brex PA, Ciccarelli O, O'Riordan JI, Sailer M, Thompson AJ, Miller DH. (2002). A longitudinal study of abnormalities on MRI and disability from multiple sclerosis. *N Engl J Med,* Vol. 346, No. 3, (January 2002), pp. 158-164, ISSN 0028-4793.

Bruhn H, Frahm J, Gyngell ML, Merboldt KD, Hänicke W, Sauter R. (1989). Cerebral metabolism in man after acute stroke: new observations using localized proton NMR spectroscopy. *Magn Reson Med,* Vol. 9, No. 1, (January 1989), pp. 126-131, ISSN 1522-2594.

Burnham JA, Wright RR, Dreisbach J, Murray RS. (1991). The effect of high-dose steroids on MRI gadolinium enhancement in acute demyelinating lesions. *Neurology,* Vol. 41, No. 9, (September 1991), pp. 1349-1354. ISSN 0028-3878.

Casanova B, Martínez-Bisbal MC, Valero C, Celda B, Martí-Bonmatí L, Pascual A, Landente L, Coret F. (2003). Evidence of Wallerian degeneration in normal appearing white matter in the early stages of relapsing-remitting multiple sclerosis: a HMRS study. *J Neurol,* Vol. 250, No. 1, (January 2003), pp. 22-28, ISSN 0340-5354.

Chard DT, Griffin CM, McLean MA, Kapeller P, Kapoor R, Thompson AJ, Miller DH. (2002). Brain metabolite changes in cortical grey and normal-appearing white matter in clinically early relapsing-remitting multiple sclerosis. *Brain,* Vol. 125, No. 10, (October 2002), pp. 2342-2352, ISSN 0006-8950.

Chataway J. (2008). When the MRI scan suggests multiple sclerosis but the symptoms do not. *J Neurol Neurosurg Psychiatry,* Vol. 79, No. 2, (February 2008), pp. 112-113, ISSN 0022-3050.

Chataway J. (2010). When confronted by a patient with the radiologically isolated syndrome. *Pract Neurol,* Vol. 10, No. 5, (October 2010), pp. 271-277, ISSN 1474-7758.

Davie CA, Hawkins CP, Barker GJ, Brennan A, Tofts PS, Miller DH, McDonald WI. (1994). Serial proton magnetic resonance spectroscopy in acute multiple sclerosis lesions. *Brain,* Vol. 117, (February 1994), pp. 49-58, ISSN 0006-8950.

Davie CA, Barker GJ, Thompson AJ, Tofts PS, McDonald WI, Miller DH. (1997). 1H magnetic resonance spectroscopy of chronic cerebral white matter lesions and normal appearing white matter in multiple sclerosis. *J Neurol Neurosurg Psychiatry,* Vol. 63, No. 6, (December 1997), pp. 736-742, ISSN 0022-3050.

De Stefano N, Matthews PM, Fu L, Narayanan S, Stanley J, Francis GS, Antel JP, Arnold DL. (1998). Axonal damage correlates with disability in patients with relapsing-remitting multiple sclerosis. Results of a longitudinal magnetic resonance spectroscopy study. *Brain,* Vol. 121, No. 8, (August 1998), pp. 1469-1477, ISSN 0006-8950.

De Stefano N, Narayanan S, Francis GS, Arnaoutelis R, Tartaglia MC, Antel JP, Matthews PM, Arnold DL. (2001). Evidence of axonal damage in the early stages of multiple sclerosis and its relevance to disability. *Arch Neurol,* Vol. 58, No. 1, (January 2001), pp. 65-70, ISSN 0003-9942.

De Stefano N, Narayanan S, Francis SJ, Smith S, Mortilla M, Tartaglia MC, Bartolozzi ML, Guidi L, Federico A, Arnold DL. (2002). Diffuse axonal and tissue injury in patients with multiple sclerosis with low cerebral lesion load and no disability. *Arch Neurol,* Vol. 59, No. 10, (October 2002), pp. 1565-1571, ISSN 0003-9942.

Engelhardt B. (2006). Molecular mechanisms involved in T cell migration across the blood-brain barrier. *J Neural Transm,* Vol. 113, No. 4, (April 2006), pp. 477-485, ISSN 0300-9564.

Falini A, Calabrese G, Filippi M, Origgi D, Lipari S, Colombo B, Comi G, Scotti G. (1998). Benign versus secondary-progressive multiple sclerosis: the potential role of proton MR spectroscopy in defining the nature of disability. *AJNR Am J Neuroradiol,* Vol. 19, No. 2, (February 1998), pp. 223-229, ISSN 0195-6108.

Filippi M, Yousry T, Campi A, Kandziora C, Colombo B, Voltz R, Martinelli V, Spuler S, Bressi S, Scotti G, Comi G. (1996). Comparison of triple dose versus standard dose gadolinium-DTPA for detection of MRI enhancing lesions in patients with MS. *Neurology,* Vol. 46, No. 2, (February 1996), pp. 379-384, ISSN 0028-3878.

Fisniku LK, Brex PA, Altmann DR, Miszkiel KA, Benton CE, Lanyon R, Thompson AJ, Miller DH. (2008). Disability and T2 MRI lesions: a 20-year follow-up of patients with relapse onset of multiple sclerosis. *Brain,* Vol. 131, No. 3, (March 2008), pp. 808-817, ISSN 0006-8950.

Floris S, Blezer EL, Schreibelt G, Döpp E, van der Pol SM, Schadee-Eestermans IL, Nicolay K, Dijkstra CD, de Vries HE. (2004). Blood-brain barrier permeability and monocyte infiltration in experimental allergic encephalomyelitis: a quantitative MRI study. *Brain,* Vol. 127, No. 3, (March 2004), pp. 616-627, ISSN 0006-8950.

Flügel A, Berkowicz T, Ritter T, Labeur M, Jenne DE, Li Z, Ellwart JW, Willem M, Lassmann H, Wekerle H. (2001). Migratory activity and functional changes of green fluorescent effector cells before and during experimental autoimmune encephalomyelitis. *Immunity,* Vol. 14, No. 5, (May 2001), pp. 547-560, ISSN 1074-7613.

Flügel A, Odoardi F, Nosov M, Kawakami N. (2007). Autoaggressive effector T cells in the course of experimental autoimmune encephalomyelitis visualized in the light of two-photon microscopy. *J Neuroimmunol,* Vol. 191, No. 1-2, (November 2007), pp. 86-97, ISSN 0165-5728.

Foong J, Rozewicz L, Davie CA, Thompson AJ, Miller DH, Ron MA. (1999). Correlates of executive function in multiple sclerosis: the use of magnetic resonance spectroscopy as an index of focal pathology. *J Neuropsychiatry Clin Neurosci,* Vol. 11, No. 1, (Winter 1999), pp. 45-50, ISN 0895-0172.

Frahm J, Bruhn H, Gyngell ML, Merboldt KD, Hänicke W, Sauter R. (1989a). Localized high-resolution proton NMR spectroscopy using stimulated echoes: initial applications to human brain in vivo. *Magn Reson Med,* Vol. 9, No. 1, (January 1989), pp. 79-93, ISSN 1522-2594.

Frahm J, Bruhn H, Gyngell ML, Merboldt KD, Hänicke W, Sauter R. (1989b). Localized proton NMR spectroscopy in different regions of the human brain in vivo. Relaxation times and concentrations of cerebral metabolites. *Magn Reson Med,* Vol. 11, No. 1, (July 1989), pp. 47-63, ISSN 1522-2594.

Fu L, Matthews PM, De Stefano N, Worsley KJ, Narayanan S, Francis GS, Antel JP, Wolfson C, Arnold DL. (1998). Imaging axonal damage of normal-appearing white matter in multiple sclerosis. *Brain,* Vol. 121, No. 1, (January 1998), pp. 103-113, ISSN 0006-8950.

Gelati M, Corsini E, De Rossi M, Masini L, Bernardi G, Massa G, Boiardi A, Salmaggi A. (2002). Methylprednisolone acts on peripheral blood mononuclear cells and endothelium in inhibiting migration phenomena in patients with multiple sclerosis. *Arch Neurol,* Vol. 59, No. 5, (May 2002), pp. 774-780, ISSN 0003-9942.

Gilmore CP, Cottrell DA, Scolding NJ, Wingerchuk DM, Weinshenker BG, Boggild M. (2010). A window of opportunity for no treatment in early multiple sclerosis? *Mult Scler,* Vol. 16, No. 6, (June 2010), pp. 756-759, ISSN 1352-4585.

Grossman RI, Lenkinski RE, Ramer KN, Gonzalez-Scarano F, Cohen JA. (1992). MR proton spectroscopy in multiple sclerosis. *AJNR Am J Neuroradiol,* Vol. 13, No. 6, (November-December 1992), pp. 1535-1343, ISSN 0195-6108.

Hawkins CP, Mackenzie F, Tofts P, du Boulay EP, McDonald WI. (1991). Patterns of blood-brain barrier breakdown in inflammatory demyelination. *Brain,* Vol. 114, No. 2, (April 1991), pp. 801-810. ISSN 0006-8950.

He J, Inglese M, Li BS, Babb JS, Grossman RI, Gonen O. (2005). Relapsing-remitting multiple sclerosis: metabolic abnormality in nonenhancing lesions and normal-appearing white matter at MR imaging: initial experience. *Radiology,* Vol. 234, No. 1, (January 2005), pp. 211-217, ISSN 0033-8419.

Henderson AP, Barnett MH, Parratt JD, Prineas JW. (2009). Multiple sclerosis: distribution of inflammatory cells in newly forming lesions. *Ann Neurol,* Vol. 66, No. 6, (December 2009); pp. 739-753, ISSN 0364-5134.

Hibberd PL. (1994). Use and misuse of statistics for epidemiological studies of multiple sclerosis. *Ann Neurol,* Vol. 36, No. Suppl. 2, (December 1994), pp. S218-230, ISSN 0364-5134.

Höftberger R, Aboul-Enein F, Brueck W, Lucchinetti C, Rodriguez M, Schmidbauer M, Jellinger K, Lassmann H. (2004). Expression of major histocompatibility complex class I molecules on the different cell types in multiple sclerosis lesions. *Brain Pathol,* Vol. 14, No. 1, (January 2004), pp. 43-50, ISSN 1015-6305.

Hohlfeld R, Kerschensteiner M, Stadelmann C, Lassmann H, Wekerle H. (2006). The neuroprotective effect of inflammation: implications for the therapy of multiple sclerosis. *Neurol Sci,* Vol. 27, No. S1, (March 2006), pp. S1-S7, ISSN 1590-1874.

Husted CA, Goodin DS, Hugg JW, Maudsley AA, Tsuruda JS, de Bie SH, Fein G, Matson GB, Weiner MW. (1994). Biochemical alterations in multiple sclerosis lesions and normal-appearing white matter detected by in vivo 31P and 1H spectroscopic imaging. *Ann Neurol.* Vol. 36, No. 2, (August 1994), pp. 157-165, ISSN 0364-5134.

IFNB Multiple Sclerosis Study Group. (11993). Interferon beta-1b is effective in relapsing-remitting multiple sclerosis. I. Clinical results of a multicenter, randomized, double-blind, placebo-controlled trial. The IFNB Multiple Sclerosis Study Group. *Neurology,* Vol. 43, No. 4, (April 1993), pp. 655-661, ISSN 0028-3878.

Jacobs L, Kinkel PR, Kinkel WR. (1986). Silent brain lesions in patients with isolated idiopathic optic neuritis. A clinical and nuclear magnetic resonance imaging study. *Arch Neurol,* Vol. 43, No. 5, (May 1986), pp. 452-455, ISSN 0003-9942.

Jackson JA, Leake DR, Schneiders NJ, Rolak LA, Kelley GR, Ford JJ, Appel SH, Bryan RN. (1985). Magnetic resonance imaging in multiple sclerosis: results in 32 cases. *AJNR Am J Neuroradiol,* Vol. 6, No. 2, (March-April 1985), pp. 171-176, ISSN 0195-6108.

Kangarlu A, Bourekas EC, Ray-Chaudhury A, Rammohan KW. (2007). Cerebral cortical lesions in multiple sclerosis detected by MR imaging at 8 Tesla. *AJNR Am J Neuroradiol,* Vol. 28, No. 2, (February 2007), pp. 262-266, ISSN 0195-6108.

Kapeller P, McLean MA, Griffin CM, Chard D, Parker GJ, Barker GJ, Thompson AJ, Miller DH. (2001). Preliminary evidence for neuronal damage in cortical grey matter and normal appearing white matter in short duration relapsing-remitting multiple sclerosis: a quantitative MR spectroscopic imaging study. *J Neurol,* Vol. 248, No. 2, (February 2001), pp. 131-138, ISSN 0340-5354.

Kapeller P, Brex PA, Chard D, Dalton C, Griffin CM, McLean MA, Parker GJ, Thompson AJ, Miller DH. Quantitative 1H MRS imaging 14 years after presenting with a clinically isolated syndrome suggestive of multiple sclerosis. *Mult Scler,* Vol. 8, No. 3, (May 2002), pp. 207-210, ISSN 0340-5354.

Kawakami N, Nägerl UV, Odoardi F, Bonhoeffer T, Wekerle H, Flügel A. (2005). Live imaging of effector cell trafficking and autoantigen recognition within the unfolding autoimmune encephalomyelitis lesion. *J Exp Med,* Vol. 201, No. 11, (June 2005), pp. 1805-1814, ISSN: 0022-1007.

Kimura H, Grossman RI, Lenkinski RE, Gonzalez-Scarano F. (1996). Proton MR spectroscopy and magnetization transfer ratio in multiple sclerosis: correlative findings of active versus irreversible plaque disease. *AJNR Am J Neuroradiol,* Vol. 17, No. 8, (September 1996), pp. 1539-1547, ISSN 0195-6108.

Kirov II, Patil V, Babb JS, Rusinek H, Herbert J, Gonen O. (2009). MR spectroscopy indicates diffuse multiple sclerosis activity during remission. J Neurol Neurosurg Psychiatry, Vol. 80, No. 12, (December 2009), pp. 1330-1336, ISSN 0022-3050.

Khan O, Shen Y, Caon C, Bao F, Ching W, Reznar M, Buccheister A, Hu J, Latif Z, Tselis A, Lisak R. (2005). Axonal metabolic recovery and potential neuroprotective effect of glatiramer acetate in relapsing-remitting multiple sclerosis. *Mult Scler,* Vol. 11, No. 6, (December 2005), pp. 646-651, ISSN 1352-4585.

Khan O, Shen Y, Bao F, Caon C, Tselis A, Latif Z, Zak I. (2008). Long-term study of brain 1H-MRS study in multiple sclerosis: effect of glatiramer acetate therapy on axonal metabolic function and feasibility of long-Term H-MRS monitoring in multiple sclerosis. *J Neuroimaging,* Vol. 18, No. 3, (July 2008), pp. 314-319, ISSN 1051-2284.

Kuhle J, Pohl C, Mehling M, Edan G, Freedman MS, Hartung HP, Polman CH, Miller DH, Montalban X, Barkhof F, Bauer L, Dahms S, Lindberg R, Kappos L, Sandbrink R. (2007). Lack of association between antimyelin antibodies and progression to multiple sclerosis. *N Engl J Med,* Vol. 356, No. 4, (January 2007), pp. 371-378, ISSN 0028-4793.

Kwon EE, Prineas JW. (1994). Blood-brain barrier abnormalities in longstanding multiple sclerosis lesions. An immunohistochemical study. *J Neuropathol Exp Neurol,* Vol. 53, No. 6, (November 1994), pp. 625-636, ISSN 0022-3069.

Lassmann H, Brück W, Lucchinetti CF. (2007). The immunopathology of multiple sclerosis: an overview. *Brain Pathol,* Vol. 17, No. 2, (April 2007), pp. 210-218, ISSN 1015-6305.

Leary SM, Davie CA, Parker GJ, Stevenson VL, Wang L, Barker GJ, Miller DH, Thompson AJ. (1999). 1H magnetic resonance spectroscopy of normal appearing white matter in primary progressive multiple sclerosis. *J Neurol,* Vol. 246, No. 11, (November 1999), pp. 1023-1026, ISSN 0340-5354.

Lebrun C, Bensa C, Debouverie M, De Seze J, Wiertlievski S, Brochet B, Clavelou P, Brassat D, Labauge P, Roullet E; CFSEP. (2008). Unexpected multiple sclerosis: follow-up of 30 patients with magnetic resonance imaging and clinical conversion profile. *J Neurol Neurosurg Psychiatry,* Vol. 79, No. 2, (February 2008), pp. 195-198, ISSN 0022-3050.

Leussink VI, Jung S, Merschdorf U, Toyka KV, Gold R. (2001). High dose methylprednisolone therapy in multiple sclerosis induces apoptosis in peripheral blood leukocytes. *Arch Neurol,* Vol. 58, No. 1, (January 2001), pp. 91-97, ISSN 0003-9942.

Lublin FD, Reingold SC. (1996).Defining the clinical course of multiple sclerosis: results of an international survey. National Multiple Sclerosis Society (USA) Advisory Committee on Clinical Trials of New Agents in Multiple Sclerosis. *Neurology,* Vol. 46, No. 4, (April 1996), pp. 907-911, ISSN 0028-3878.

Lumsden CE. (1970). The neuropathology of multiple sclerosis, In: *Handbook of Clinical Neurology,* Vinken PJ, and Bruyn GW (Eds.), Vol. 9, pp. 217-309, Elsevier, ISSN 0072-9752, Amsterdam, North-Holland.

Mathiesen HK, Tscherning T, Sorensen PS, Larsson HB, Rostrup E, Paulson OB, Hanson LG. (2005). Multi-slice echo-planar spectroscopic MR imaging provides both global and local metabolite measures in multiple sclerosis. *Magn Reson Med,* Vol. 53, No. 4, (April 2005), pp. 750-759, ISSN 1522-2594.

Matthews PM, Pioro E, Narayanan S, De Stefano N, Fu L, Francis G, Antel J, Wolfson C, Arnold DL. (1996). Assessment of lesion pathology in multiple sclerosis using quantitative MRI morphometry and magnetic resonance spectroscopy. *Brain,* Vol. 119, No. 3, (June 1999), pp. 715-722, ISSN 0006-8950.

McDonald WI, Sears TA. (1970). The effects of experimental demyelination on conduction in the central nervous system. *Brain,* Vol. 93, No. 3, (March 1970), pp. 583-598. ISSN 0006-8950.

McDonald WI, Compston A, Edan G, Goodkin D, Hartung HP, Lublin FD, McFarland HF, Paty DW, Polman CH, Reingold SC, Sandberg-Wollheim M, Sibley W, Thompson A, van den Noort S, Weinshenker BY, Wolinsky JS. (2001). Recommended diagnostic criteria for multiple sclerosis: guidelines from the International Panel on the diagnosis of multiple sclerosis. *Ann Neurol,* Vol. 50, No. 1, (July 2001), pp121-127, ISSN 0364-5134.

Miller DH, Grossman RI, Reingold SC, McFarland HF. (1998). The role of magnetic resonance techniques in understanding and managing multiple sclerosis. *Brain,* Vol. 121, No. 1, (January 1998), pp. 3-24, ISSN 0006-8950.

Miller DH, Weinshenker BG, Filippi M, Banwell BL, Cohen JA, Freedman MS, Galetta SL, Hutchinson M, Johnson RT, Kappos L, Kira J, Lublin FD, McFarland HF, Montalban X, Panitch H, Richert JR, Reingold SC, Polman CH. (2008). Differential diagnosis of suspected multiple sclerosis: a consensus approach. *Mult Scler,* Vol. 14, No. 9, (November 2008), pp. 1157-1174, ISSN 1352-4585.

Narayanan S, Fu L, Pioro E, De Stefano N, Collins DL, Francis GS, Antel JP, Matthews PM, Arnold DL. (1997). Imaging of axonal damage in multiple sclerosis: spatial distribution of magnetic resonance imaging lesions. *Ann Neurol,* Vol. 41, No. 3, (March 1997), pp. 385-391, ISSN 0364-5134.

Pascual AM, Martínez-Bisbal MC, Boscá I, Valero C, Coret F, Martínez-Granados B, Marti-Bonmati L, Mir A, Celda B, Casanova B. (2007). Axonal loss is progressive and partly dissociated from lesion load in early multiple sclerosis. *Neurology,* Vol. 69, No. 1, (July 2007), pp. 63-67, ISSN 0028-3878.

Paty DW, Li DK. (1993). Interferon beta-1b is effective in relapsing-remitting multiple sclerosis. II. MRI analysis results of a multicenter, randomized, double-blind, placebo-controlled trial. UBC MS/MRI Study Group and the IFNB Multiple Sclerosis Study Group. *Neurology,* Vol. 43, No. 4, (April 1993), pp. 662-667, ISSN 0028-3878.

Peters AR, Geelen JA, den Boer JA, Prevo RL, Minderhoud JM, 's Gravenmade EJ. (1995). A study of multiple sclerosis patients with magnetic resonance spectroscopic imaging. *Mult Scler,* Vol. 1, No. 1, (April 1995), pp. 25-31, ISSN 1352-4585.

Polman CH, Reingold SC, Edan G, Filippi M, Hartung HP, Kappos L, Lublin FD, Metz LM, McFarland HF, O'Connor PW, Sandberg-Wollheim M, Thompson AJ, Weinshenker BG, Wolinsky JS. (2005). Diagnostic criteria for multiple sclerosis: 2005 revisions to the "McDonald Criteria". *Ann Neurol,* Vol. 58, No. 6, (December 2005), pp. 840-846, ISSN 0364-5134.

Polman CH, Reingold SC, Banwell B, Clanet M, Cohen JA, Filippi M, Fujihara K, Havrdova E, Hutchinson M, Kappos L, Lublin FD, Montalban X, O'Connor P, Sandberg-Wollheim M, Thompson AJ, Waubant E, Weinshenker B, Wolinsky JS. (2011)

.Diagnostic criteria for multiple sclerosis: 2010 revisions to the McDonald criteria. *Ann Neurol*, Vol. 69, No. 2, (February 2011), pp. 292-302, ISSN 0364-5134.

Poser CM, Paty DW, Scheinberg L, McDonald WI, Davis FA, Ebers GC, Johnson KP, Sibley WA, Silberberg DH, Tourtellotte WW. (1983). New diagnostic criteria for multiple sclerosis: guidelines for research protocols. *Ann Neurol,* Vol. 13, No. 3, (March 1983), pp. 227-231, ISSN 0364-5134.

Prat A, Biernacki K, Lavoie JF, Poirier J, Duquette P, Antel JP. (2002). Migration of multiple sclerosis lymphocytes through brain endothelium. *Arch Neurol,* Vol. 59, No. 3, (March 2002), pp. 391-397, ISSN 0003-9942.

Richards TL. Proton MR spectroscopy in multiple sclerosis: value in establishing diagnosis, monitoring progression, and evaluating therapy. (1991). *AJR Am J Roentgenol,* Vol. 157, No. 5, (November 1991), pp. 1073-1078, ISSN 1546-3141.

Rooney WD, Goodkin DE, Schuff N, Meyerhoff DJ, Norman D, Weiner MW. (1997). 1H MRSI of normal appearing white matter in multiple sclerosis. *Mult Scler,* Vol. 3, No. 4, (August 1997), pp. 231-237, ISSN

Roser W, Hagberg G, Mader I, Brunnschweiler H, Radue EW, Seelig J, Kappos L. (1995). Proton MRS of gadolinium-enhancing MS plaques and metabolic changes in normal-appearing white matter. *Magn Reson Med,* Vol. 33, No. 6, (June 1995), pp. 811-817, ISSN 1522-2594.

Ruiz-Peña JL, Piñero P, Sellers G, Argente J, Casado A, Foronda J, Uclés A, Izquierdo G. (2004). Magnetic resonance spectroscopy of normal appearing white matter in early relapsing-remitting multiple sclerosis: correlations between disability and spectroscopy. *BMC Neurol,* Vol. 10, No. 6, (June 2004), pp. 4-8, ISSN 1471-2377.

Sarchielli P, Presciutti O, Tarducci R, Gobbi G, Alberti A, Pelliccioli GP, Orlacchio A, Gallai V. (1998). 1H-MRS in patients with multiple sclerosis undergoing treatment with interferon beta-1a: results of a preliminary study. *J Neurol Neurosurg Psychiatry,* Vol. 64, No. 2, (February 1998), pp. 204-212, ISSN 0022-3050.

Sarchielli P, Presciutti O, Pelliccioli GP, Tarducci R, Gobbi G, Chiarini P, Alberti A, Vicinanza F, Gallai V. (1999). Absolute quantification of brain metabolites by proton magnetic resonance spectroscopy in normal-appearing white matter of multiple sclerosis patients. *Brain,* Vol 122, No. 3, (March 1999), pp. 513-521, ISSN 0006-8950.

Sastre-Garriga J, Ingle GT, Chard DT, Ramió-Torrentà L, McLean MA, Miller DH, Thompson AJ. (2005). Metabolite changes in normal-appearing gray and white matter are linked with disability in early primary progressive multiple sclerosis. Arch Neurol, Vol. 62, No. 4, (April 2005), pp. 569-573, ISSN 0003-9942.

Schiepers C, Van Hecke P, Vandenberghe R, Van Oostende S, Dupont P, Demaerel P, Bormans G, Carton H. (1997). Positron emission tomography, magnetic resonance imaging and proton NMR spectroscopy of white matter in multiple sclerosis. *Mult Scler,* Vol. 3, No. 1, (February 1997), pp. 8-17, ISSN 1352-4585.

Schubert F, Seifert F, Elster C, Link A, Walzel M, Mientus S, Haas J, Rinneberg H. (2002). Serial 1H-MRS in relapsing-remitting multiple sclerosis: effects of interferon-beta therapy on absolute metabolite concentrations. MAGMA, Vol. 14, No. 3, (June 2002), pp. 213-222,

Schuhmacher GA, Beebe G, Kibler RF, Kurland LT, Kurtzke JF, McDowell F, Nagler B, Sibley WA, Tourtellotte WW, Willmon TL. (1965). Problems of experimental trials of therapy in multiple sclerosis: report by the panel on the evaluation of experimental trials of therapy in multiple sclerosis. *Ann N Y Acad Sci,* Vol. 31., no. 122, (March 1965), pp. 552-556, ISSN 0077-8923.

Sellner J, Schirmer L, Hemmer B, Mühlau M. (2010). The radiologically isolated syndrome: take action when the unexpected is uncovered? *J Neurol,* Vol. 257, No. 10, (October 2010), pp. 1602-1611, ISSN 0340-5354.

Serbecic N, Aboul-Enein F, Beutelspacher SC, Graf M, Kircher K, Geitzenauer W, Brannath W, Lang P, Kristoferitsch W, Lassmann H, Reitner A, Schmidt-Erfurth U. (2010). Heterogeneous pattern of retinal nerve fiber layer in multiple sclerosis. High resolution optical coherence tomography: potential and limitations. *PLoS One.* Vol.5, No. 11, (November 2010), e19843, ISSN 1932-6203.

Serbecic N, Aboul-Enein F, Beutelspacher SC, Vass C, Kristoferitsch W, Lassmann H, Reitner A, Schmidt-Erfurth U. (2011). High resolution spectral domain optical coherence tomography (SD-OCT) in multiple sclerosis: the first follow up study over two years. *PLoS One.* Vol. 6, No. 5, (May 2011), e19843, ISSN 1932-6203.

Siger-Zajdel M, Selmaj K. (2006). Proton magnetic resonance spectroscopy of normal appearing white matter in asymptomatic relatives of multiple sclerosis patients. *Eur J Neurol,* Vol. 13, No. 3, (March 2006), pp. 296-298, ISSN 1351-5101.

Simone IL, Federico F, Trojano M, Tortorella C, Liguori M, Giannini P, Picciola E, Natile G, Livrea P. (1996). High resolution proton MR spectroscopy of cerebrospinal fluid in MS patients. Comparison with biochemical changes in demyelinating plaques. *J Neurol Sci,* Vol. 144, No. 1-2, (December 1996), pp. 182-190, ISSN 1300-1817.

Siva A, Saip S, Altintas A, Jacob A, Keegan BM, Kantarci OH. (2009) Multiple sclerosis risk in radiologically uncovered asymptomatic possible inflammatory-demyelinating disease. *Mult Scler,* Vol. 15, No. 8, (August 2009), pp. 918-927, ISSN 1352-4585.

Sijens PE, Mostert JP, Oudkerk M, De Keyser J. (2006). (1)H MR spectroscopy of the brain in multiple sclerosis subtypes with analysis of the metabolite concentrations in gray and white matter: initial findings. *Eur Radiol,* Vol. 16, No. 2, (February 2006), pp. 489-495, ISSN 0938-7994.

Smith KJ, Lassmann H. (2002). The role of nitric oxide in multiple sclerosis. *Lancet Neurol,* Vol. 1, No. 4, (August 2002), pp. 232-241, ISSN 1474-4422.

Smith KJ. (2007). Sodium channels and multiple sclerosis: roles in symptom production, damage and therapy. *Brain Pathol,* Vol. 17, No. 2, (April 2007), pp. 230-242, ISSN 1015-6305.

Sriram S, Steiner I. (2005). Experimental allergic encephalomyelitis: A misleading model of multiple sclerosis. *Ann Neurol,* Vol. 58, No. 6, (December 2005), pp. 939–945, ISSN 0364-5134.

Srinivasan R, Sailasuta N, Hurd R, Nelson S, Pelletier D. (2005). Evidence of elevated glutamate in multiple sclerosis using magnetic resonance spectroscopy at 3 T. *Brain,* Vol. 128, No. 5, (May 2005), pp. 1016-1025, ISSN 0006-8950.

Staffen W, Zauner H, Mair A, Kutzelnigg A, Kapeller P, Stangl H, Raffer E, Niederhofer H, Ladurner G. (2005). Magnetic resonance spectroscopy of memory and frontal brain region in early multiple sclerosis. *J Neuropsychiatry Clin Neurosci,* Vol. 17, No. 3, (Summer 2005), pp. 357-363, ISSN 0895-0172.

Suhy J, Rooney WD, Goodkin DE, Capizzano AA, Soher BJ, Maudsley EE, Waubant E, Andersson PB, Weiner MW. (2000). 1H MRSI comparison of white matter and lesions in primary progressive and relapsing-remitting MS. *Mult Scler,* Vol. 6, No. 3, (January 2000), pp. 148-155, ISSN 1352-4585.

Tedeschi G, Bonavita S, McFarland HF, Richert N, Duyn JH, Frank JA. (2001). Proton MR spectroscopic imaging in multiple sclerosis. *Neuroradiology,* Vol. 44, No. 1, (January 2002), pp. 37-42, Jan;44(1):37-42, ISSN 0028-3940.

Tiberio M, Chard DT, Altmann DR, Davies G, Griffin CM, McLean MA, Rashid W, Sastre-Garriga J, Thompson AJ, Miller DH. (2006). Metabolite changes in early relapsing-remitting multiple sclerosis. A two year follow-up study. *J Neurol,* Vol. 253, No. 2, (February 2006), pp. 224-230, ISSN 1351-5101.

Tourbah A, Stievenart JL, Iba-Zizen MT, Zannoli G, Lyon-Caen O, Cabanis EA. (1996). In vivo localized NMR proton spectroscopy of normal appearing white matter in patients with multiple sclerosis. *J Neuroradiol,* Vol. 23, No. 2, (September 1996), pp. 49-55, ISSN 0150-9861.

Tourbah A, Stievenart JL, Gout O, Fontaine B, Liblau R, Lubetzki C, Cabanis EA, Lyon-Caen O. (1999). Localized proton magnetic resonance spectroscopy in relapsing remitting versus secondary progressive multiple sclerosis. *Neurology,* Vol. 53, No. 5, (September 1999), pp. 1091-1097, ISSN 0028-3878.

van Walderveen MA, Barkhof F, Pouwels PJ, van Schijndel RA, Polman CH, Castelijns JA. (1999). Neuronal damage in T1-hypointense multiple sclerosis lesions demonstrated in vivo using proton magnetic resonance spectroscopy. *Ann Neurol,* Vol. 46, No. 1, (July 1999), pp. 79-87, ISSN 0364-5134.

Vrenken H, Barkhof F, Uitdehaag BM, Castelijns JA, Polman CH, Pouwels PJ. (2005). MR spectroscopic evidence for glial increase but not for neuro-axonal damage in MS normal-appearing white matter. *Magn Reson Med,* Vol. 53, No. 2, (February 2005), pp. 256-266, ISSN 1522-2594.

Wattjes MP, Harzheim M, Lutterbey GG, Bogdanow M, Schmidt S, Schild HH, Träber F. (2008). Prognostic value of high-field proton magnetic resonance spectroscopy in patients presenting with clinically isolated syndromes suggestive of multiple sclerosis. *Neuroradiology,* Vol. 50, No. 2, (February 2008), pp. 123-129, ISSN 0028-3940.

Wattjes MP, Harzheim M, Lutterbey GG, Bogdanow M, Schild HH, Träber F. (2008). High field MR imaging and 1H-MR spectroscopy in clinically isolated syndromes suggestive of multiple sclerosis: correlation between metabolic alterations and diagnostic MR imaging criteria. *J Neurol,* Vol. 255, No. 1, (January 2008), pp. 56-63, ISSN 0340-5354.

Waubant E. (2006). Biomarkers indicative of blood-brain barrier disruption in multiple sclerosis. *Dis Markers,* Vol. 22, No. 4, (November 2006), pp. 235-244, ISSN 0278-0240.

Weinshenker BG, Bass B, Rice GP, Noseworthy J, Carriere W, Baskerville J, Ebers GC. (1989a). The natural history of multiple sclerosis: a geographically based study. I. Clinical course and disability. *Brain,* Vol. 112, No. 1, (February 1989), pp. 133-146, ISSN 0006-8950.

Weinshenker BG, Bass B, Rice GP, Noseworthy J, Carriere W, Baskerville J, Ebers GC. (1989b). The natural history of multiple sclerosis: a geographically based study. 2. Predictive value of the early clinical course. *Brain,* Vol. 112, No. 6, (December 1989), pp. 1419-1428, ISSN 0006-8950.

Young IR, Hall AS, Pallis CA, Legg NJ, Bydder GM, Steiner RE. (1981). Nuclear magnetic resonance imaging of the brain in multiple sclerosis. *Lancet.* Vol. 318, No. 8255 (November 1981), pp. 1063-1066, ISSN 0140-6736.

4

Wilson's Disease in Brain Magnetic Resonance Spectroscopy

Beata Tarnacka
Mazovian Center of Rehabilitation, Konstancin Jeziorna
Poland

1. Introduction

Wilson's disease (WD) is an inherited disorder of copper metabolism first defined by Dr Samuel Alexander Kinnier Wilson in 1912 (Wilson, 1912). WD is caused by mutations to the gene coding for ATPase copper transporting beta polypeptide (ATP7B), which is located on 13 chromosome 13 and expressed in the liver (Bull et al.,1993; Loudianos et al.,1999; Yamaguchi et al.,1993; Frydman et al., 1985). The disease is inherited in an autosomal recessive manner.

WD is present worldwide in most populations, and particularly in those in which consanguineous marriage is common. The disease frequency is estimated to be between 1 in 5,000 and 1 in 30,000, and the heterozygous carriers (Hzc) frequency is approximately 1 in 90 (Figus et al., 1995).

In the ATP7B gene of WD a variety of mutations were defected. These defects include insertion, deletion, splice site and point mutations. In most ethnic groups, one or a small number of these ATP7B gene mutations are predominant, in addition to many other rare mutations. In Europeans and North Americans, two ATP7B point mutations: His1069Gln and Gly1267Arg account for 38% of mutations described in WD (Thomas et al., 1995). There is still no favorable correlation between phenotype and genotype, but frame shift deletions and nonsense mutations that cause a truncation of the translated protein product usually result in a severe form of the disease because of loss of the functional protein. The knowledge of the prevalence of mutations is helpful in achieving rapid mutational screening. Mutations in ATP7B cause a reduction in the conversion of apoceruloplasmin into ceruloplasmin, which, is therefore present at low levels in WD patients.

A failure to excrete copper into the biliary canaliculi leads to its toxic accumulation in the hepatocytes (Schilsky&Tavill, 2003). The copper excess may damage hepatic mitochondria and oxidative damage to hepatic cells and cause the spillage of copper into the blood, thereby overloading other organs such as the brain, kidney and red blood cells, initiating toxic damage (Schilsky&Tavill, 2003). In the early stages of WD diffuse cytoplasmic copper accumulation can be seen only by special immunohistochemical stains for copper detecting. The early accumulation of copper is associated with hepatic steatosis. The ultrastructural abnormalities range from enlargement and separation of the mitochondrial inner and outer membranes with widening of the intercristal spaces, to increases in the density and granularity of the matrix. During the disease progression periportal inflammation mononuclear cellular infiltration lobular necrosis and bridging fibrosis occur. The areas of the brain main affected in WD are the basal ganglia (lenticular nuclei), which macroscopically appear brown in color because of copper deposition (Scheinberg& Sternlieb, 1984). In the early stages of the WD, proliferation of large protoplasmic astrocytes such as Opalski cells and Alzheimer cells occurs. During the disease progression the degeneration occurs leading to necrosis, gliosis and cystic changes. The degeneration can be seen in the brainstem, thalamus, cerebellum and cerebral cortex. During the WD progression, copper deposits can lead to vacuolar degeneration in proximal renal tubular cells, appearance of the 'Kayser–Fleischer' (KF) ring in Descemet's membrane. Copper from the hepatic cells degradation can be released into the circulation and can damage red blood cells, thereby inducing hemolysis (Schilsky&Tavill, 2003).

The majority of patients with WD present or with hepatic or neuropsychiatric symptoms, and with either clinically asymptomatic or symptomatic liver involvement. The remaining patients, may present with symptoms attributable to the involvement of other organs, as acute non-immunological hemolytic anemia, osteoarthritis, arrhythmias, rheumatic-fever-like manifestation, renal function abnormalities, primary or secondary amenorrhea, repeated and unexplained spontaneous abortions. Patients with hepatic WD (hWD) usually present in late childhood or adolescence, and exhibit features of acute hepatitis, fulminant hepatic failure, or progressive chronic liver disease in the form of either chronic active hepatitis or cirrhosis of the macronodular type (Schilsky&Tavill, 2003;. Hoogenraad, 1997). The mean age of onset of neurological WD (nWD) is the second to third decade (Hoogenraad, 1997). Most of patients present with extrapyramidal, cerebellar and cerebral-related symptoms. Tremor, gait and speech disturbances are the most common initial presentation symptoms. Patients may present also present with dystonia. About 30% of patients experience psychiatric disturbances (Hoogenraad, 1997). These disturbances can manifest as changes in school-related or work-related performance, attention deficit hyperactivity disorder, impulsivity, paranoid psychosis, obsessive behavior, depression, suicidal tendencies or bizarre behavior, and can occur early or late in the disease course.

The WD diagnosis and monitoring is based on history, physical, biochemical, liver biopsy and genetic mutations and imaging assessment. The KF ring is an important marker in nWD examination. The WD is biochemically characterized by low ceruloplasmin and total serum copper levels, increased 24-hour urinary copper excretion, and abnormally high hepatic copper content in the liver biopsy particularly in children performed. Another noninvasive method for assessing copper metabolism is incorporation of radioactive copper into the hepatocytes used with favorable results in Poland specially in presymptomatic gene mutation carriers, siblings of WD patients diagnosis (Członkowska et al. , 1973). The mutation screening to identify defects in the ATP7B gene can confirmation of WD diagnosis, but will not necessarily detect all disease producing mutations.

2. Neuroimaging

2.1 Magnetic resonance imaging

Neuroimaging plays an important role in the diagnosis and monitoring of WD patients. In brain CT scans hypodensities and atrophy of the bilateral basal ganglia, brainstem, cerebellum and cerebral cortex can be seen (Hoogenraad, 1997). MRI is much more sensitive method for revealing abnormalities in WD (Hoogenraad, 1997;. Sinha et al., 2006). On T1-weighted images, generalized brain atrophy is seen in about 75% of cases, and hypointensities in the basal ganglia. On T2-weighted images, hyperintensity in the basal ganglia, white matter, thalamus or brainstem can be seen (Figure 1). These abnormalities are caused by neuronal loss, gliosis, degeneration of fibers, and vacuolization associated with increased water content in the brain. Signal abnormalities vary according to the stage of the disease, and can be reversible with therapy in the early stages. In some cases, T2-weighted images show hypointensity in the basal ganglia (globus pallidus) region may be as a result of deposition of iron in exchange for copper after chelation (Figure 2).

In some WD patients with WD MRI shows a typical pallidal hyperintensity on T1-weighted images (Cordoba et al., 2003) (Figure 3). This abnormality appears to be secondary to the accumulation of manganese in basal ganglia because of portal-systemic shunting (Cordoba et al., 2003).

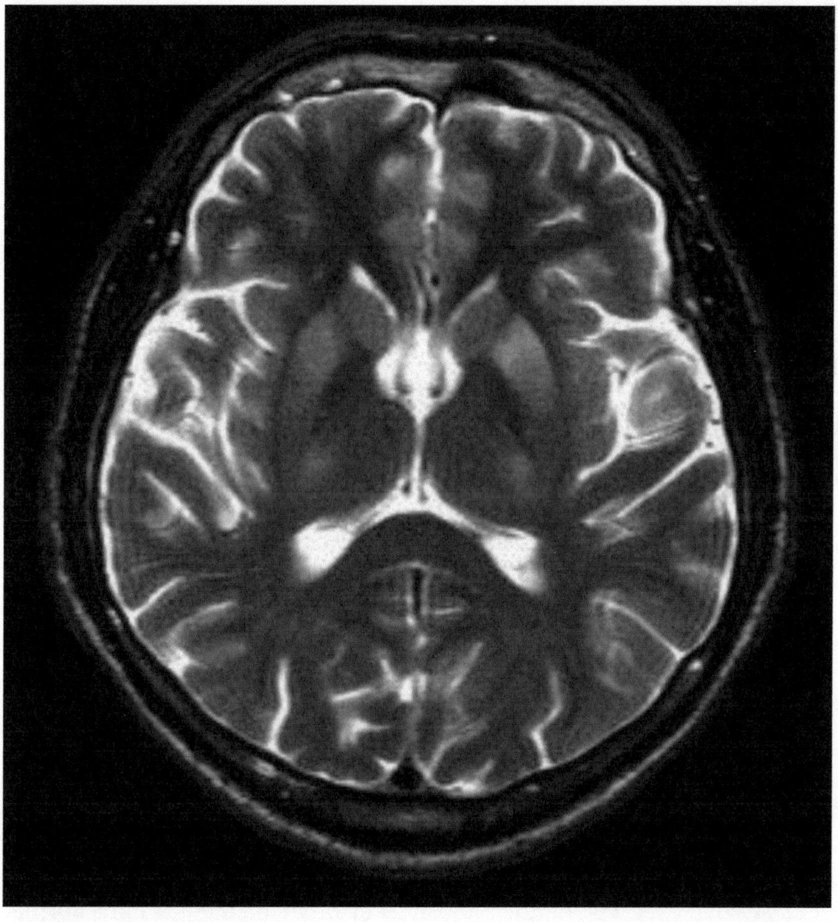

Fig. 1. Axial T2 - weighed MRI image of a 31- years – old men with WD, MRI was done before treatment. The picture shows bilateral hyperintensities in putamen, caudatum and thalami and degree of diffuse brain atrophy.

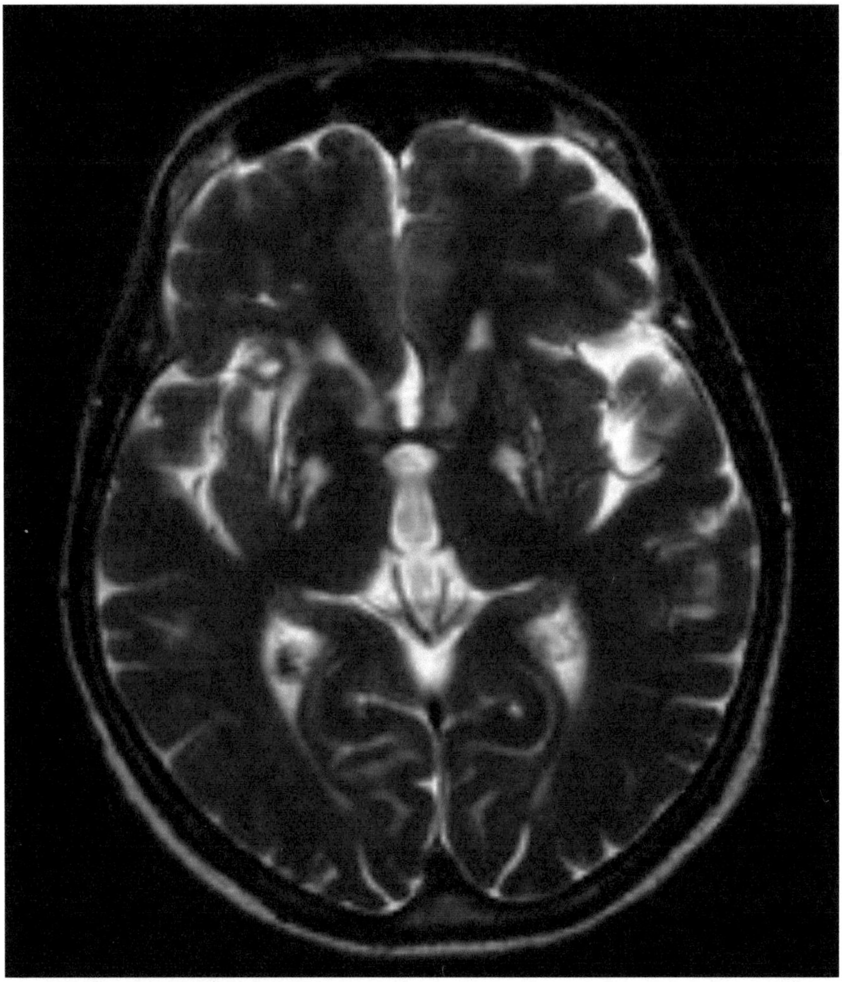

Fig. 2. Axial T2 - weighed MRI image of a 47- years – old women with WD treated for more than 10 years. The picture shows persistent hyperintensities in putamen, caudatum globus pallidus and degree of diffuse brain atrophy and hypointensity in the basal ganglia.

Proton Magnetic Resonance spectroscopy (^{1}H-MRS) is a practical research tool for elucidating the pathophysiology underlying certain diseases (Rudkin & Arnold, 1999). In patients with hepatic encephalopathy (HE), ^{1}H-MRS has been used to detect metabolic abnormalities in the brain with very high sensitivity (Ross et al., 1999). The biochemical alterations that were detected in HE included an increase in cerebral glutamine compounds (Glx) and a decrease in myoinositol (mI) and choline (Cho) metabolites (Cordoba et al., 2002). Other metabolites detectable in vivo by ^{1}H-MRS are N-acetylaspartate (NAA), considered to be a marker of neuronal health, and creatine (Cr), often used as an internal standard against which the resonance intensities of other metabolites are normalized. The role of NAA in nervous system can be related to: action as an organic osmolyte that counters the "anion deficit" in neurons, or a cotransport substrate for a proposed "molecular water pump" that removes metabolic water from neurons; NAA is a precursor for the enzyme-mediated neuronal dipeptide N-acetylaspartylglutamate biosynthesis; NAA provides a source of acetate for myelin lipid synthesis and is involved in energy metabolism in neuronal mitochondria-reflect improvement of neuronal energetic (Moffett et al.,2007).

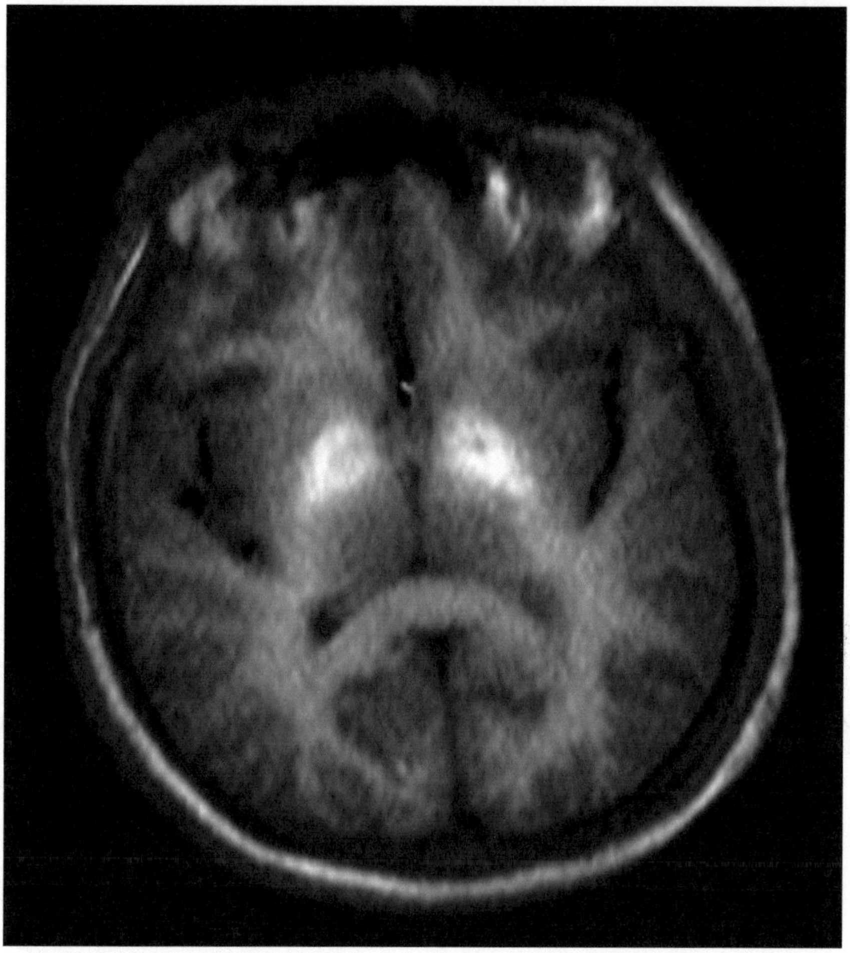

Fig. 3. Axial T1 - weighed MRI image of a 45- years – old WD patient with hepatic cirrhosis with subclinical hepatic encephalopathy.

^{1}H-MRS is a technique that could help distinguish between brain changes caused by HE and those related to copper toxicosis in WD. To elucidate the pathomechanism of the cerebral pathology of WD a study using ^{1}H-MRS in 37 newly diagnosed WD patients in the globus pallidus and thalamus examined bilaterally was performed (Tarnacka et al, 2009a). The calculations were performed for: mI, Cho, creatine (Cr), NAA, lipid (Lip), Glx. In all WD patients a significantly decreased mI/Cr and NAA/Cr ratio level and an increased Lip/Cr ratio in the pallidum was observed. Analysis revealed a significantly increased Glx/Cr and Lip/Cr ratio in the thalamus. In the pallidum of nWD patients, Cho/Cr and Glx/Cr and Lip/Cr ratios were higher than in control subjects, and the NAA/Cr was significantly lower (Table 1). In hWD patients, the mI/Cr and Cho/Cr and NAA/Cr ratio levels were lower than in controls (Table 1). The Cho/Cr and Lip/Cr ratios were higher in the thalami of nWD patients, and Lip/Cr ratios were higher than controls' in patients only with hWD. On the Figure 4 the examples of ^{1}H-MRS spectra in nWD and hWD and presymptomatic patients compared with control subjects are provided.

Patients:	mI/Cr	Cho/Cr	Glx/Cr	NAA/Cr	Lip/Cr
nWD	0,66 ± 0,31	0,89 ± 0,30*	1,26 ± 0,51*	1,43 ± 0,42 ¥¶	0,94 ± 0,46*
hWD	0,50 ± 0,27¶¥	0,68 ± 0,24¶	1,38 ± 0,39*	1,36 ± 0,39¶¥	0,81 ± 0,31*
presymptomatic	0,35 ± 0,10	0,66 ± 0,09	1,37 ± 0,24	1,59 ± 0,14	0,65 ± 0,08
Control group	0,72 ± 0,15	0,78 ± 0,15	1,11 ± 0,25	1,61 ± 0,26	0,47 ± 0,20

^{1}H-MRS study pallidum

Patients:	mI/Cr	Cho/Cr	Glx/Cr	NAA/Cr	Lip/Cr
nWD	0,74± 0,30	1.01 ± 0,27*	1,19 ± 0,32	1,91 ± 0,56	0,74 ± 0,32*
hWD	0,85 ± 0,27	1.07 ± 0,24	1.21 ± 0,39	1,73 ± 0,39	0.78 ± 0,31*
presymptomatic	0,76±0,21	0,91±0,23	1,13±0,20	1,69±0,32	0,50±0,22
Control group	0,82 ± 0.20	0,83 ± 0,14	1,11 ± 0,21	1,68 ± 0,24	0,50 ± 0,20

^{1}H-MRS.thalamus

*statistically higher than in control group
¶ statistically lower than in control group
¥ statistically lower compared with thalami

Table 1. The mean relative metabolic ratios in (left and right) pallidum and (right and left) thalamus in neurological (nWD) and hepatic (hWD) and presymptomatic subgroups.

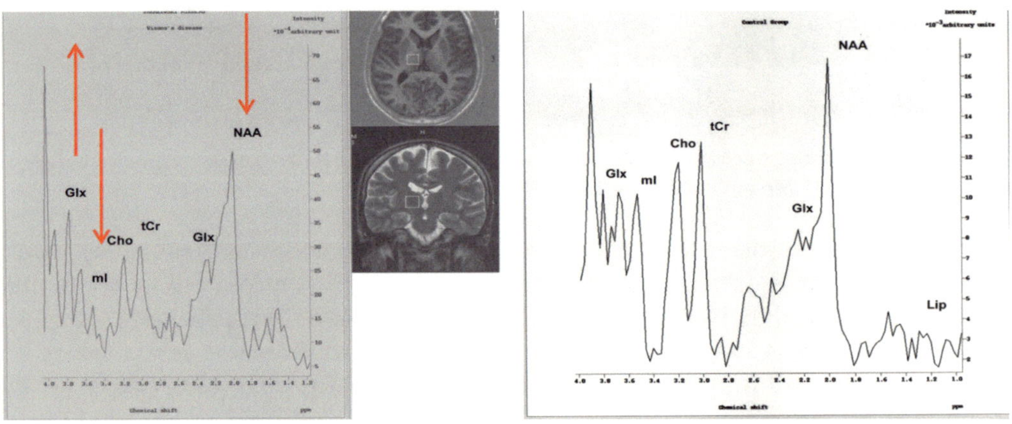

hWD patient WD (32 years old), **Control subject (36 years old)**

Fig. 4. a. ^{1}H-MRS images of patient with hepatic WD presentation compared with control subject. Proton spectrum shows expression of Glx; Cho and NAA were significantly reduced. The axial image shows the inset from where the spectrum was recorded.

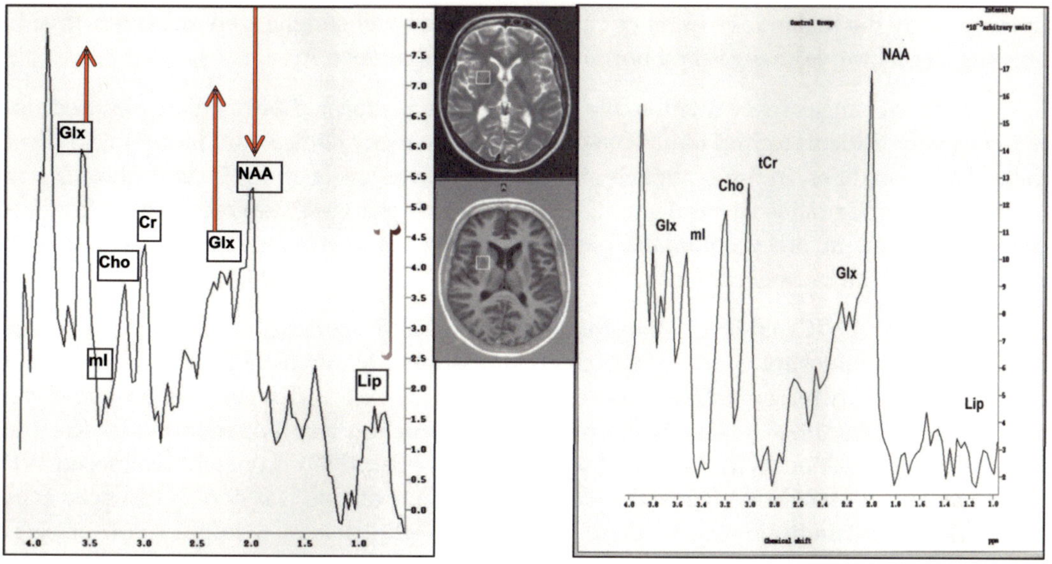

nWD patient (41 years old) **Control subject (36 years old)**

Fig. 4. b. ^{1}H-MRS images of patient with neurological WD presentation compared with control subject. Proton spectrum shows expression of Glx, Lip; NAA was significantly reduced. The axial image shows the inset from where the spectrum was recorded.

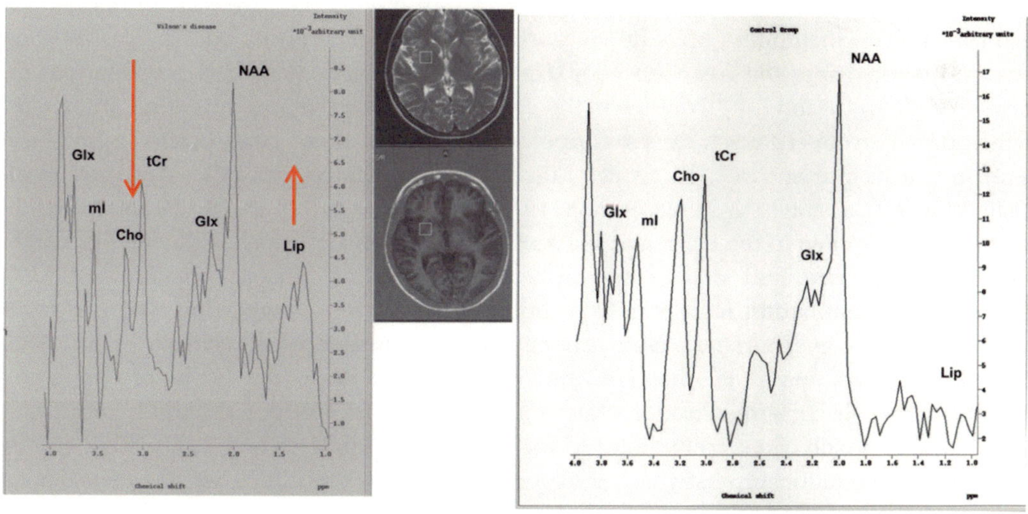

Patient presymptomatic (32 years old) **Control subject (36 jears old)**

Fig. 4. c. ^{1}H-MRS images of presymptomatic WD patients compared with control subject. Proton spectrum shows expression of Lip; Cr was significantly reduced. The axial image shows the inset from where the spectrum was recorded.

In those study the thalamic changes compared with the basal ganglia were more sensitive to ongoing degenerative changes and portal-systemic encephalopathy.

Spectroscopic changes in presymtomatic patients were performed only on 4 cases, because of it was very difficult to find patients, who did not have any clinical and biochemical (liver failure) abnormalities. In those patients significantly lower levels of ml/Cr and Cho/Cr and increase of Glx/Cr ratios in basal ganglia. In thalami no changes were seen. Those findings can suggest that in presymptomatic patients in MRS early encephalopatic changes with decrease of ml can be noticed.

The decreased Cho/Cr and ml/Cr in the pallidum of hWD patients could be indicative of minimal HE. Mioinositol is one of the chief compatible organic osmolytes responsible for equilibrating an increased intracellular tonicity (Cho, is believed to be also an osmolyte) (Danielsen & Ross, 1999). The ml/Cr and Cho/Cr reduction was also reported by Kraft in one *de novo* WD patient with hepatic disease (Kraft E et al.,1999). In newly diagnosed WD patients a reduction of NAA/Cr in the pallidum of hWD patients was noted (Tarnacka et al, 2009). This could indicate that in these patients, ^{1}H-MRS detects a combination of early encephalopathic and neurodegenerative changes, if NAA can be considered a neuronal marker.

Newly diagnosed WD patients with neurological impairment showed an increased level of Cho/Cr and Lip/ Cr in the pallidum and thalamus; furthermore, Glx/Cr was increased and NAA/Cr was decreased in the pallidum. The Cho peak is considered a potential biomarker for the status of membrane phospholipid metabolism (Danielsen & Ross, 1999), so that an elevated Cho signal most likely reflects an increase in membrane turnover. In pathologies characterised by membrane breakdown, such as neurodegeneration, bound Cho moieties may be liberated into the free Cho pool (Danielsen & Ross, 1999). It is possible that the increase of Cho/Cr and Lip/Cr ratios in the pallidum and the thalami can reflect an increase in membrane turnover caused by free copper accumulation, or can be associated with gliosis because Cho is present in high concentrations in oligodendrocytes (Van der Hart et al., 2000). In nWD patients, the increased level of Glx/Cr in the pallidum, can be related to the shunting of ammonia to the brain and glutamine accumulation. The elevation of Glx, can be also related to neuronal energy impairment. Removal of glucose greatly accelerates glutamate transamination to aspartate in brain synaptosomes, suggesting that glutamate could be an energy source in brain under some circumstances (Erecinska et al, 1988). Aspartate transaminase is the enzyme that accomplishes the task of glutamate transamination. It consumes oxaloacetate and glutamate to produce aspartate and alpha-ketoglutarate, which can directly enter to the TCA cycle (Moffett et al, 2007). Most studies concerning the relationship between neurospectroscopic abnormalities and the neurological HE manifestation found an association between the presence of HE and Glx/Cr level (Kreis et al., 1992;. Cordoba et al., 2001). In nWD patients no other metabolite changes specific for HE such as ml/Cr and Cho/Cr reduction was detected, so it is conceivable that because of chronic liver failure, in nWD patients the compensatory mechanism to counteract intracellular hypertonicity can take place, with no ml depletion, but with an increase of Glx. This finding, could indicate, that in newly diagnosed nWD patients an HE could exist. Patients with liver cirrhosis do present with parkinsonian signs including: tremor, bradykinesia, dysarthria, hypomimia, or rigidity. Some authors have speculated that the neurological symptoms of WD can be caused by concomitant liver disease (Victor, 1999).

These MRS findings can prove that in newly diagnosed nWD patients in the brain a porto-systemic shunting changes, but also neurodegenerative pattern associated with Cho, Lip and NAA/Cr depletion nWD can coexist. Verma compared brain metabolite alternations in patients with acute liver failure, acute-on-chronic liver failure and chronic liver disease (Verma et al, 2008). He found that NAA/Cr ratio was significantly decreased in acute-on-chronic liver failure and chronic liver disease. This fact can prove that in chronic liver disease an mitochondrial dysfunction can be detected due to neurotoxic effect. It is also worthy to mentioned that in patients with hepatic and neurological impairment in WD a significant negative correlation in the pallidum between the clinical status and the NAA/Cr was detected (Tarnacka et al, 2009).

From the 37 patients newly diagnosed, we followed 17WD cases for more than one year period (Tarnacka et al, 2008). In the ^{1}H-MRS done during the follow-up of all WD patients, significantly lower levels of mI/Cr and higher levels of Lip/Cr compared to the control group were persistently noted (Figure 5a). In patients with hepatic signs with improvement, a statistically significant increase of mI/Cr and Glx/Cr in follow- up ^{1}H-MRS was observed (about one year post-treatment, Figure 5b). In patients with neurological improvement after treatment in the follow-up ^{1}H-MRS, a statistically significant increase of NAA/Cr was noted (Table 5c). During neurological deterioration in one case, a decrease of Glx/Cr and NAA/Cr was seen, in contrast to another neurologically impaired patient with liver failure exacerbation, where a decrease of mI/Cr and increase of Glx/Cr was observed (Tarnacka et al, 2009).

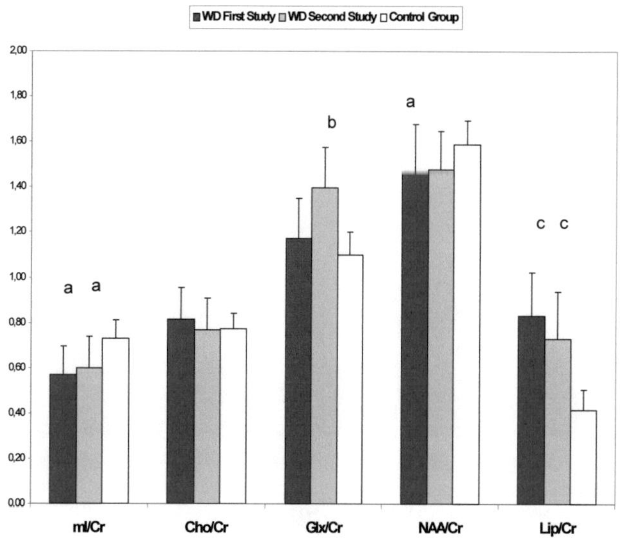

a. significantly lower than in controls ($p<0.005$),
b. significantly higher than in controls ($p<0.0001$) and compared with first study $p<0.005$,
c. significantly higher than in controls ($p<0.005$),

(a)

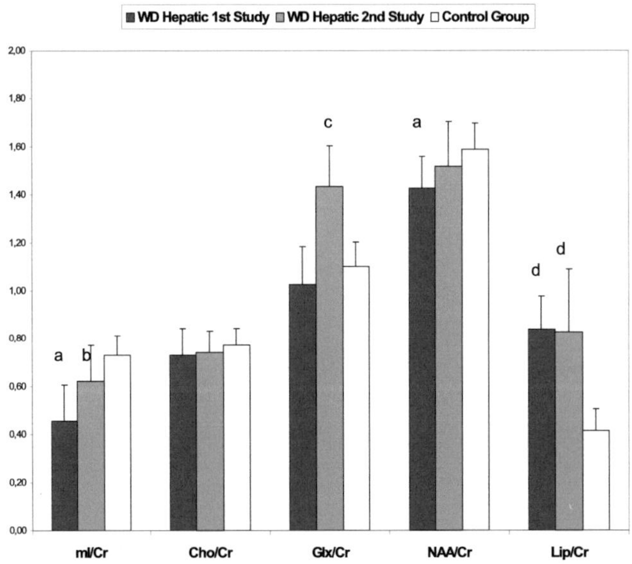

a. significantly lower than in controls, p<0.005,
b. significantly higher compared with first study p<0.04,
c. significantly higher than in controls, p<0.00006 and compared with first study p<0.002,
d. significantly higher than in controls, p<0.005

(b)

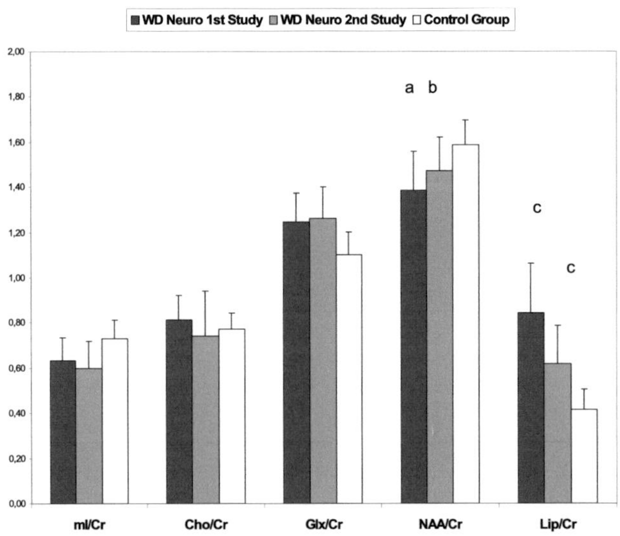

a. significantly lower than in controls, p<0.05,
b. significantly higher compare with first study, p<0.01
c. significantly higher than in controls, p<0.02

(c)

Fig. 5. The mean metabolic ratios in patients with improvement: a) all 15 WD patients b) hepatic subgroup (n=9), c) neurological subgroup (n=6), in the first and second ^{1}H-MRS test compared to the age-matched control subjects. Statistical analysis in text.

The alternations of NAA/Cr ratio in neurologically impaired patients and mI/Cr and Glx/Cr in patients with liver failure could be a sensitive marker of the clinical recovery and deterioration in those WD patients.

A decrease in relative NAA concentrations has been observed in pathological processes known to involve neuronal loss (Rudkin & Arnold, 1999). NAA is synthesized by neuronal mitochondria, which are sensitive to injury (Bates et al., 1996). A reversible decrease of NAA could well be caused by mitochondrial toxin 3-nitropropionate (Dauntry et al., 2000). Mitochondrial proteins seem to be the target of copper toxicity, because a decrease in the

	mI/Cr	Cho/Cr	Glx/Cr	NAA/Cr	Lip/Cr
All	0.66±0.30	0.89±0.21[a]	1.35±0.20[b]	1.44±0.35	0.93±0.48[c]
CS	0.83±0.14	0.75±0.16	1.09±0.31	1.61±0.22	0.45±0.18
hWD	0.63±0.33	0.79±0.38	1.33±0.47	1.47±0.38	0.99±0.57[d]
CS	0.66±0.14	0.76±0.16	1.09±0.31	1.58±0.22	0.43±0.18
nWD	0.72±0.21	0.96±0.36[e]	1.36±0.44[f]	1.41±0.42	0.89±0.48[g]
CS	0.95±0.41	0.75±0.12	1.09±0.23	1.63±0.28	0.46±0.22

a. significantly higher than in controls (p<0.0002)
b. significantly higher than in controls (p<0.0005)
c. significantly higher than in controls (p<0.00002)
d. significantly higher than in controls (p<0.000000)
e. significantly higher than in controls (p<0.00002)
f. significantly higher than in controls (p<0.004)
g. significantly higher than in controls (p<0.0003)

(a)

	mI/Cr	Cho/Cr	Glx/Cr	NAA/Cr	Lip/Cr
All	0.68±0.30	0.79±0.36	1.10±0.37	1.36±0.26[a]	0.94±0.31[b]
CS	0.71±0.18	0.76±0.16	1.13±0.21	1.65±0.21	0.47±0.16
hWD	0.64±0.22	0.58±0.21[c]	1.31±0.18	1.45±0.50	0.87±0.50[d]
CS	0.78±0.28	0.93±0.24	1.20±0.27	1.56±0.31	0.50±0.22
nWD	0.75±0.34	1.03±0.30[e]	1.18±0.32	1.30±0.25[f]	0.86±0.29[g]
CS	0.71±0.17	0.65±0.16	1.03±0.22	1.60±0.29	0.47±0.20

a. significantly lower than in controls (p<0.01),
b. significantly higher than in controls (p<0.003)
c. significantly lower than in controls (p<0.001)
d. significantly higher than in controls (p<0.0003)
e. significantly higher than in controls (p<0.0003)
f. significantly lower than in controls (p<0.002)
g. significantly higher than in controls (p<0.003)

(b)

Table 2. The mean metabolites ratios compared with control subjects (CS) in all WD patients, in hWD and nWD subgroups in: a) patients with improvement of clinical status, b) patients with no improvement of clinical status.

levels of the subunits of some of the complexes of the respiratory chain occurs (complex I being the most affected) (Aricello et al., 2005). It is possible that in WD, functional changes in neurons affecting oxidative metabolism may result in the reversible changes in relative concentration of NAA are reported in those study here. These findings suggest, that the early diagnosis and treatment of WD patients can reduce neurons metabolic disturbances and avoid their degeneration process. It is a very useful information which can prove that in nWD patients with improvement of clinical signs in the brain reversible functional changes of neurons could be detected.

In WD patients treated for long time in nWD and hWD subgroups with improvement or no improvement of clinical status the MRS findings in Table 2 are provided (Tarnacka et al., 2010). In those study we investigated 4 hWD patients, with no improvement and 8 with marked improvement; and 8 nWD patients with marked improvement and 7 with no improvement of clinical status. In hWD patients with improvement the MRS did not show any important pathological changes and in the nWD with improvement significantly higher Cho/Cr, Glx/Cr and Lip/Cr ratios levels compared with controls were noted (Table 2a). In hWD patients with no improvement the lower Cho/Cr and in nWD significantly lower NAA/Cr and higher Cho/Cr and Lip/Cr ratios were detected (Table 2b).

In all WD patients who showed improvement after treatment, MRS revealed a higher level of Cho/Cr, Glx/Cr and Lip/Cr ratios. In our previous study, we demonstrated a decrease in NAA/Cr ratio in all symptomatic patients, which increased after one year of treatment (Tarnacka et al, 2008). In patients treated for a longer time with improvement of clinical status no NAA/Cr decrease was seen; this could suggest that in WD patients the NAA/Cr depletion is reversible during the first few years of treatment and that treatment with z-s or d-p can protect them from further WD progression. The Cho/Cr and Glx/Cr elevation may mirror the glial proliferation that can be detected in patients even after long-term treatment (Horoupian et al., 1988). In this study, the persistence of NAA/Cr was related to a lack of improvement in neurological status (Tarnacka et al., 2010), what is in concordance with earlier reports in the literature showing a lower level of NAA in the striatum in neurologically impaired patients who received treatment (Page et al,.2004; Lucato et al., 2005). The lower level of NAA/Cr in the pallidum in these patients may suggest that, in patients with neurological involvement, persistent neuronal dysfunction may occur as a result of copper and/or iron deposition. NWD patients with no improvement initially had lower ceruloplasmin levels compared with those in whom neurological recovery was noted. It is possible that in these patients the iron metabolism could also be disturbed because of ceruloplasmin deficiency, which can be enhanced during chelation treatment (Medici et al.,2007).

2.1.1 MRS in heterozygous WD gene carriers

Wilson's disease a genetic disease due to mutation of both alleles of "Wilson's disease" gene ATP7b. The number of heterozygotes - having only one faulty copy of the gene - is high, around 1-2% of the human population (Johnson, 2001). Heterozygote carriers should not have symptoms of hepatic, neurological dysfunctions, but in other recessive disorders such as phenyloketonuria, some deviations in brain function in the literature were reported (Vogel, 1984). Because ^{1}H-MRS is able to detect brain abnormalities that are invisible in clinical assessment and MRI a study using this method to investigate the probability of brain changes in Hzc was performed (Tarnacka et.al, 2009b). We observed statistically significant higher ratios of Glx/Cr and Lip/Cr in ^{1}H-MRS in Hzc in the pallidum (Table 3). Glx is a glial marker; the increase of Glx/Cr could correlate with the glial proliferation as a result of the protective function of the astrocytes to copper and iron accumulation. The significantly higher level of Lip/Cr may reflect the liberation of lipids from membranes during their breakdown as a reaction to copper and iron overload. Our results may instead suggest that WD Hz carriers accumulate free copper or iron or both in basal ganglia and thalami. Hzc in our study were much older than WD cases are and in an animal model of WD copper and iron levels were found to be augmented during aging in striatum and substantia nigra (Kim et al., 2001). It is possible that during aging in Hz there is an increase of copper and iron accumulation because of ATP7b and ceruolplasmin impairment. There is accumulating evidence that ceruloplasmin, a copper protein with ferroxidase activity, plays an important role in iron metabolism and is also the principal plasma copper-binding protein (Harris et al., 1998). In our Hz the ceruloplasmin level was lower in only four cases, but ceruloplasmin levels in the blood are influenced by acute-phase reactions. The copper accumulation in the brain can also be caused by disruption in its excretion. In animal models, heterozygous mice have a reduced ability to excrete copper, which may indicate that half of the normal liver ATP7b copper transporter activity is insufficient to deal with a large amount of copper intake (Cheach et al., 2007). Like iron, copper is a heavy metal that can induce the Fenton reaction via production of free radicals and copper and iron accumulation increased with aging might have deleterious of liver and brain via oxidative stress.

	mI/Cr	Cho/Cr	Glx/Cr	NAA/Cr	Lip/Cr
^{1}H-MRS study Gp Hz:	0.73±0,19	0.81±0,13	1.38±0,30*	1.5±0,28	0.96±0,40**
Control subjects	0.82 ± 0,82	0.78 ± 0,16	1.11 ± 0,26	1.62 ± 0,27	0.48 ± 0,20
^{1}H-MRS study Th Hz	0.90 ± 0,27	0. 95 ± 0,23	1.44± 0,40¥	1.93± 0,35	1.08± 0,40¶
Control subjects	0.82± 0,21	0.84 ± 0,15	1.12 ± 0,21	1.69 ± 0,25	0.51 ± 0,20

*significantly higher than in controls, p<0.00006
** significantly higher than in controls, p<0.00002
¥ significantly higher than in controls, p<0.0006
¶ significantly higher than in controls, p<0.000001

Table 3. The mean metabolites ratios in heterozygotes (Hz) and control subjects from left and right globus pallidus (Gp) and right and left thalamus (Th) with standard deviations.

2.1.2 MRS versus Wilson's disease treatment

The treatment of WD patients may take many forms, from drug therapy (chelating agents as d-penicillamine (d-p) or trientine, zinc therapy, tetrathiomolibdate) to liver transplantation

(LT). The aim of medical treatment for WD is to remove the toxic deposit of copper from the body to produce a negative copper balance, and to prevent its reaccumulation. Successful therapy is measured in terms of a restoration of normal levels of free serum copper and its excretion in the urine. In 9 patients treated for more than one year with d-p in author's preliminary study, statistically significant increase of Glx/Cr and NAA/Cr ratios was noticed in contrary to 8 patients treated with zinc sulphate (z-s) were decrease of ml/Cr and NAA/Cr was detected (Figure 6a,b). D-penicillamine seams to be more effective (increase of NAA/Cr) during one year treatment, compared with z-s, but those study was performed on a quite small sample of patients. Those findings can also confirm Brewers observations, that zinc compounds are slow acting drugs and the decrease of mI/Cr can reflect the metabolic deterioration during zinc therapy (Brewer, 2005).

Current therapeutic strategies are often effective in the treatment of WD and provide a negative copper balance, however the course of WD in some treated patients may be unpredictable (Członkowska et al., 2005). The effectiveness of chelation or zinc therapy should therefore be monitored. So far, the only useful tests of monitoring the treatment efficiency are laboratory and imaging methods. Biochemical tests used in monitoring WD treatment include plasma liver tests, caeruloplasmin, copper and zinc in serum, and urinary copper and zinc excretion tests. These methods may sometimes be not sufficiently in particular at the beginning of the treatment when most of treatment side-effects occur as iatrogenic worsening during d-p therapy. In this stage wee postulated that ^{1}H-MRS can be used in early stages of treatment monitoring when the alternations of NAA, mI and Glx can mirror therapeutic response or deterioration (Tarnacka et al, 2008). We think that ^{1}H-MRS can also be helpful in differential diagnosis of clinical deterioration in patients with WD.

In patients with progressive liver failure or acute liver failure from fulminant hepatitis with or without intravenous hemolysis, orthotropic hepatic transplantation is an efficient treatment (Hoogenraad, 1997). Hepatic transplantation is also indicated in the absence of liver failure in patients with neurological WD in whom chelation therapy has proved ineffective, and significant improvements in neurological features have been reported (Polson et al., 1987). We presented a study of spectroscopic changes in globus pallidus in 3 patients with WD undergoing LT. The first case was a patient with neurological and hepatic impairment who was undergoing LT because of liver cirrhosis exacerbation. The second and third patients were subjects only with hepatic signs and the LT was performed because of liver failure. In the patient with neurological signs the MRS was performed 4 months after LT because there was no neurological improvement, and again one year after that. In the first MRS in those patient there was an increase in Glx/Cr, NAA/Cr and Lip/Cr ratios levels compared with the controls (Figure 7a). After one year's observation time an improvement of clinical status was observed and no changes of metabolites ratios were seen(Figure 7a). Before LT in the patient with liver cirrhosis mI/Cr ratio level was very low, in both patients with liver failure a decreased level of Glx/Cr, NAA/Cr and increased Lip/Cr ratios levels compared with controls were found (Figure 7b,c). After LT in those patients an increase of mI, Glx/Cr and NAA/Cr was seen (Figure 7.bc). Those data provide that after LT in those WD patients a renormalization of brain metabolites changes detected in ^{1}H-MRS could be seen.

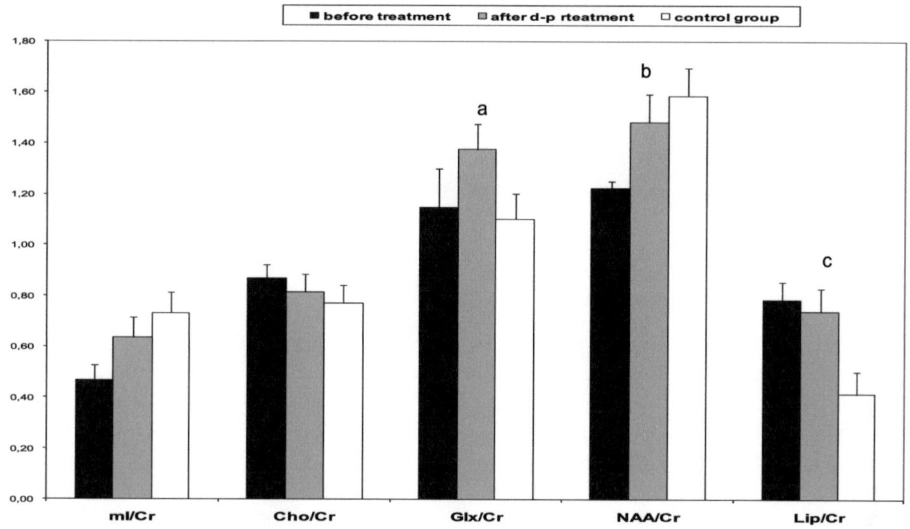

a. statistically higher than in controls (p<0,0003),
b. statistically higher than before treatment (p<0,01),
c. statistically higher than in controls (p<0,00004),

a)

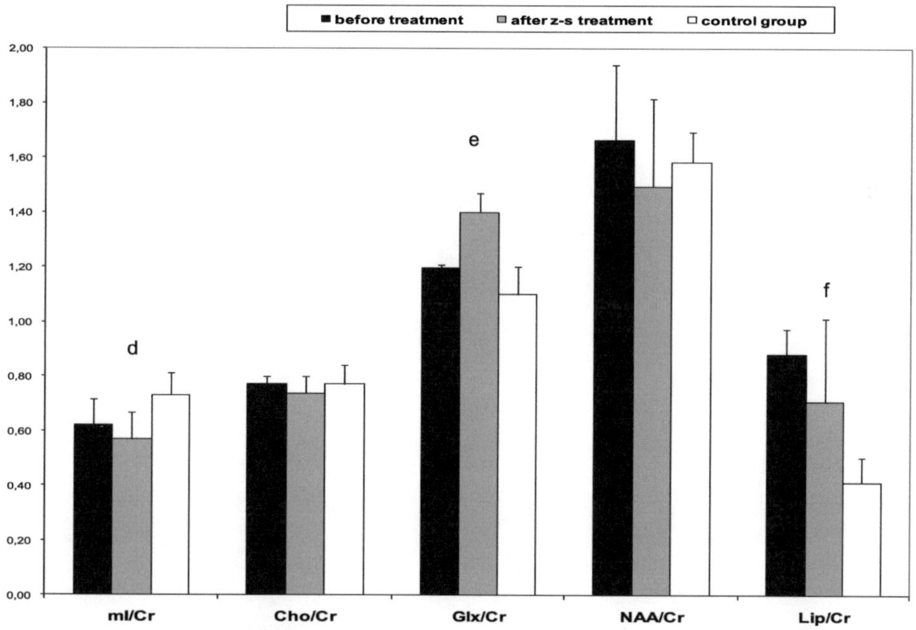

a. significantly higher than in controls (p<0,003),
b. significantly higher than in controls (p<0,0002),
c. significantly higher than in controls (p<0,001).

b)

Fig. 6. The mean metabolites ratios before treatment with d-p (a) and z-s (b), after minimum one year of treatment and in control subjects.

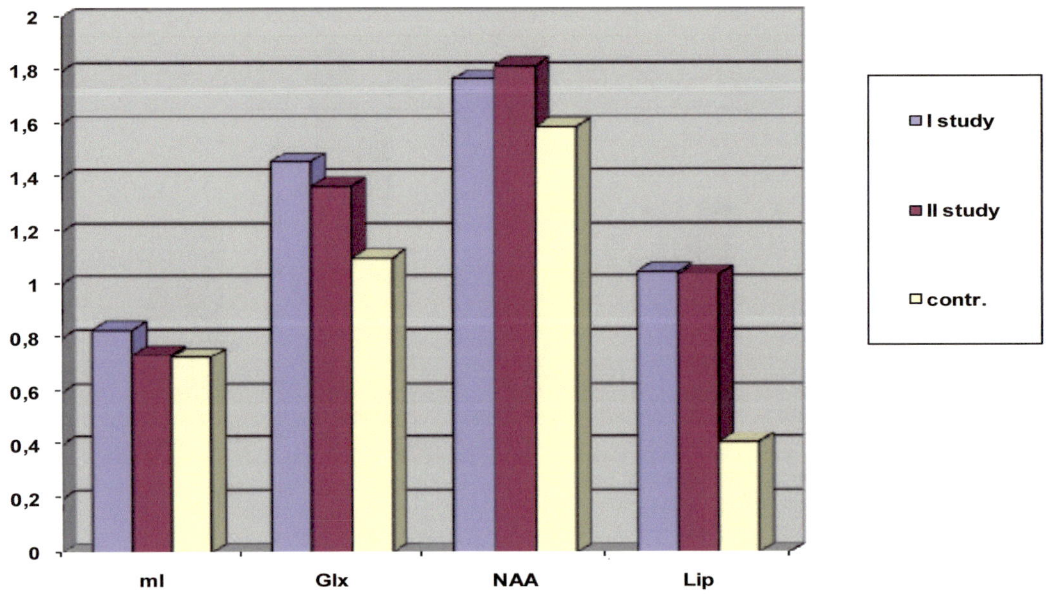
2
1,8
1,6
1,4
1,2
1
0,8
0,6
0,4
0,2
0
mI
Glx
NAA
Lip
I study
II study
contr.

a)

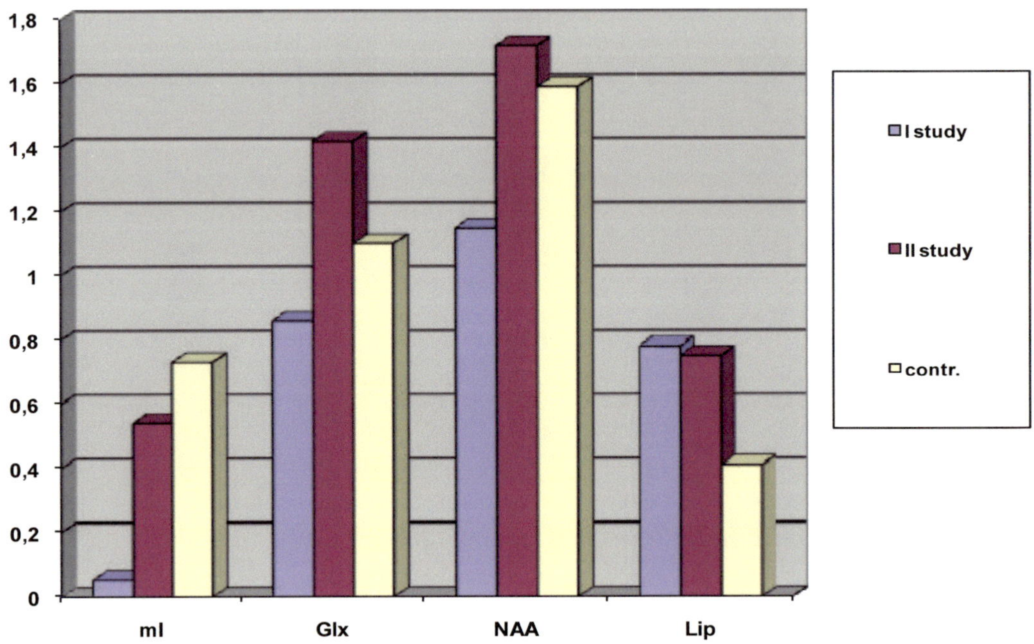
1,8
1,6
1,4
1,2
1
0,8
0,6
0,4
0,2
0
mI
Glx
NAA
Lip
I study
II study
contr.

b)

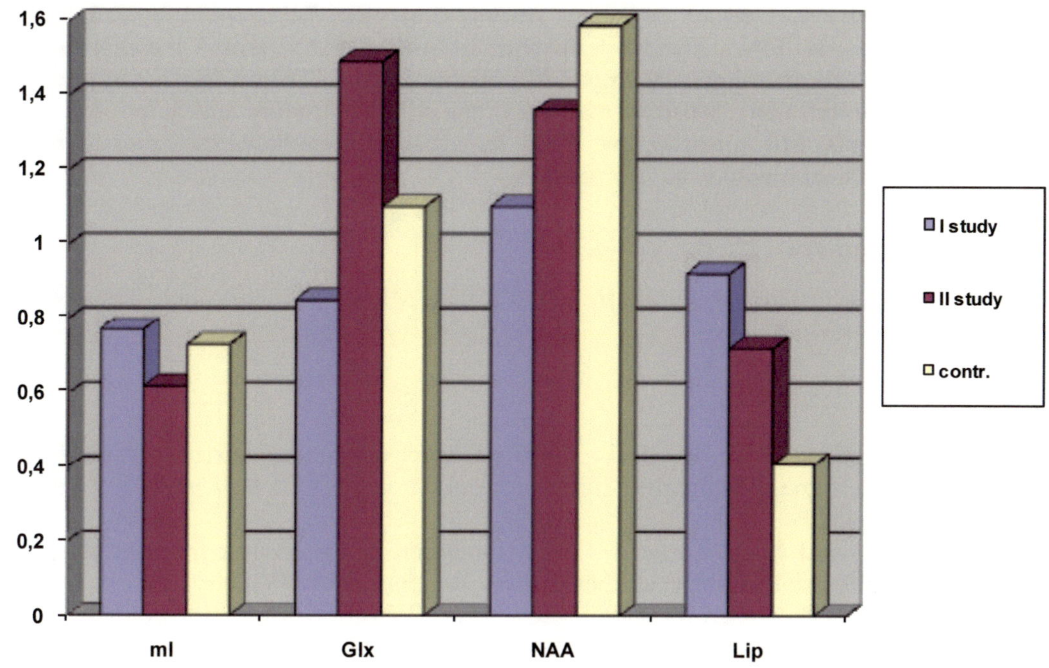

c)

Fig. 7. The mean metabolites ratios in globus pallidus in 3 patients undergoing liver transplantation, in first patient a) second- b) third- c), explanation in the text.

3. Conclusion

In conclusion, the results of the present studies appear to prove that in WD the astrocytic abnormalities occur primarily with dysfunction of the astrocytic-neuronal interactions. This process leads to metabolic derangement in neurons. During the disease progression and increasing copper deposition in the brain the compensation reactions as metallothionein synthesis become inefficient and the degenerative changes of astrocytes prevail over their detoxicative possibilities. The copper liberates from damaged astrocytes, and can also damage the neurons directly. Free copper can induce the neuronal mitochondria dysfunction causing the impaired NAA synthesis, but on this stage the destructive process can be reversible, because the increase of NAA/Cr can be observed in most treated patients. This is a very important conclusion, because it shows that the first year of treatment are pivotal in the therapeutic process. In majority of patients in this stage the central nervous system damage can be reversible. These findings emphasize the need for early diagnosis and treatment of WD. Effective antioxidant therapy introduced in early stages of WD might have modifying effect of metabolic disturbances in neurons. The neuronal dysfunction lasting longer can cause non reversible degenerative process like in patients treated for long time with no neurological improvement. Irreversible astrocytic dysfunction caused by copper can be related with disturbed ceruloplasmin synthesis causing iron overload and lead to lack of neurological improvement in some WD patients. The ^{1}H-MRS technique can be useful in treatment monitoring in patients with WD in early stages (until one year). MRS seems to be more effective method in comparison with MRI in monitoring effectiveness of treatment during first year. MRS could be helpful in differential diagnosis of the clinical deterioration in treated WD patients. The alternations of NAA/Cr ratio in neurologically impaired patients and ml/Cr and Glx/Cr in patients with liver failure could be a sensitive markers of the clinical recovery and deterioration in those WD patients. MR spectroscopy could be a useful complementary tool in other monitoring treatment methods in WD patients.

4. Acknowledgment

This work was supported by grant from the Polish Ministry of Education and Science (3P05B/119/23).

5. References

Aricello, M.; Rotillo, G. & Rossi, L. (2005). Copper-dependent toxicity in SH-SY5Y neuroblastoma cells involves mitochondrial damage. *Biochem Biophys Res Commun* 327:454-459.

Bates, T.; Strangward M. & Keelan J. (1996). Inhibition of N-acetylaspartate production: implications for 1 H-MRS studies in vivo. *Neuroreport* 7:1397-1400.

Brewer, G. (2005). Neurologically presenting Wilson's disease: epidemiology, pathophysiology and treatment. *CNS Drugs*;19:185-92.

Bull, P.; Thomas, G. & Rommens, J. et al. (1993) The Wilson disease gene is a putative copper transporting P-type ATPase similar to the Menkes gene. *Nat Genet* 5: 327–337

Cheach, D.; Deal, Y. & WRIGHT, P. et al. Heterozygous tx mice have an increased sensitivity to copper loading: Implications for Wilson's disease carriers. *Biometals* 2007;20:751-760 .

Cordoba, J.; Alonso, J. & Rovira, A. et al. (2001). The development of low grade cerebral edema in cirrhosis is supported by the evolution of 1H magnetic resonance abnormalities after liver transplantation. *J Hepatol* 3:596-604.

Cordoba, J.; Sanpedro, F. & Alonso, J. et al. (2002). 1 H magnetic resonance in the study of hepatic encephalopthy in humans. *Metabolic Brain Disease* 17:415-29.

Członkowska, A.; Galewicz, A. & Rodo M et al. (1973). Observation on copper metabolism in Wilson's disease. Acta Univ Caro Med 56:175-178.

Członkowska, A.; Tarnacka, B. & Litwin, T. et al (2005). Wilson's disease - cause of mortality in 164 patients during 1992-2003 observation period. *J Neurol* 252:698-703.

Danielsen, E. & Ross B. (1999). Magnetic resonance spectroscopy diagnosis of neurological diseases. New York: *Marcel Dekker,*

Dauntry, C.; Vaufrey, F. & Brouillet, E. et al. (2000). Early N-acetylaspartate depletion is a marker of neuronal dysfunction in rats and primates chronically treated with the mitochondrial toxin 3-nitropropionic acid. *J Cereb Blood Flow Metab* 20:789-799.

Erecinska, M.; Zaleska, M. & Nissim, I. et al. (1988). Glucose and synaptosomal glutamate metabolizm: studies with [15N] glutamate. *J Neurochem* 51:892-902.

Figus, A.; Angius, A. & Loudianos, G. et al. (1995) Molecular pathology and haplotype analysis of Wilson disease in Mediterranean populations. *Am J Hum Genet* 57: 1318–1324.

Frydman, M.; Bonne-Tamir, B. & Farrer, L. et al. (1985) Assignment of the gene for Wilson disease to chromosome 13: linkage to the esterase D locus. *Proc Natl Acad Sc USA* 82: 1891–1821

Harris, L.; Klomb, L. & Giltin J. (1998). Aceruloplasminemia: an inherited neurodegenerative disease with impairment of iron homeostasis. *Am J Clin Nutr* 67 (suppl):972S-977S.

Hoogenraad, T. (1997). Wilson's Disease. London Philadelphia Toronto Sydney Tokyo: *WB. Saunders Company* Ttd.

Horoupian, D.; Sternlieb, I. & Scheinberg, I. (1988). Neuropathological findings in penicillamine - treated patients with Wilson's disease. Clinical *Neuropathology* 7:62-67.

Johnson, S. (2001). Is Parkinson's disease the heterozygote form of Wilson's disease: PD=1/2 WD? *Medical Hypotheses*;56:171-173.

Kim, H.; Kim, D. & Lee, B. et al. (2001). Diffusion-weighted image and MR spectroscopic analysis of a case of MELAS with repeated attacks. *Yonsei Med J* 42:128-33.

Kraft, E. Trenkwalder, C. & Then Berg, F. et al. (1999). Magnetic resonance proton spectroscopy of brain in Wilson's disease. *J Neurol* 246:693-9.

Kreis, R.; Ross. B. &, Farrow, N. et al. (1992). Metabolic disorders of the brain in chronic hepatic encephalopathy detected with H-1 MR spectroscopy. *Radiology* 182:19-27.

Loudianos, G.; Dessi, V. & Lovicu, M. et al. (1999) Molecular characterization of Wilson disease in the Sardinian population—evidence of a founder effect. *Hum Mutat* 14: 294–303.

Lucato, L.; Barbosa, M. & Machado, A. et al. (2005). Proton MR spectroscopy in Wilson disease: analysis of 36 cases. *Am J Neuroradiol* 26:1066-1071.

Medici, V.; Di Leo, V. & Lamboglia, F. et al. (2007). Effect of penicillamine and zinc on iron metabolizm in Wilson's disease. *Scand J Gastroenterol* 42:1495-1500.

Moffett, J.; Ross, B. & Arun, P. et al. (2007). N -acetylaspartate in CNS: from neurodiagnostic to neurobiology. *Progress in Neurobiol* 81:89-131.

Page, R.; Davie, F. & MacManus, D. et al. (2004). Clinical correlation of brain MRI and MRS abnormalities in patients with Wilson's disease. *Neurology* 63:638-643.

Polson, R.; Rolles, K. & Calne, R. et al. (1994). Reversal of severe neurological manifestations of Wilson's disease following orthoptic liver transplantation. *Q J Med* 244:685-691.

Ross, B.; Jacobson, S. , & Villami, F. et al. (1994). Subclinical hepatic encephalopathy: proton MR spectroscopic abnormalities. *Radiology* 93:457-63.

Rudkin, T. & Arnold, D. (1999). Proton magnetic resonance spectroscopy for the diagnosis and management of cerebral disorders. *Arch Neurol* 56:919-26.

Scheinberg, I. & Sternlieb, I. (1984) Wilson disease. Philadelphia: *WB Saunders*

Schilsky, M. & Tavill, A. (2003) Wilson disease. In Disease of the Liver, edn 9, 1169–1186 (Eds Schiff ER et al.) Philadelphia: *Lippincott Williams & Wilkins*

Sinha, S.; Taly, A. & Ravishankar, S. et al. (2006). Wilson's disease: cranial MRI observations and clinical correlation. *Neuroradiology* 48:613-21.

Tarnacka, B.; Szeszkowski, W. & Gołębiowski, M. et al. (2008). MR spectroscopy in monitoring the treatment of Wilson's disease patients. *Mov Disord* 23:1560-6.

Tarnacka, B.; Szeszkowski, W. & Gromadzka, G. et al. (2010). Brain Proton Magnetic Spectroscopy in long-term treatment of Wilson's disease patients. *Metab Brain Dis* 25:325-9.

Tarnacka, B.; Szeszkowski, W. & Gołębiowski, M. et al. (2009). Metabolic changes in 37 newly diagnosed Wilson's disease patients assessed by Magnetic Resonance Spectroscopy. *Park Rel Dis* 15:582-6.

Tarnacka, B.; Szeszkowski, W. & Gromadzka, G. et al. (2009). Heterozygous carriers for Wilson's disease - magnetic spectroscopy changes in the brain. *Metab Brain Dis* 24:463-8.

Thomas, G.; Forbes, J. & Roberts E. et al. (1995) The Wilson disease gene: spectrum of mutations and their consequences. *Nat Genet* 9: 210–217.

Van der Hart, M.; Czeh, B. & Biurrun, G. et al. (2000). P receptor antagonist an cloimipramine prevent stress-induced alternations in cerebral metabolites, cytogenesis in the dentate gyrus and hippocampal volume. *Molecular Psychiatry* 7:933-41.

Victor, M. (1999). Neurologic manifestation of gastrointestinal diseases. In Asbury AK. McKann CM, McDonald W. Diseases of the nervous system. Clinical Neurobiology, *Saunders, Philadelphia,* pp 1470-82.

Vogel, F. (1984). Clinical consequences of heterozygosity for autosomal-recessive diseases. *Clinical Genetics* 25:381-415.

Wilson, S. (1912) Progressive lenticular degeneration: a familial nervous disease associated with cirrhosis of the liver. *Brain* 34: 295–509

Yamaguchi, Y.; Heiny, M. & Gitlin, J. et al. (1993) Isolation and characterization of a human liver cDNA as a candidate gene for Wilson disease. *Biochem Biophys Res Common* 197: 271–277

5

MRS in MS, With and Without Interferon Beta 1a Treatment, to Define the Dynamic Changes of Metabolites in the Brain, and to Monitor Disease Progression

Münire Kılınç Toprak[1,*], Banu Çakir[2],
E.Meltem Kayahan Ulu[2] and Zübeyde Arat[3]
[1]Baskent University, Faculty of Medicine, Department of Neurology, Fevzi Cakmak Caddesi, Bahcelievler, Ankara
[2]Baskent University, Faculty of Medicine, Department of Radiology, Ankara
[3]Baskent University, Faculty of Medicine, Department of Internal Medicine, Ankara
Turkey

1. Introduction

Multiple sclerosis (MS) is a common cause of chronic neurological disability in young adults. Magnetic Resonance Imaging (MRI) readily identifies multifocal white matter lesions(WML) that represent areas of demyelination and is thus useful in supporting the diagnosis of MS, even after a single clinical episode(McDonald et al., 2001). MRI is also widely used to monitor disease progression in natural history and in therapeutic trial studies. However, conventional MRI does not detect the subtle histopathological changes that are described in the normal-appearing white matter (NAWM) in patients with MS(Allen & McKeown, 1979; Bitsch et al., 1999). MRS has been used in the evaluation of MS to help further define the nature of the lesions revealed by T2-weighted MRI(Arnold, Matthews, Francis, O'Connor, & Antel, 1992; Arnold et al., 1994; Bitsch et al., 1999; Davie et al., 1997; De Stefano et al., 1995; Fu et al., 1998; Gonen et al., 2000; Matthews et al., 1996; Narayana, Doyle, Lai, & Wolinsky, 1998; Pan et al., 1996; Rooney et al., 1997; Sarchielli et al., 1999; Tourbah et al., 1999; van Walderveen, Barkhof et al., 1999). The measurement of N-acetly aspartic acid (NAA) is thought to be a marker of axonal loss, damage or dysfunction. Many studies (Arnold et al., 1992; Arnold et al., 1994; Davie et al., 1997; De Stefano et al., 1995; Husted et al., 1994; Narayana et al., 1998,(Allen & McKeown, 1979; De Stefano et al., 1995; Fu et al., 1998; Husted et al., 1994; Narayana et al., 1998) have shown a reduction in the absolute concentration of NAA or the NAA/Cr ratio in MS lesions. However, pathological(Allen & McKeown, 1979) and quantitative MRSI studies(Armspach, Gounot, Rumbach, & Chambron, 1991; Filippi et al., 1995; Gasperini et al., 1996; Loevner et al., 1995) have shown that in patients with clinically definite MS, abnormalities also occur in the NAWM(Arnold et al., 1992; Davie et al., 1997; Davie et al.,

* Corresponding Author

1994; Fu et al., 1998; Husted et al., 1994; Narayana et al., 1998). Although the principal finding of MRS studies in patients with MS was a decrease in the NAA peak area, opposite results were obtained for other metabolites(Davie et al., 1994; Davies, Newcombe, Williams, McDonald, & Clark, 1995; De Stefano et al., 1995; Husted et al., 1994; Larsson et al., 1991). Despite the difficulties in interpreting data obtained in vivo, MRS provides direct information about metabolic variations and the damage to or integrity of myelin and axons, which are not revealed by traditional MRI(Arnold et al., 1994; Ferguson, Matyszak, Esiri, & Perry, 1997; Fernando et al., 2004).

In patients with relapsing remitting multiple sclerosis (RRMS), interferons reduce the attack frequency of the disease, the mean attack duration, the annual lesion burden, and the frequency of gadolinium (Gd) enhancement on MRI. However the mechanism of action of interferons in patients with MS and the effect of interferons on axonal injury remain undefined. We questioned whether treatment with interferon beta-1a (INFβ-1a) would enable the recovery of injured axons. To determine this, we used MRSI to examine changes in the metabolic peaks of neuronal markers NAA, Cho(Choline), and Cr(Creatine) after treatment with INFβ-1a(Rebif 44 μg) in a small group of patients with RRMS. An untreated group was studied for comparison, and healthy volunteers were used as controls.

2. Materials and methods

2.1 Patients and methods

We studied 10 patients (7 women 3 men) with clinically definite RRMS (median age, 39 years; age range 22-50 years). The median expanded status scale score (EDSS) was 2.1 (range 1.0-3.0), and the median duration of disease was 4.7 years (range, 1-20 years). In the 2 years before their participation in the study, all patients had had at least one relapse. None of the patients had undergone immunosuppressant therapy ever before, or corticosteroid treatment within 2 months before the initiation of the study. Five patients elected not to be

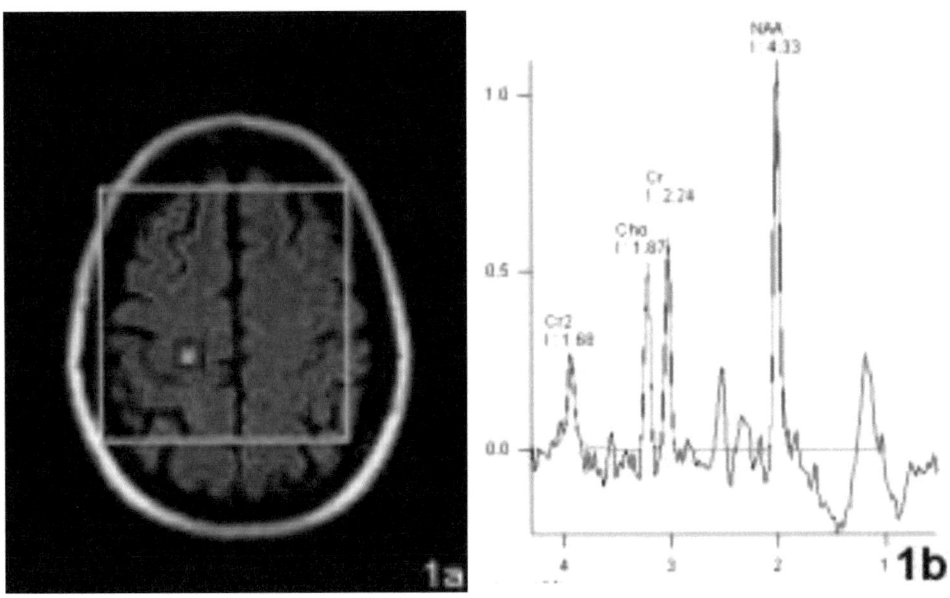

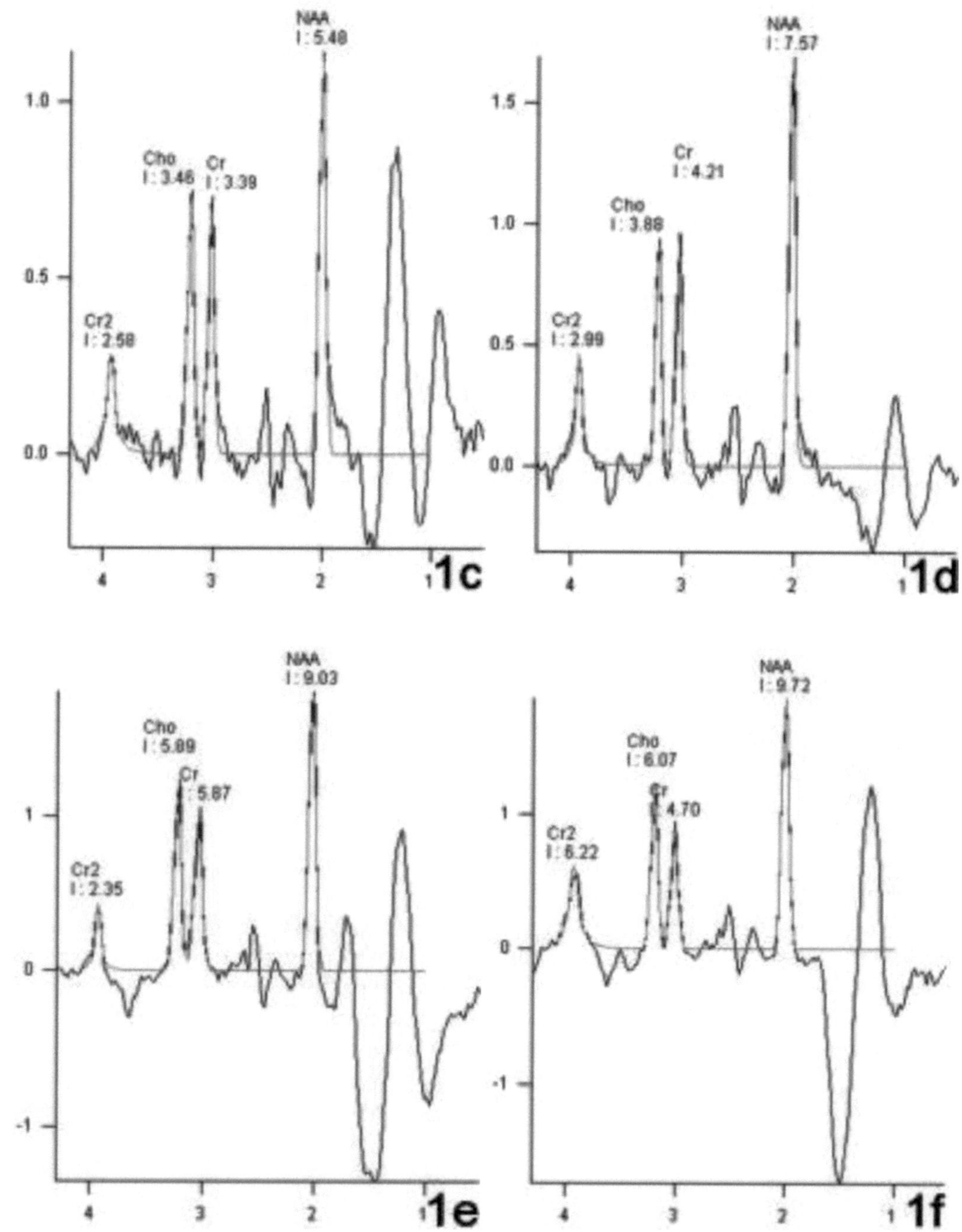

Fig. 1. a-f: Axial fluid-attenuated, inversion recovery (FLAIR) MR image of a 50-year-old woman receiving INFβ-1a treatment shows a voxel placed over a WM lesion in the right centrum semiovale (1a). The multivoxel CSI MRI spectrum of this lesion is obtained during study months zero, 1, 3, 6, and 12 (b-f). The results of proton MRSI show that there is a statistically significant increment in absolute NAA and Cho values.

treated. Five other patients received INFβ-1a treatment. All patients were evaluated at the beginning of the study and during the first, third, sixth, and twelfth month. During their follow-up evaluations, neurological examinations that included EDSS assessment were performed in addition to MR studies with gadopentetate dimegluminelinium (Gd) 0,1 mmol/kg intravenously, and MRSI (Figure 1a-f). A relapse was defined as the appearance of new neurological symptoms or worsening of prior neurological symptoms of 48 hours' duration in addition to objective evidence of a change in neurological status of a patient who has been clinically stable for the 4 prior weeks. All patients suspected of having an attack were examined within 7 days of the onset of symptoms and were treated with intravenous methyprednisolone (IVMP) at a dose of 1 g/day for 5 days. At the beginning of the study, MRI and MRSI studies were also performed on 6 healthy, age-matched and sex-matched control subjects (4 women, 2 men; median age, 33.6 years, age range, 27-48 years) who had neither systemic nor neurologic disease. The local ethics committee approved the study.

2.1.1 MRI studies

All MRI and MRSI studies were performed with a 1.5 Tesla MR unit (Siemens Magnetom Symphony, Erlangen, Germany) with a standard quadrature head coil. To detect focal WM lesions, we used conventional MRI, including axial T1 weighted (TR 586 ms, TE 15 ms, 5 mm slice thickness), fluid-attenuated, inversion recovery (FLAIR) (TR 9000 ms, TE 98 ms, 5 mm slice thickness), axial and sagittal proton density (TR 2200 ms, TE 30 ms, 5 mm slice thickness), T2-weighted spin echo sequences (TR 2200 ms, TE 80 ms, 5 mm slice thickness) and post-gadolinium axial and sagittal T1 weighted (TR 779 ms, TE 15 ms, 5 mm slice thickness) spin echo sequences. MRI images were acquired with a matrix size of 145x256 mm and FOVof 230x230 mm. During the same session, water-suppressed proton MRSI was performed by means of multivoxel chemical shift imaging (TR/TE: 1500/135, voxel volume 1 cm^3). Metabolite peaks of NAA, Cho, and Cr were assessed in both WML -without Gd enhancement- and in NAWM.

2.1.2 Statistics

SPSS 11 for Windows was used for statistical analysis. The Kruskal-Wallis Test was used to compare the basal NAWM metabolite peaks among treated, untreated and healthy control subjects. The Mann-Whitney U test was used to compare the basal WML metabolite peaks in treated and untreated patients. Then, multivariate analysis of variance (MANOVA) was used to compare the NAWM and WML metabolite peaks in treated and untreated patients throughout the study period. The Wilcoxon signed rank test was used to compare changes in the NAWM and WML metabolite peaks during study months zero, 1, 3, 6, and 12. Results with $p < .05$ were considered as significant.

3. Results

3.1 Treatment effect as assessed by relapse rate, and new T2 lesions with and without GD enhancement

Five patients (3 women and 2 men) elected not to be treated. Four of those 5 patients experienced no attacks during the 12 months of the study. However, the results of MRI examination revealed new Gd-enhancing lesions without a trace of an accompanying clinical MS attack at the initiation of the study in 3 patients during the sixth month of the study. The results of serial MR examinations of another patient revealed new T2 lesions without Gd-enhancement that were present without evidence of a clinical MS attack from the initiation of the study until the twelfth study month. However, during the twelfth month, that patient experienced a clinical MS attack (moderate paresis [4/5] of the left leg), and a new Gd-enhancing lesion was identified. And only that patient received pulse steroid therapy once daily for 5 days.

Five other patients received INFβ-1a treatment (subcutaneous INFβ-1a 44 μg -Rebif-3 times per week). Among the subjects who received INFβ, two patients had Gd-enhancing new T2 lesions on almost every MRI examination, another patient had a Gd-enhancing lesion only on the last MRI examination of the study, and the remaning patients exhibited no new lesions. None of those patients experienced a clinical MS attack accompanying the MRI activities. There was no significant change in the EDSS scores of the patients in either group throughout the study.

3.2 MRSI results

There was no statistically significant difference between the basal metabolite levels in the NAWM of patients with MS and the healthy control subjects (*P*> .005) (Table 1). There was also no statistically significant difference between the basal metabolite peaks in the WML between the untreated and treated MS patients (Table 2).

NAWM metabolic peaks		NAA Basal	CHO Basal	CR Basal
Untreated	Mean	6,5±4,6	4,3±1,9	3,9±1,8
	Median	4,8950	3,4650	3,1650
Treated	Mean	7,1±2,3	4,5±1,4	4,3±1,3
	Median	7,8100	4,7550	4,5200
Control	Mean	6,8±0,4	4,1±0,7	4,0±0,2
	Median	6,9250	4,2900	3,9800
WML metabolic peaks		**NAA Basal**	**CHO Basal**	**CR Basal**
Untreated	Mean	6,0±3,7	4,4±1,9	3,8±1,8
	Median	4,8900	4,6700	3,1900
Treated	Mean	6,8±2,5	4,8±1,6	3,9±1,2
	Median	5,4800	5,0950	3,7900

NAA: N-acetyl aspartate, Cho: Choline, Cr: Creatine

Table 1. Basal normal-appearing white matter and white matter metabolite levels in treated and untreated patients and controls

We analyzed whether any difference emerged in the NAWM metabolite peaks between the treated and untreated patients throughout the study period and found that a significant difference existed in NAWM NAA peaks (P = .003); Cho peaks (P = .001); and Cr peaks (P = .006) beginning from the first month of the study. When we evaluated the groups separately to assess when that difference emerged between the basal and the following months' NAA, Cho and Cr peaks we noted that in the treatment group, the NAA peaks began to increase during the sixth month (P = .000); Cho peaks increased during the sixth and twelfth months (P = .000); and an increment in the Cr peak was found in the third (P< .04), sixth (P = .001), and twelfth study months (P = .00). However, in the untreated group, none of the NAA, Cho or Cr peaks (in NAWM) varied significantly during the entire study period (P> .05) (Graphic 1).

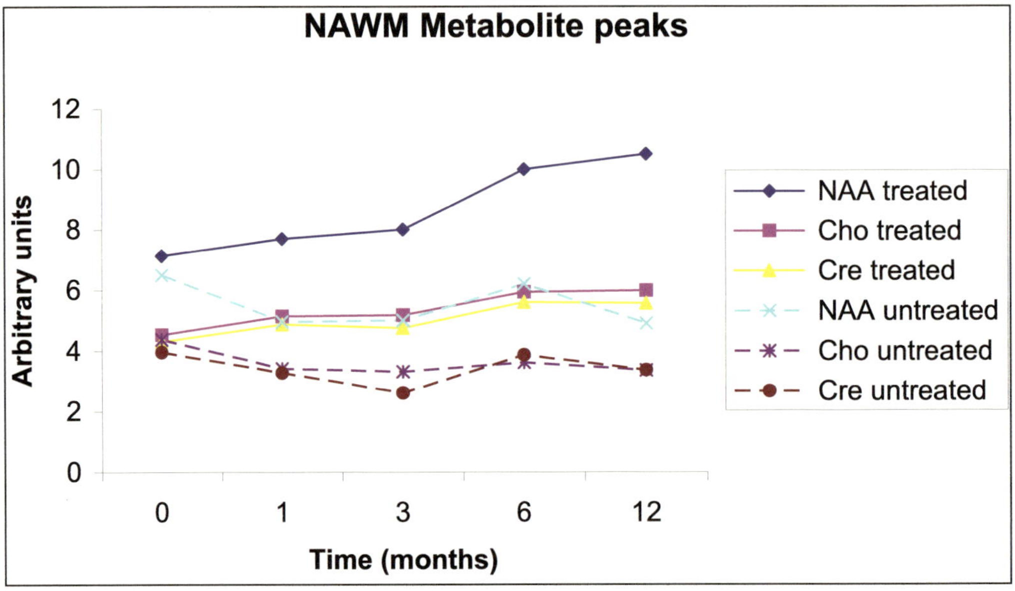

Graphic 1.

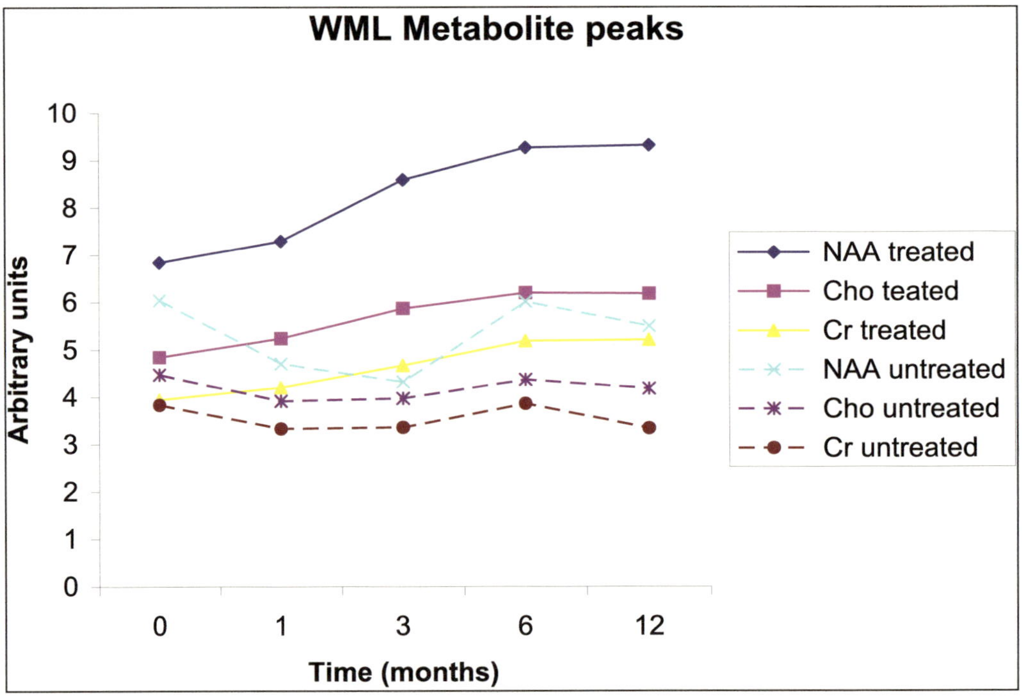

Graphic 2.

We found a significant difference between the changes in WML NAA (*P*= .001), Cho (*P* = .025); and Cr (*P* = .031) peaks of untreated and treated patients, beginning from the first month. When we evaluated the groups separately to determine when the difference emerged between the basal WML NAA peaks and the following months' NAA peaks, we noted that the NAA peaks started to increase during the sixth month in the treatment group (*P* = .001); the Cho peak started to increase during the first month (*P* = .03); and the Cr peak began to increase during the third month in the treatment group (*P* = .04). However, NAA, Cho or Cr peaks did not vary significantly in WML over the entire period of study in the untreated group (*P* > .05) (Graphic 2).

4. Discussion

In this study, variations in cerebral metabolites were assessed during treatment with INFβ-1a in a small group of patients with RRMS, and the results were compared with those in untreated patients matched for age and disability. We used the absolute quantification of the metabolites. The use of ratios is potentially less sensitive to the effects of disease in MS than is the use of absolute values; measurement error may be increased when two measures rather than one are required(Fernando et al., 2004). The use of the ratio to Cr also requires the assumption that Cr is normal in the patients' NAWM. However, there have been reports of abnormalities of Cr levels in demyelinating lesions and in the NAWM in patients with MS(Brex et al., 1999; Pan et al., 1996; Rooney et al., 1997; Suhy et al., 2000; van Walderveen, Truyen et al., 1999). Pan and colleagues found an isolated increase in Cr without a change in the level of Cho or NAA in the NAWM(Pan et al., 1996)of patients with MS. An increase in Cr was also found in a clinically isolated syndrome (CIS) group(Fernando et al., 2004). In that study, an increase in Cr was found in a subgroup of subjects with abnormal T2-weighted MRI results and in those with MS defined according to the McDonald criteria(Fernando et al., 2004). Those studies suggest that Cr may not be a reliable internal standard for use in the investigation of the effects of demylinating disease upon metabolite concentrations.

We have found no significant difference between the basal metabolite peak areas of NAA, Cho and Cr in the NAWM of patients with MS and that of healthy controls (*P* >.005). This was attributed to the patients' having been on relatively early stages of the disease (primarily 2-5 years after diagnosis) and their low EDSS levels. Those factors indicate that widespread axonal damage either had not occurred or was not detectactable at this stage and that the reduced NAA found in established MS is acquired later in the disease course. In a study, when 15 clinically isolated syndrome patients with T2 abnormalities were considered separately, their NAWM NAA concentrations were not found to be significantly different from those in controls(Brex et al., 1999). In our study, there was no significant difference between NAWM metabolite peaks of the treated and untreated groups in the results of the initial MRSI (*P*> .005) showing that the 2 patient groups were homogenous. We found that in the treatment group, NAWM NAA and Cho peaks began to increase during the sixth month, and that Cr peaks began to increase during the third month. No change was observed in the untreated group. When we evaluated WML metabolite changes, we found that in the treatment group, NAA and Cr peaks began to increase during the third month and Cho peaks began to increase during the first month. No changes in the metabolite peak areas of WML were observed in the untreated group.

There are a number of possible explanations for the increase in NAA that occurred between the sixth and twelfth months of treatment. Chronic low-grade encephalitis is probably present in patients with MS. There is pathological evidence of an increase in inflammatory cells in the NAWM of such patients(Allen & McKeown, 1979). The results of studies using Gd-enhanced MRI suggest that the blood-brain barrier is diffusely impaired in patients with MS. This chronic, low-level inflammation could result in widespread, partially reversible axonal damage and loss, and INFβ could induce its reversal.

A number of tissue injury mediating factors have been implicated in the production of the symptoms of MS(Moreau et al., 1996). INFβ directly or indirectly inhibits both the production of a number of those associated inflammatory factors (including interferon gamma) and the ability of those factors to stimulate nitric oxide release from astrocytes(Stewart et al., 1997). Elevated nitric oxide production and the consequent damage to mitochondria in surrounding neurons may be mitigated by INFβ and this could be a mechanism of action of INFβ in patients with MS(Stewart, Land, Clark, & Heales, 1998). NAA is produced by neuronal mitochondria(Patel & Clark, 1979), this could explain the recovery of NAA in patients with MS who are treated with INFβ. The increase in NAA could also be associated with the reversal of axonal metabolic dysfunction that is associated with in apparent myelin pathology in the NAWM.

In this study, one of the principal effects, which seems to be due to INFβ-1a, was an increase in the total Cho peak, which in the NAWM became evident during the sixth month of treatment and persisted through the twelfth month, and in the WML became evident during the first month of treatment then persisted throughout the study period. Choline-containing compounds are considered to be turnover products of cell membranes, and an increase in the level of Cho seems to be related primarily to inflammatory and glial cell proliferation rather than to myelin destruction. This observation was confirmed in a histopathological and spectroscopic correlative study in EAE, the results of which showed that a high Cho was associated with inflammation and not with demyelination. Furthermore, glial proliferation in bioptic samples from patients with MS was consistent with an in vivo increase in Cho(Brenner et al., 1993). An increased level of Cho has been described in MS lesions in a variety of studies(Bitsch et al., 1999; Davie et al., 1994; Kapeller et al., 2001; Narayana et al., 1998). Myelin and membrane constituents make a major contribution to the constituent of Cho; therefore, increased lesion cellularity and turn over may account for the observed increase in the level of Cho. However, an increase in Cho has been interpreted as an index of active or recent demyelination by some authors(Confort-Gouny et al., 1993; Davie et al., 1994; Kapeller et al., 2001; Larsson et al., 1991), an association suggested by the finding of an abundance of Cho-containing compounds in myelin and in all cell membranes, including those of inflammatory cells, in patients with MS(Brenner et al., 1993). This increase in the level of Cho may occur without significant clinical deterioration or disease activity. In a recent study, an increase in metabolite concentrations of Cho and Cr was found in CIS NAWM(Fernando et al., 2004). H-MRS-visible Cho containing compounds are derived primarily from cell membranes and may be elevated when there is increased cell turnover. Because the relation between the variations in Cho levels and the pathological changes in underlying lesions is not very well known at the moment, it cannot be excluded that the rise in Cho peak could express an increased turnover of myelin in the plaques and NAWM examined, a turnover that may not be the result of new demyelination, but the consequence of the remodeling of plaques or the effects of a remyelination process.

Although an increase in the Cr level has been found in the NAWM of patients with MS(Brex et al., 1999; Rooney et al., 1997; Suhy et al., 2000; van Walderveen, Barkhof et al., 1999), some experts do not agree on the fluctuations of that metabolite in MS lesions. However, some authors have reported a decrease in total Cr(van Walderveen, Barkhof et al., 1999); others have reported an increase(Kapeller et al., 2001; Suhy et al., 2000). It has been suggested that apart from the axonal damage occurring in the NAWM of patients with MS, there is a proliferation of glial cells that produces an increase in the Cr level(Pan et al., 1996; van Walderveen, Barkhof et al., 1999). When working at 4.1tesla with 0.5 voxels, Pan and colleagues found an isolated increase in the Cr level without concomitant changes in Cho or NAA levels in the WM far from the WM lesions and suggested that in NAWM, there may have been reactive astrocytosis without inflammatory changes. It has been postulated that an increase in the Cr level may reflect an astrocytic (gliotic) or oligodendrocytic remyelinating process. Histological evidence confirms that gliosis is the most common abnormality in macroscopically normal WM of patients with MS. Thus the MRSI abnormalities observed in such patients may be due to the effect of microscopic lesions below the resolution of the images(Rooney et al., 1997; Suhy et al., 2000). However, the increase in Cr along with Cho levels in NAWM and WM may also be accounted for an increase in metabolism, which might be expected to occur with inflammatory or glial reactive features like those in the NAWM of patients with MS.

There are some limitations of our study: The small number of patients, the short duration of study, an open label design, and the patients' being either in relatively early stages of disease or experiencing a relatively benign course of MS. However the numbers of patients in relatively early stages of the disease are more or less similar between the groups, and again the ones with a relatively benign form are again similarly distributed between the groups. Therefore we do not consider that this would have caused a bias in our results. It would have been better if the study were performed with a greater number of patients along with a longer study period. However we could not perform such a more desirable study design because of ethical problems.

5. Conclusions

Our results showed that NAA, Cho and Cr in a VOI that predominantly contains NAWM increased in patients with MS after 1 year of treatment with INFβ-1a. The same effect was also observed in WML after treatment. This evidence supports the theory that although axonal pathology begins early in the course of MS, INFβ-1a therapy may reverse part of that early axonal and metabolic dysfunction, and thus inhibit permanent axonal loss. Follow-up studies could help to define the dynamic changes of metabolites in MS plaques and to monitor the disease progression in MS.

6. References

Allen, I. V., & McKeown, S. R. (1979). A histological, histochemical and biochemical study of the macroscopically normal white matter in multiple sclerosis. *J Neurol Sci, 41*(1), 81-91.

Armspach, J. P., Gounot, D., Rumbach, L., & Chambron, J. (1991). In vivo determination of multiexponential T2 relaxation in the brain of patients with multiple sclerosis. *Magn Reson Imaging, 9*(1), 107-113.

Arnold, D. L., Matthews, P. M., Francis, G. S., O'Connor, J., & Antel, J. P. (1992). Proton magnetic resonance spectroscopic imaging for metabolic characterization of demyelinating plaques. *Ann Neurol, 31*(3), 235-241.

Arnold, D. L., Riess, G. T., Matthews, P. M., Francis, G. S., Collins, D. L., Wolfson, C., et al. (1994). Use of proton magnetic resonance spectroscopy for monitoring disease progression in multiple sclerosis. *Ann Neurol, 36*(1), 76-82.

Bitsch, A., Bruhn, H., Vougioukas, V., Stringaris, A., Lassmann, H., Frahm, J., et al. (1999). Inflammatory CNS demyelination: histopathologic correlation with in vivo quantitative proton MR spectroscopy. *AJNR Am J Neuroradiol, 20*(9), 1619-1627.

Brenner, R. E., Munro, P. M., Williams, S. C., Bell, J. D., Barker, G. J., Hawkins, C. P., et al. (1993). The proton NMR spectrum in acute EAE: the significance of the change in the Cho:Cr ratio. *Magn Reson Med, 29*(6), 737-745.

Brex, P. A., Gomez-Anson, B., Parker, G. J., Molyneux, P. D., Miszkiel, K. A., Barker, G. J., et al. (1999). Proton MR spectroscopy in clinically isolated syndromes suggestive of multiple sclerosis. *J Neurol Sci, 166*(1), 16-22.

Confort-Gouny, S., Vion-Dury, J., Nicoli, F., Dano, P., Donnet, A., Grazziani, N., et al. (1993). A multiparametric data analysis showing the potential of localized proton MR spectroscopy of the brain in the metabolic characterization of neurological diseases. *J Neurol Sci, 118*(2), 123-133.

Davie, C. A., Barker, G. J., Thompson, A. J., Tofts, P. S., McDonald, W. I., & Miller, D. H. (1997). 1H magnetic resonance spectroscopy of chronic cerebral white matter lesions and normal appearing white matter in multiple sclerosis. *J Neurol Neurosurg Psychiatry, 63*(6), 736-742.

Davie, C. A., Hawkins, C. P., Barker, G. J., Brennan, A., Tofts, P. S., Miller, D. H., et al. (1994). Serial proton magnetic resonance spectroscopy in acute multiple sclerosis lesions. *Brain, 117 (Pt 1)*, 49-58.

Davies, S. E., Newcombe, J., Williams, S. R., McDonald, W. I., & Clark, J. B. (1995). High resolution proton NMR spectroscopy of multiple sclerosis lesions. *J Neurochem, 64*(2), 742-748.

De Stefano, N., Matthews, P. M., Antel, J. P., Preul, M., Francis, G., & Arnold, D. L. (1995). Chemical pathology of acute demyelinating lesions and its correlation with disability. *Ann Neurol, 38*(6), 901-909.

Ferguson, B., Matyszak, M. K., Esiri, M. M., & Perry, V. H. (1997). Axonal damage in acute multiple sclerosis lesions. *Brain, 120 (Pt 3)*, 393-399.

Fernando, K. T., McLean, M. A., Chard, D. T., MacManus, D. G., Dalton, C. M., Miszkiel, K. A., et al. (2004). Elevated white matter myo-inositol in clinically isolated syndromes suggestive of multiple sclerosis. *Brain, 127*(Pt 6), 1361-1369.

Filippi, M., Campi, A., Dousset, V., Baratti, C., Martinelli, V., Canal, N., et al. (1995). A magnetization transfer imaging study of normal-appearing white matter in multiple sclerosis. *Neurology, 45*(3 Pt 1), 478-482.

Fu, L., Matthews, P. M., De Stefano, N., Worsley, K. J., Narayanan, S., Francis, G. S., et al. (1998). Imaging axonal damage of normal-appearing white matter in multiple sclerosis. *Brain, 121 (Pt 1)*, 103-113.

Gasperini, C., Horsfield, M. A., Thorpe, J. W., Kidd, D., Barker, G. J., Tofts, P. S., et al. (1996). Macroscopic and microscopic assessments of disease burden by MRI in multiple sclerosis: relationship to clinical parameters. *J Magn Reson Imaging, 6*(4), 580-584.

Gonen, O., Catalaa, I., Babb, J. S., Ge, Y., Mannon, L. J., Kolson, D. L., et al. (2000). Total brain N-acetylaspartate: a new measure of disease load in MS. *Neurology, 54*(1), 15-19.

Husted, C. A., Goodin, D. S., Hugg, J. W., Maudsley, A. A., Tsuruda, J. S., de Bie, S. H., et al. (1994). Biochemical alterations in multiple sclerosis lesions and normal-appearing white matter detected by in vivo 31P and 1H spectroscopic imaging. *Ann Neurol, 36*(2), 157-165.

Kapeller, P., McLean, M. A., Griffin, C. M., Chard, D., Parker, G. J., Barker, G. J., et al. (2001). Preliminary evidence for neuronal damage in cortical grey matter and normal appearing white matter in short duration relapsing-remitting multiple sclerosis: a quantitative MR spectroscopic imaging study. *J Neurol, 248*(2), 131-138.

Larsson, H. B., Christiansen, P., Jensen, M., Frederiksen, J., Heltberg, A., Olesen, J., et al. (1991). Localized in vivo proton spectroscopy in the brain of patients with multiple sclerosis. *Magn Reson Med, 22*(1), 23-31.

Loevner, L. A., Grossman, R. I., Cohen, J. A., Lexa, F. J., Kessler, D., & Kolson, D. L. (1995). Microscopic disease in normal-appearing white matter on conventional MR images in patients with multiple sclerosis: assessment with magnetization-transfer measurements. *Radiology, 196*(2), 511-515.

Matthews, P. M., Pioro, E., Narayanan, S., De Stefano, N., Fu, L., Francis, G., et al. (1996). Assessment of lesion pathology in multiple sclerosis using quantitative MRI morphometry and magnetic resonance spectroscopy. *Brain, 119 (Pt 3)*, 715-722.

McDonald, W. I., Compston, A., Edan, G., Goodkin, D., Hartung, H. P., Lublin, F. D., et al. (2001). Recommended diagnostic criteria for multiple sclerosis: guidelines from the International Panel on the diagnosis of multiple sclerosis. *Ann Neurol, 50*(1), 121-127.

Moreau, T., Coles, A., Wing, M., Isaacs, J., Hale, G., Waldmann, H., et al. (1996). Transient increase in symptoms associated with cytokine release in patients with multiple sclerosis. *Brain, 119 (Pt 1)*, 225-237.

Narayana, P. A., Doyle, T. J., Lai, D., & Wolinsky, J. S. (1998). Serial proton magnetic resonance spectroscopic imaging, contrast-enhanced magnetic resonance imaging, and quantitative lesion volumetry in multiple sclerosis. *Ann Neurol, 43*(1), 56-71.

Pan, J. W., Hetherington, H. P., Vaughan, J. T., Mitchell, G., Pohost, G. M., & Whitaker, J. N. (1996). Evaluation of multiple sclerosis by 1H spectroscopic imaging at 4.1 T. *Magn Reson Med, 36*(1), 72-77.

Patel, T. B., & Clark, J. B. (1979). Synthesis of N-acetyl-L-aspartate by rat brain mitochondria and its involvement in mitochondrial/cytosolic carbon transport. *Biochem J, 184*(3), 539-546.

Rooney, W. D., Goodkin, D. E., Schuff, N., Meyerhoff, D. J., Norman, D., & Weiner, M. W. (1997). 1H MRSI of normal appearing white matter in multiple sclerosis. *Mult Scler, 3*(4), 231-237.

Sarchielli, P., Presciutti, O., Pelliccioli, G. P., Tarducci, R., Gobbi, G., Chiarini, P., et al. (1999). Absolute quantification of brain metabolites by proton magnetic resonance spectroscopy in normal-appearing white matter of multiple sclerosis patients. *Brain, 122 (Pt 3)*, 513-521.

Stewart, V. C., Giovannoni, G., Land, J. M., McDonald, W. I., Clark, J. B., & Heales, S. J. (1997). Pretreatment of astrocytes with interferon-alpha/beta impairs interferon-gamma induction of nitric oxide synthase. *J Neurochem, 68*(6), 2547-2551.

Stewart, V. C., Land, J. M., Clark, J. B., & Heales, S. J. (1998). Pretreatment of astrocytes with interferon-alpha/beta prevents neuronal mitochondrial respiratory chain damage. *J Neurochem, 70*(1), 432-434.

Suhy, J., Rooney, W. D., Goodkin, D. E., Capizzano, A. A., Soher, B. J., Maudsley, A. A., et al. (2000). 1H MRSI comparison of white matter and lesions in primary progressive and relapsing-remitting MS. *Mult Scler, 6*(3), 148-155.

Tourbah, A., Stievenart, J. L., Gout, O., Fontaine, B., Liblau, R., Lubetzki, C., et al. (1999). Localized proton magnetic resonance spectroscopy in relapsing remitting versus secondary progressive multiple sclerosis. *Neurology, 53*(5), 1091-1097.

van Walderveen, M. A., Barkhof, F., Pouwels, P. J., van Schijndel, R. A., Polman, C. H., & Castelijns, J. A. (1999). Neuronal damage in T1-hypointense multiple sclerosis lesions demonstrated in vivo using proton magnetic resonance spectroscopy. *Ann Neurol, 46*(1), 79-87.

van Walderveen, M. A., Truyen, L., van Oosten, B. W., Castelijns, J. A., Lycklama a Nijeholt, G. J., van Waesberghe, J. H., et al. (1999). Development of hypointense lesions on T1-weighted spin-echo magnetic resonance images in multiple sclerosis: relation to inflammatory activity. *Arch Neurol, 56*(3), 345-351.

6

Magnetic Resonance Spectroscopy (MRS) in Kidney Transplantation: Interest and Perspectives

Bon Delphine, Seguin François and Hauet Thierry
Inserm U927, Poitiers
Université de Poitiers, Faculté de Médecine et de Pharmacie, Poitiers
CHU Poitiers, Pole UBM, Service de Biochimie, Poitiers
IBISA, Domaine Expérimental du Magneraud, Surgères
France

1. Introduction

Currently, in biology, Magnetic Resonance Spectroscopy (MRS) is widely used in metabonomics for diagnosis and prognostication in a wide range of studies from brain (Blasco et al., 2010) to leg (Borel et al., 2009) pathologies. Between both, the topic of interest in this section: the kidney. We will especially focus on kidney transplantation. Indeed, in France as well as in Europe, the number of patients awaiting transplant is still rising while the number of transplantations performed remains stable and even decreases (Figure 1.).

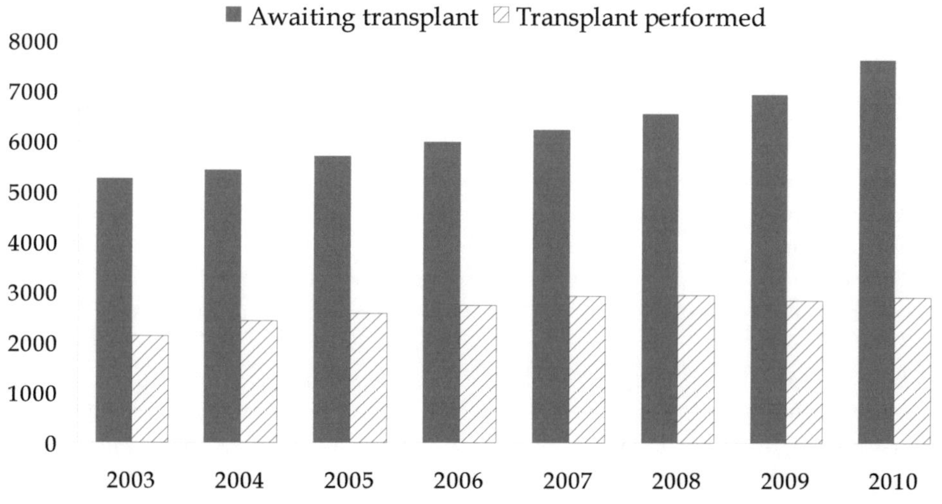

Fig. 1. Evolution of the number of patients on the waiting list for transplant and the number of transplantations performed between 2003 and 2010 in France (from Agence de la Biomédecine Rapport annuel 2011).

Although campaigns for organ donation increase the number of donors, donated organs are most often in marginal conditions because the donors often present co-morbidity factors (diabetes, obesity, cardiovascular disease, hypertension, poor renal function). In the case of the kidney, the percentage of successful grafts tends to decrease. These factors weaken the organ and render it more susceptible to develop lesions following ischemia reperfusion, the unavoidable syndrome encountered during organ preservation. As the extend of these lesions is correlated to graft outcome, it is necessary to improve the entire sequence of ischemia-reperfusion and in particular to find ways to improve storage conditions and decrease the rate of delayed graft function after kidney transplantation.

In kidney transplantation, delayed graft function is mainly due to the intensity of ischemia reperfusion lesions associated with the hypothermic and hypoxic conditions during preservation. These lesions are exacerbated at the moment of transplantation with reoxygenation that occurs during the reperfusion. In this light, tissue damages identified by the detection of endogenous metabolic changes in plasma and urine would permit a better estimation of graft quality and improved management of the graft, to the direct benefit of the patient. High Resolution Magnetic Resonance Spectroscopy (HR MRS) in these fluids could permit the identification of biomarkers indicative of specific kidney lesions occurring during an ischemia-reperfusion sequence.

The purpose of the chapter is to make a mini-review about thematics involving kidney transplantation from animals, mainly large white pig, to humans in order to highlight the potential of MRS, high resolution or imaging, and what perspectives could be envisioned to improve comprehension of kidney transplantation.

2. High resolution NMR

2.1 Kidney analysis

Before considering transplantation, it is important to review nephrologic situations and nephropathologies that have been widely analyzed by MRS to find biomarkers of pathologies associated to kidney.

In 1999, Garrod and al. established the biochemical composition of normal inner and outer renal cortex and renal papilla from rats (Garrod et al., 1999). This work realised with ^1H liquid NMR spectroscopy on tissue extracts and with ^1H hrmas (high resolution magic angle spining) NMR spectroscopy on crude tissue allowed the direct observation of metabolites into kidney and showed the metabolic composition of the 3 main areas of the kidney. They established the $_1H$ (hydrogen-1) and $_{13}C$ (carbon-13) chemical shift assignments of metabolites found in cortex and/or papilla. Still with ^1H hrmas NMR spectroscopy, a team realised the metabolic profiling of normal and hypertensive rat kidney (Huhn et al., 2004). They showed that better differentiation between both groups occurred in the kidney cortex. It has also been shown that NMR can be used to compare intact kidney, blood plasma and urine of 4 species of rodent. They thus showed that metabolic data acquired on laboratory animals can only be extended to wild species with the use of a lot of precaution (Griffin et al., 2000).

On those bases, and among pathologies affecting the kidney, diabetic nephropathy is one of the lethal manifestations of diabetic systemic disease (Zhao et al., 2011). Using a rat model of diabetic nephropathy induced by streptozotocin, the authors performed a holistic metabolic analysis in order to elucidate the mechanism of this disease. For that purpose, they realised ^{1}H liquid NMR spectra of urine on one hand and kidney extracts on the other. Elevated level of glucose in diabetic rats affected the ketone pathway, fatty acid oxidation, tricarboxylic acid cycle and glycolosis. Those metabolic changes led to decrease of energy production, hence aggravating kidney damage. Moreover, in this study the authors assessed osmolyte metabolism.

Another cause of kidney failure is autosomal dominant polycystic kidney diseases (ADPKD). Some candidate urinary protein biomarkers such as KIM1 or NGAL have already been evaluated for this nephropathology. However, to improve the quality of diagnosis for ADPKD, complete ^{1}H and ^{13}C NMR fingerprint of urine were put in place (Gronwald et al., 2011). Elevated levels of proteins and methanol were found in patients with ADPKD receiving medication against hypertension.

NMR is well suited for the study of neprotoxicity. In 1998, the team of Nicholson reported urine metabolic profiles in 15 groups of animal treated with nephrotoxic molecules and compared spectra with control. They thus highlighted endogenous biomarkers of nephrotoxic insult (Holmes et al., 1998). Citrate, 2-oxoglutarate and hippurate were the most discriminating metabolites between treated group and control group whereas formate and dimethylamine showed almost not change. Other studies on administration of nephrotoxic compounds realised with urine and plasma of Sprague-Dawley rats focused on lanthanum, a rare earth compound used as fertilizer with a higher accumulation rate and a lower metabolic rate (Feng et al., 2002) or thioacetamide (Waters et al., 2005). In the first study, the authors showed that a 6-months long ingestion of La^{3+}-induced nephro- and hepato-toxicity which could be highlighting by using NMR. From a dose of 10 mg/kg of $La(NO_3)^{3+}$, all the evolving quantified metabolites involved Krebs cycle intermediates or amino acids that are potential NMR markers for La^{3+}-induced proximal tubular lesions. Moreover, decrease of creatinine in urine highlighted a low glomerular filtration. A second study focused on energy intermediairy (citrate, lactate, succinate) and lipid metabolisms. The work also realised on intact kidney tissue using hrmas NMR spectroscopy (Garrod et al., 2001; Wang et al., 2006) established changes in the spectral profile of renal papilla involved the marked depletion of several renal osmolytes such as glycerophosphocholine, betaine, and myo-inositol.

Finally, the effects of cyclosporine A, the basis for most immunosuppressive protocols and used for allograft recipients on kidneys were evaluated (Lenz et al., 2004; Serkova et al., 2003). This treatment is well known for its nephrotoxicity. Cyclosporine A induced a decrease of poly unsaturated fatty acid and an increase of lipid peroxidation which suggests the use of an alternative pathway for energy production when the oxidative mitochondrial pathway is inhibited. This lipid peroxidation is responsive for kidney damage especially in the cortex and medulla. Cyclosporine A also leads to osmolyte regulation (taurine, betaine and trimethylamine-N-oxide (TMAO)).

2.2 Kidney transplantation analysis

2.2.1 Isolated Perfused Kidney (IPK) of pig

The isolated perfused pig kidney (IPK) was used to mimic the ischemia reperfusion episode occurring during transplantation. This model was destined to assess initial renal function after different preservation condition. The schematic diagram of the isolated perfusion method is illustrated in the Figure 2. Based on an isolated perfused kidney, HR MRS injury biomarkers of an ischemia-reperfusion sequence were identified in the urine. Spectra modifications compared to histological or biochemical analysis showed changes of some metabolites excretion.

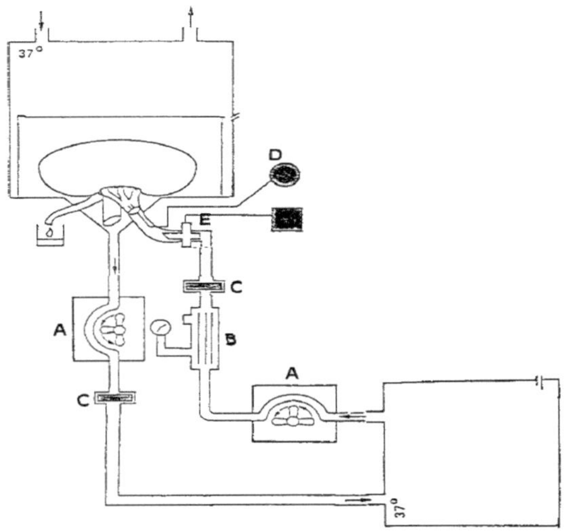

Fig. 2. Schematic diagram illustrating the isolated perfusion method in which A is the peristaltic pump, B, the oxygenator, C, the filter, D, the pressure transducer, E, the flow meter and electromagnetic flow probe (Hauet et al., 2000d).

One of the first studies using HR MRS on this model was performed to mimic the non-heart-beating donor situation. The kidney underwent a warm ischemic period before the hypothermic period of conservation and reperfusion (Hauet et al., 1997b). In this study, 3 groups of pigs were used. In the control group, kidneys were flushed with cold heparinized saline and immediately perfused. Kidney of a second group underwent a cold flush and 24 hours of cold-storage preservation (CSP) and finally reperfusion. The last group was composed of kidneys with 30 minutes of warm ischemia, 24 hours of CSP and reperfusion. The reperfusion occurred at 37°C and was performed with Kreb's solution supplemented with 22 amino acids. Among the interesting metabolites, TMAO and lactate were higher in the group with warm ischemia and related to damage of medullar cells and to tubular dysfunction respectively. Another study performed with the IPK was performed to assess the effect of cold storage conservation time with EuroCollins solution (EC) (Hauet et al., 1997a). Perfusion time was pushed to 72 hours and the degree of proximal tubule cell damage was increased with prolonged cold ischemia (Goujon et al., 1999). Urine content after a delay of 24 hours of perfusion was not significantly different from urine content at the beginning of the perfusion. After 48 hours, urine profile was significantly different. Rises of TMAO/creatinine and lactate/creatinine ratio measured with NMR were in accordance with elevated levels of beta-N-acetylglucosaminidase and lactate dehydrogenase. The same protocol was used to compare EC to University of Wisconsin solution (UW) (Hauet et al., 2000c; Hauet et al., 1999). Metabolites released into the conservation solution analyzed with NMR also confirmed classical biochemical parameters such as perfusion flow rate, glomerular filtration rate (GFR), tubular reabsortion of sodium and lactate dehydrogenase levels (Hauet et al., 2000d).

2.2.2 In vivo autotransplantation pig model

The IPK model, which provided ex vivo information, was converted to a preclinical model with 3-months old large white pig. Briefly, the basic model was to remove the kidney, preserve it 24 hours and then transplant it in the same animal with a contralateral nephrectomy. We followed the animal for 3 months after transplantation and we studied biochemical parameter in order to correlate them with MRS data.

In this model, damage biomarkers appearing after an ischemia reperfusion episode were analyzed in order to confirm their pertinence with the follow up of the recovery of function. To summarize, metabolites quantified with liquid NMR were TMAO, correlated to medullar lesions, acetate correlated to cortical lesions and lactate linked to global ischemia. Amino acids such as alanine or valine could be associated with proximal tubules dysfunction. Creatinine measured in both plasma and urine allowed the determination of GFR. All these metabolites were highlighted in different studies summarized below.

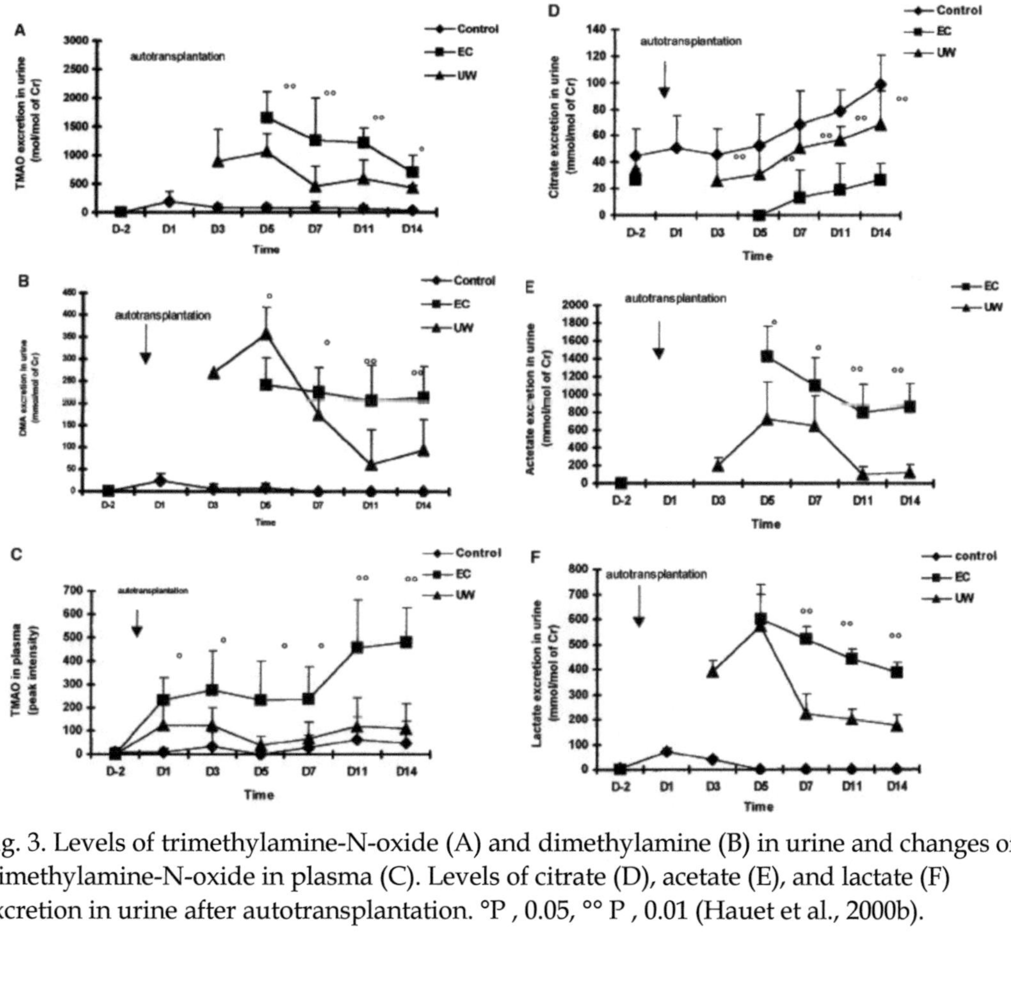

Fig. 3. Levels of trimethylamine-N-oxide (A) and dimethylamine (B) in urine and changes of trimethylamine-N-oxide in plasma (C). Levels of citrate (D), acetate (E), and lactate (F) excretion in urine after autotransplantation. °P , 0.05, °° P , 0.01 (Hauet et al., 2000b).

In 2000, comparison of EC and UW solution with CSP, already performed on IPK of pig, was performed on this preclinical model of kidney autotransplantation (Hauet et al., 2000b). The control group, undergoing uninephrectomy, presented 100% survival at day 14 whereas only 75% and 66 % of UW and EC pigs survived, respectively. Glutathione-S-transferase and creatinine clearance were significantly different between EC and UW groups with a light advantages for UW compared to control. Results obtained with MRS on urine and plasma are presented in figure 3. Delayed graft function was associated with the release of osmolytes such as TMAO in urine and in plasma. Moreover, dimethylamine, acetate, citrate and lactate level in the UW group were always closer to control group levels compared to levels in the EC group. These data outline the effect of UW preservation against renal medullar injury and impairment of oxidative metabolism. Here, strength of MRS was highlighted: in one experiment, with a 200 to 500 µL volume of sample, detection and quantitation of large number of metabolites can be made. This allows for a multivariable analysis which is an important factor for diagnostic and prognostic purpose.

Using the same experimental design, the impact of the preservation solution was demonstrated and the addition of colloids (polyethylene glycol (PEG)) into an extracellular solution showed better results (Faure et al., 2002). Indeed, in the urine spectra, TMAO/creatine ratio were significantly higher in kidney preserved with EC, UW or a solution containing PEG-50 than in kidney preserved with a solution containing PEG-30. This demonstrated that PEG reduced damages to the renal medulla during conservation, in a dose-dependent manner. Citrate was not detected during the first postoperative week in urine from kidneys preserved in EC. Its excretion was detected significantly earlier in urine from the ICPEG30 group than from the UW and ICPEG50 groups. This suggested that PEG associated to an intracellular solution improved oxidative metabolism and reduced renal medulla injury, also in a concentration-dependent manner. Furthermore, the addition of antioxidative (Baumert et al., 1999) or anticoagulant (Favreau et al., 2010) molecules, trimetazidine and melagatran respectively, into the preservation solution increased the performance of the hypothermic conservation. The effect of trimetazidine during conservation with EC or UW showed interesting results. The early excretion of acetate in the trimetazidine supplemented group demonstrated an efficient function recovery of the citric acid cycle compared with standard solutions (Hauet et al., 2000a). Combination of PEG and trimetazidine in conservation solution was the next step of long term time study which included 18 groups also exploring cold ischemia time (Doucet et al., 2004). Biological parameters indicated that reduced delayed graft was found when combining PEG and trimetazidine during CSP. Histological staining for CD4+ positive cells indicated that PEG reduced CD4+ positive cells infiltration and trimetazidine was efficient in reducing the inflammatory reaction. The NMR analysis was again in accordance with these results. Acetate excretion between day 1 and day 14 was improved in all experimental group preserved with trimetazidine while urinary TMAO was reduced in all trimetazidine group and we noticed presence of TMAO in plasma in all group except from control. Combination of trimetazidine with PEG seemed to be the best option for kidney conservation and MRS brought supplementary information to classical biochemical parameters such as GFR or sodium excretion. In addition, this study underlined that MRS permits the performance of a multivariate analysis in a single experiment.

Use of conditioning drugs before conservation was also investigated. Donor pretreatment with N-acetylcysteine (NAC) has been shown to ameliorate acute renal failure. Extractions with perchloric acid of kidney tissue samples 24 hours after transplantation were performed and hydrosoluble metabolites were analyzed with ^{1}H liquid NMR spectroscopy. In parallel, blood samples were analyzed. TMAO again gave the best results. Its decreased levels in the blood of NAC group compared to control group were associated with a decrease of allantoin in the blood and kidney tissue. This latter metabolite results from the free radical action of urate and its presence indicates free radical activities. Pretreatment with NAC reduced radical excretion, hence reduced free radical activity and thus tissue damages (Fuller et al., 2004).

2.2.3 Application to Human

Use of HR MRS in Human to follow transplanted kidney recovery of function highlighted several issues. The main problem came from the drug treatment received by patients after transplantation. We observed overlapping between the signals of the metabolites of interest and of the drugs. In these conditions it is often difficult to extract information about the kidney function. Moreover a high variability, in addition of the individual variability, is often observed. This variability, mainly due to diet, may cause urine profile modifications which can hide variations of the metabolite of interest in relation with the kidney injuries. One solution could be to introduce a 2-days controlled diet before each sampling to minimise those environmental variation. However, an older study performed on 33 patients who underwent primary renal allograft transplantation, using the same immunosuppressive regiment and of which 57.6% achieve immediate graft function, showed that patients with good graft function and normal patients had urinary TMAO/creatinine level inferior to 200 µmol/mM while patients with graft dysfunction had urinary TMAO/creatinine level of 410 ± 102 µmol/mM (Foxall et al., 1993).

2.3 Perspectives

2.3.1 Perfusate analysis

Hypothermic machine perfusion (MP) is increasingly being preferred to CSP. Indeed, MP has been showed to offer protection to the organ since the 80's (Alijani et al., 1985; Kwiatkowski et al., 2007; Wight et al., 2003) with benefits such as reduction of delayed graft function and increased survival. However, the mechanisms involved in these improvements are still unclear and need to be elucidated. Biomarkers such as lactate dehydrogenase, total glutathione-S-transferase or N-acetyl-β-D-glucosaminidase measured at the end of the perfusion in the machine perfusates are used by clinicians. Even if those markers are independently efficient to predict graft outcome, they are not efficient enough to be taken into account in the decision to transplant or discard a donation after brain death or controlled donation after cardiac death (Moers et al., 2010; Siew et al., 2011). Again the potential of multivariate analysis offered by NMR could be used to predict graft outcome. In a recent study in a pig model of autotransplantation of livers, the effect of warm ischemia on metabolites contents into perfusats was measured (Liu et al., 2009).

Currently, our team is attempting to answer the question: can ^{1}H HR NMR metabonomic analysis during machine perfusion be used to predict graft outcome? We thus work on perfusates from different protocols of kidney transplantation using MP. We evaluate the effect of warm ischemia, duration of ischemia, types of solution and temperatures of preservation and finally effect of adjuvant in the perfusion solution. We showed, in a small cohort of pig with two distinct graft outcomes, that a correlation between creatininemia at day 7 after transplantation and choline concentration after 24 hours of perfusion existed. Other metabolites like TMAO, lactate or glutathione showed the same correlation (Figure 4.). Metabonomic NMR analysis of machine perfusates could thus be use to predict graft outcome. A larger study is required to validate this finding, especially since this technique is easily transposable to the clinic.

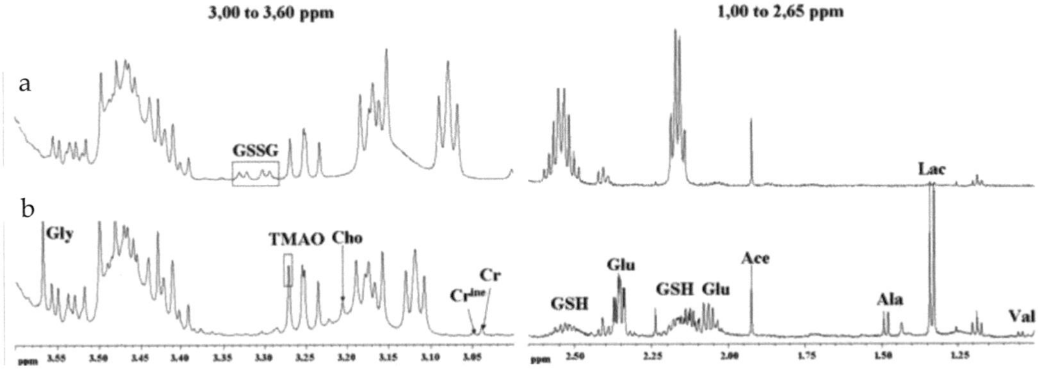

Fig. 4. ^{1}H HR NMR spectra of kidney perfusion solution (a) at the beginning of the perfusion and (b) after 24 hours of perfusion. (Ace: acetate, Ala: alanine, Cho: choline, Cr: creatine, Cr^{ine}: creatinine, Glu: glutamate, GSH: reduced glutathione, GSSG: oxidized glutathione, TMAO: trimethylamine-N-oxide, Val: valine).

2.3.2 ^{1}H hrmas NMR on kidney tissue or cells

In an hrmas probe, adapted for classical spectrometer, samples are spun with high speed (2000 - 5000 Hz) at a 54.7° angle. This rotation leads to decreased heterogeneity of samples and allows direct sample analysis. ^{1}H hrmas NMR is thus particularly adapted for tissue or cells without sample pre-treatment (Desmoulin et al., 2008). Addition of deuterated water into phosphate buffer solution is the only required modification of the samples.

In regards to the in vitro analysis of ischemia reperfusion injuries, our team developed an endothelial cell model mimicking transplantation through a hypoxia-reoxygenation episode in which conditions of hypoxia and/or reoxygenation can be modulated by changing temperature of hypoxia, atmosphere or conservation solutions. ^{1}H hrmas NMR is a precious tool for this application but needs improvement for cell analysis. Indeed, the main problem resides on cell quantity, especially after hypoxia when cell number is inferior to 1 million as it is the case in our experiments. Use of the rotor allows for limitation of volume inside the tube and is one of the solutions we are examining. On the other hand, after 30 minutes spinning at 2500 Hz at 4°C, when cells were replaced into culture medium, 40 to 60 % of cells were still alive and restarted growing normally after 24 hours. Thus, we could imagine the use of ^{1}H hrmas NMR to study all hypoxia-reoxygenation sequence on the same cells. In parallel, supernatant can also been analyzed in order to follow the cell metabolism.

Concerning tissue analysis, care has to be taken during tissue collection. Indeed, as already mentioned, because of its histological heterogeneity the kidney has different metabolites composition depending on the area (Garrod et al., 1999). For autotransplantation models as in clinical studies, a defined protocol for biopsy must be respected by all involved parties.

3. Magnetic resonance in vivo

3.1 MRI

Magnetic resonance imaging (MRI) is a non invasive technique bringing essential information in the diagnostic of kidney transplant rejection since it can provide data on the anatomic and functional status of the transplanted kidney (Beckmann et al., 2000). Briefly, anatomic MRI is applied to evaluate the transplanted organ by assessing structural and anatomical changes or by measuring the graft volume. The most popular imaging sequences are the T1- and T2-weighted spin echo sequences and the T1-weighted gradient echo sequence. However, it would really be informative to add other acquisition sequences to obtain functional information about the transplanted kidney, if the magnet system is available during enough time to perform these exams. Indeed, further information can be obtained on perfusion and functionality of the graft and the integrity of the tissue.

In addition of the magnetic resonance angiography to image blood vessels, quantification of the renal blood flow can be performed with dynamic MRI (Montet et al., 2003). Using a contrast agent, an association of a lower MRI perfusion with chronic allograft nephropathy severity was found (Pereira et al., 2011). Perfusion was determined in chosen area of the kidney, by measuring enhanced signal in the region of interest during the injection of the contrast agent. These results led to an homogeneous estimation of the perfusion, and the ability to evaluate the entire kidney with perfusion MRI may have benefits in establishing which areas of the transplant have a reduction in perfusion. The limitation in obtaining an entire kidney image is the necessity to use a cardiac gating to avoid pulsatility in the arterial curve. Another problem is the potential nephrotoxicity of the gadolinium which is generally used as contrast agent in a chelated form. Using low dose three dimensional magnetic resonance renography, the mean transit time of the tracer for the different compartment of the kidney (vascular, tubular and collecting system) was measured different in normal kidneys, transplanted kidneys with acute tubular necrosis and transplanted kidney with acute rejection (Yamamoto et al., 2011) indicating that a multicompartimental tracer kinetic renal model may help to differentiate acute rejection from acute tubular necrosis in transplanted kidney.

Ultra-small superparamagnetic particles of iron oxides (USPIO) could be used as contrast agent in clinical medicine for in vivo MRI due to their properties to locally perturb magnetic field and novel particles are in development (Mills et al., 2011). Their toxicity is not well known and liquiq ^{1}H NMR analysis of plasma and urine demonstrated metabolic changes (Feng et al., 2010). Energenetic and lipidic pathways such as glucose and amino acid metabolisms were affected by USPIO administration. Whereas no change has been found in histopathological analysis of tissue between two types of USPIO administration, coated with dextran or uncoated, coated-USPIO administration led to acetate, unsaturated fatty acids and some amino acids elevation in the ^{1}H hrmas kidney profile. It also led to decrease of triacylglycerol, myo-niositol or taurine, for instance (Feng et al., 2011). Hence, this sort of tracer has to be used with precaution.

A noninvasive magnetic resonance arterial spin labeling (ASL) technique has been performed to evaluate kidney perfusion without contrast agents (Artz et al., 2011). ASL uses the blood as an endogenous contrast agent allowing perfusion measurements without gadolinium injection. Using a flow-sensitive alternating inversion recovery (FAIR) sequence, inflowing blood is selectively labeled to have an opposite magnetization compared to the destination tissue. The difference between a labeled image and a non labeled image can be used to calculate tissue perfusion. The first results obtained indicated that medullar perfusion was systematically lower in transplanted versus native kidneys irrespectively of estimated glomerular filtration rate (eGFR). Cortical perfusion was lower for transplanted kidneys when eGFR was > 60 ml/min per 1.73 m^2 and correlated with eGFR in both native and transplanted kidneys. These results were obtained with a one model compartment requiring rapid water exchange assumption between the intravascular and extravascular space. A two compartments model would allow more accurate perfusion quantification, but would require measurements which are not possible in a clinically feasible scan time.

Diffusion weighted (DW) MRI, which was established for the tissue characterization and lesion detection (Thoeny &De Keyzer, 2011), is particularly interesting for kidney function exploration because of its high blood flow and water transport functions. Simple acquisition is performed with a bipolar gradient (diffusion gradient) dedicated to the assessment of fluid movements. When molecules of water moves, the absence of rephasement of the nuclear spin appears as a loss of signal intensity on the image. If diffusion is restricted, molecules of water reduce their movement and may be refocused by the second gradient impulse (Palmucci et al., 2011). Different intensities of diffusion gradient can be used to determine the Apparent Diffusion Coefficient (ADC). The DW MRI techniques yields a total ADC in each voxel explored that provides information on diffusion properties of water, including contribution from micro-circulation (Le Bihan et al., 1988). Thus image processing allows to separate the micro-circulation information, quantified with the perfusion fraction (F_P) which reflects micro-circulation of blood and movement of fluids in predefined structure such as tubules and glomeruli, and the primarily pure diffusion with the perfusion-free diffusion (ADC_D) (Eisenberger et al., 2010). The potential of ADC has been studied in kidney transplantation to determined modification in case of graft rejection or acute tubular necrosis. In patients with stable allograft function (posttransplant time between 8 and 10 months), total ADC and ADC_D were found identical in the cortex and medulla of the transplanted kidney while values were higher in cortex than in medulla of healthy volunteers. Cortical total ADC and ADC_D were higher in native kidneys than in transplanted kidneys (Thoeny et al., 2006), and a difference in ADC_D was observed between patients with normal clearance (>60 mL/min) and low clearance (>30 mL/min) where ADC_D were the lowest (Palmucci et al., 2011). In allografts with stable function early after transplantation (posttransplantation time of 10 days) ADC_D and F_P were also found identical in cortex and medulla, but the F_P was strongly reduced in the cortex and medulla of renal transplants with allograft rejection and acute tubular necrosis. F_P correlated with eGFR, while no correlation were found between eGFR and ADC_D or total ADC (Eisenberger et al., 2010). These results show that DW MRI is a promising non-invasive method for detection or monitoring of functional derangements early after kidney transplantation.

The blood oxygen level dependent (BOLD) MRI is a functional MRI technique allowing assessment of the tissue oxygenation. When the kidney is the explored organ, it allows the differentiation of specific anatomical regions (I.E cortex, inner and outer medulla). BOLD MRI is based on susceptibility differences between oxyhemoglobin and deoxyhemoglobin which induce image contrast differences, generally obtained with a gradient echoes sequence. Oxyhemoglogin is diamagnetic, and has no effect on the NMR signal of the surrounding water, by contrast deoxyhemoglobin is paramagnetic, increasing its magnetic properties and modifying the signal relaxation of the surrounding water molecules. Higher concentrations of deoxyhemoglobin induces shorter apparent T2 relaxation time, which is in relation with the oxygen consumption in the tissue. In a murine model, BOLD MRI of a clamped kidney showed the decreased oxygenation of all regions. 24 hours after reperfusion, a lower reoxygenation of the outer medulla than control was found, and a higher reoxygenation of the cortex and an identical reoxygenation of the inner medulla were determined (Oostendorp et al., 2011). These results highlighted the potential of BOLD MRI for the detection of change in kidney tissue oxygenation. Non invasive exploration of human kidneys showed that oxygenation was lower in medulla than in the cortex, confirming a physiological medullar hypoxia (Malvezzi et al., 2009; Thoeny et al., 2006). A few days post transplantation, this technique showed an increase of T2 relaxation times in the cortex and medulla of the transplanted kidney, compared to the donated kidney of living donor before collection, demonstrating increased oxygenation (Malvezzi et al., 2009). A few months after transplantation, an increased oxygen content in the medulla was observed despite an unchanged perfusion fraction (Thoeny et al., 2006). Comparing allografts with normal function or acute tubular necrosis, a decreased blood flow and an increased oxygen bioavailability in the medulla of acutely rejecting kidneys were observed, suggesting a greater decrease in oxygen use (Sadowski et al., 2010). No significant modification of BOLD and DW MRI were observed in patients with acute tubular necrosis compared to normal functioning allografts. These results indicate the potential of these MRI techniques to longitudinally follow transplanted kidneys and obtain information on function.

As an anecdote, MRI was tested for the counting the kidney glomerules number and size distribution in normal rat kidneys using ferritin as labeling and compared to standard stereological evaluation (Heilmann et al., 2011). This study showed that this ex vivo analysis of entire kidney was less time consuming than stereological method.

3.2 ^{31}P MRS

Magnetic resonance spectroscopy of Phosphorus-31 (^{31}P) can be performed in kidney during the preservation period and in vivo after transplantation. In these two cases, ^{31}P MRS brings information about the energetic metabolism. This non invasive methods allows the observation of a limited number of metabolites which are mainly: adenosine triphospate (ATP) which gives three signals corresponding to the three phosphorus nuclei in the ATP molecule (α, β and γ phosphorus corresponding to the position of the phosphorus nucleus in the molecule); inorganic phosphate (Pi) which has a chemical shift varying with the intracellular pH; phosphomonoesters (PME), mainly including phosphocholine and phosphoethanolamine that is highly concentrated in the renal cortex; phosphodiesters (PDE), corresponding to the resonances of glycerophosphocholine (GPC) and glycerol-phosphoethanolamine (GPE) which can be used as an indicator of the physiological integrity of the organ (Wolff &Balaban, 1988). Phosphocreatine is not seen in NMR spectrum of kidney, and when it appears in vivo, it comes from the surrounding tissues.

Ex vivo or in vivo, ^{31}P MRS does not allow an absolute quantification thus only signal ratios can be used. These ratios were studied in the preservation period and after the transplantation of the kidney, and compared with the kidney graft function. During the preservation period, ^{31}P MRS was performed ex vivo with the kidney in the preservation solution and in the apparatus of conservation. The ATP disappeared quickly after the collection and perfusion with a cold preservation solution, in spite of the fact that the kidney was immediately cooled to 4°C and maintained to this temperature. The most significant indicator of graft quality was the ratio of PME to Pi (PME/Pi), determined in human cadaveric kidneys prior to planned transplantation, which has been correlated with tubular necrosis and delayed graft function (Bretan et al., 1989; Hene et al., 1994). A high PME/Pi ratio was associated with the best renal function after transplantation; a decrease of this ratio (decrease of PME and/or increase of Pi) correlated with prolonged acute tubular necrosis. In regards to the determination of this ratio in the preserved kidney, the difficulty was the presence of a phosphate buffer in the preservation solution, this Pi signal overlapping the intracellular inorganic phosphate. Determination of this ratio can be obtained using Chemical Shift Imaging (CSI). This technique uses spatial resolution to obtain a 2D-CSI spectra, where each spectrum comes from a voxel. The interest is to minimize the Pi signal of the preservation solution in the voxel's content. In these conditions, a better correlation was obtained between PME/Pi ratio and serum creatinine 14 days after transplantation (Niekisch et al., 2004). A decrease of the PME/Pi ratio was shown as a monoexponential time dependent function in pig kidneys (von Elverfeldt et al., 2007). This decrease shows the influence of preservation time on transplantation outcome, and the authors determined a different decay constant with the preservation solution (comparison between two solutions) suggesting a predictive indicator of the preservation quality with time. This PME/Pi ratio indicator can be obtained with the kidney staying in its preservation container, at preservation temperature. No injection or biopsy is necessary, allowing easy integration of this exam in the period between collection and transplantation; the only condition being a non-magnetic container to be introduced in the magnet of a magnetic resonance apparatus (whole body scanner MR for this exam).

After transplantation it is possible to perform an in vivo ^{31}P MRS of the kidney, which remains fully non invasive as it does not require injection nor anesthesia. More information can be obtained from the ^{31}P spectrum of kidney since in addition to the PME and PDE signals, ATP signals can be observed and intracellular pH can be determined with the chemical shift of the Pi. When spectrum is obtained from the whole kidney, β-ATP to Pi ratio measured 2 or 3 years after transplantation has been shown to be an excellent indicator of long term survival of the transplanted kidney (3 years when ratio > 1.2 and 5 years when ration > 2.5) (Seto et al., 2001). When MRS was performed in the 4 weeks after transplantation, the PME to PDE ratio seemed to be an indicator of allograft function (Klemm et al., 1998), showing a good correlation with serum creatinine levels. High PME/PDE ratio reflects the cell membrane regeneration process occurring during the first weeks after ischemia; PME level is considered as a reflection of the membrane phospholipid metabolism with the degree of cell growth and regeneration, while in contrast PDE level correspond to intermediate metabolites formed during cell membrane degradation. A decreased PME/PDE ratio was found in patients with delayed graft function due to acute tubular necrosis, but was not observed in patient with allograft rejection. A better localization of the voxel for ^{31}P MRS could be obtained with CSI technique (Vyhnanovska et al., 2011), allowing the discard of surrounding tissue from the kidney signal in the spectra and the reduction in result dispersion, even if resolution did not permit to distinguish cortex from medulla in the spectra. In these conditions it is possible to distinguish different types of kidney failure after transplantation: (i) acute tubular necrosis, characterized by a decrease of PDE/β-ATP, PDE/Pi and PME/Pi compared to controls; (ii) acute rejection episodes (ARE), characterized by an increase of PME/β-ATP and PME/Pi ratio compare to controls. This method permitted the demonstration that late kidney graft dysfunction patients exhibited a higher Pi/β-ATP and lower PDE/Pi and PME/Pi ratio compared with ARE patients.

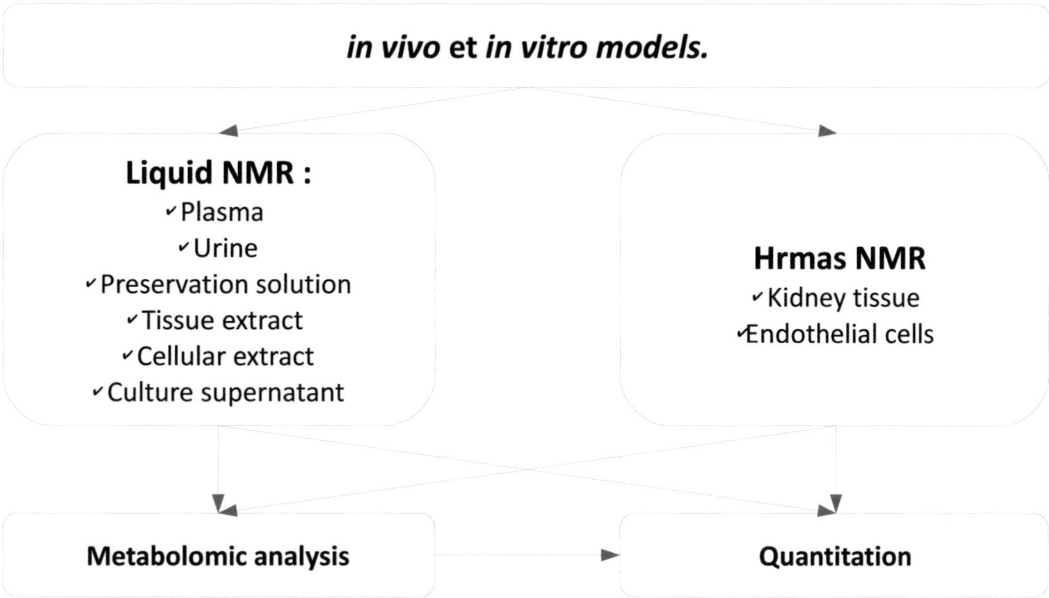

Fig. 5. Summary of samples for liquid or hrmas MRS analysis to study ischemia-reperfusion phenomena occurring during kidney transplantation.

4. Conclusion

From liquid NMR analysis of urine in IPK or perfusate in an autotransplantation model of large white pig, to hrmas analysis of cell culture or biopsy from Human (abstracted in the figure 5.) through imaging, MRS, combined with metabolomic analysis is a powerful tool for the study of transplantation. Despite all the difficulties in regards to kidney heterogeneity or low detection limit for cell analysis, MRS is still an interesting implement deserving of amelioration. Advances concerning imaging and contrast agents as well as transposition of hrmas to imaging are also the key for better diagnosis, prognosis and transplantation comprehension.

5. Acknowledgment

We thank all people working in the INSERM U927 unit and allow us to access in vitro or in vivo samples: William Hebrard, Sébastien Giraud, Frédéric Favreau, Nicolas Chatauret and Raphael Thuillier, for his grammatical help especially. Thank to Nadège Boildieu, technician performed almost all the NMR acquisition in the team.

6. Abbreviations

^{1}H	Hydrogen-1
^{13}C	Carbon-13
^{31}P	Phosphorus-31
ADC	Apparent Diffusion Coefficient
ADC_D	Perfusion-free diffusion
ADPKD	Autosomal dominant polycystic kidney diseases

ARE	Acute rejection episode
ASL	Arterial spin labeling
ATP	Adenosine triphospate
BOLD	Blood oxygen level dependent
CSI	Chemical Shift Imaging
CSP	Cold-storage preservation
DW	Diffusion weighted
EC	EuroCollins solution
eGFR	Estimated glomerular filtration rate
F_P	Perfusion fraction
GFR	Glomerular filtration rate
GPC	Glycerophosphocholine
GPE	Glycerophosphoethanolamine
hrmas	High resolution magic angle spinning
IPK	Isolate perfused kidney
MP	Machine perfusion
MRI	Magnetic resonance imaging
MRS	Magnetic Resonance Spectroscopy
NAC	N-acetylcysteine
NMR	Nuclear Magnetic Resonance
PDE	Phosphodiesters
PEG	Polyethylene glycol
Pi	Inorganic phosphate
PME	Phosphomonoesters
TMAO	Trimethylamine-N-oxide
USPIO	Ultra-small superparamagnetic particles of iron oxides
UW	University of Wisconsin solution

7. References

Alijani, M.R., Cutler, J.A., DelValle, C.J., Morres, D.N., Fawzy, A., Pechan, B.W., & Helfrich, G.B. (1985). Single-donor cold storage versus machine perfusion in cadaver kidney preservation. Transplantation *40*, 659-661.

Artz, N.S., Sadowski, E.A., Wentland, A.L., Grist, T.M., Seo, S., Djamali, A., & Fain, S.B. (2011). Arterial spin labeling MRI for assessment of perfusion in native and transplanted kidneys. Magnetic resonance imaging *29*, 74-82.

Baumert, H., Goujon, J.M., Richer, J.P., Lacoste, L., Tillement, J.P., Eugene, M., Carretier, M., & Hauet, T. (1999). Renoprotective effects of trimetazidine against ischemia-reperfusion injury and cold storage preservation: a preliminary study. Transplantation *68*, 300-303.

Beckmann, N., Hof, R.P., & Rudin, M. (2000). The role of magnetic resonance imaging and spectroscopy in transplantation: from animal models to man. NMR in biomedicine *13*, 329-348.

Blasco, H., Corcia, P., Moreau, C., Veau, S., Fournier, C., Vourc'h, P., Emond, P., Gordon, P., Pradat, P.F., Praline, J., *et al.* (2010). 1H-NMR-based metabolomic profiling of CSF in early amyotrophic lateral sclerosis. PloS one *5*, e13223.

Borel, M., Pastoureau, P., Papon, J., Madelmont, J.C., Moins, N., Maublant, J., & Miot-Noirault, E. (2009). Longitudinal profiling of articular cartilage degradation in osteoarthritis by high-resolution magic angle spinning 1H NMR spectroscopy: experimental study in the meniscectomized guinea pig model. Journal of proteome research *8*, 2594-2600.

Bretan, P.N., Baldwin, N., Novick, A.C., Majors, A., Easley, K., Ng, T., Stowe, N., Rehm, P., Sreem, S.B., & Steinmuller, D.R. (1989). Pretransplant assessment of renal viability by phosphorus-31 magnetic resonance spectroscopy: clinical experience in 40 recipient patients. Transplantation *48*, 48-53.

Desmoulin, F., Bon, D., Martino, R., & Malet-Martino, M. (2008). Étude critique de l'utilisation de la RMN HR-MAS pour l'analyse des tissus biologiques, HR-MAS NMR analysis of biological tissues: a critical report. CR Chimie *11*, 423-433.

Doucet, C., Dutheil, D., Petit, I., Zhang, K., Eugene, M., Touchard, G., Wahl, A., Seguin, F., Milinkevitch, S., Hauet, T., *et al.* (2004). Influence of colloid, preservation medium and trimetazidine on renal medulla injury. Biochimica et biophysica acta *1673*, 105-114.

Eisenberger, U., Thoeny, H.C., Binser, T., Gugger, M., Frey, F.J., Boesch, C., & Vermathen, P. (2010). Evaluation of renal allograft function early after transplantation with diffusion-weighted MR imaging. European Radiology *20*, 1374-1383.

Faure, J.P., Hauet, T., Han, Z., Goujon, J.M., Petit, I., Mauco, G., Eugene, M., Carretier, M., & Papadopoulos, V. (2002). Polyethylene glycol reduces early and long-term cold ischemia-reperfusion and renal medulla injury. The Journal of pharmacology and experimental therapeutics *302*, 861-870.

Favreau, F., Thuillier, R., Cau, J., Milin, S., Manguy, E., Mauco, G., Zhu, X., Lerman, L.O., & Hauet, T. (2010). Anti-thrombin therapy during warm ischemia and cold preservation prevents chronic kidney graft fibrosis in a DCD model. Am J Transplant *10*, 30-39.

Feng, J., Li, X., Pei, F., Chen, X., Li, S., & Nie, Y. (2002). 1H NMR analysis for metabolites in serum and urine from rats administrated chronically with La(NO3)3. Analytical biochemistry *301*, 1-7.

Feng, J., Liu, H., Bhakoo, K.K., Lu, L., & Chen, Z. (2011). A metabonomic analysis of organ specific response to USPIO administration. Biomaterials.

Feng, J., Liu, H., Zhang, L., Bhakoo, K., & Lu, L. (2010). An insight into the metabolic responses of ultra-small superparamagnetic particles of iron oxide using metabonomic analysis of biofluids. Nanotechnology *21*, 395101.

Foxall, P.J., Mellotte, G.J., Bending, M.R., Lindon, J.C., & Nicholson, J.K. (1993). NMR spectroscopy as a novel approach to the monitoring of renal transplant function. Kidney international *43*, 234-245.

Fuller, T.F., Serkova, N., Niemann, C.U., & Freise, C.E. (2004). Influence of donor pretreatment with N-acetylcysteine on ischemia/reperfusion injury in rat kidney grafts. The Journal of urology *171*, 1296-1300.

Garrod, S., Humpfer, E., Spraul, M., Connor, S.C., Polley, S., Connelly, J., Lindon, J.C., Nicholson, J.K., & Holmes, E. (1999). High-resolution magic angle spinning 1H NMR spectroscopic studies on intact rat renal cortex and medulla. Magn Reson Med *41*, 1108-1118.

Garrod, S., Humpher, E., Connor, S.C., Connelly, J.C., Spraul, M., Nicholson, J.K., & Holmes, E. (2001). High-resolution (1)H NMR and magic angle spinning NMR spectroscopic investigation of the biochemical effects of 2-bromoethanamine in intact renal and hepatic tissue. Magn Reson Med *45*, 781-790.

Goujon, J.M., Hauet, T., Menet, E., Levillain, P., Babin, P., & Carretier, M. (1999). Histological evaluation of proximal tubule cell injury in isolated perfused pig kidneys exposed to cold ischemia. The Journal of surgical research *82*, 228-233.

Griffin, J.L., Walker, L.A., Garrod, S., Holmes, E., Shore, R.F., & Nicholson, J.K. (2000). NMR spectroscopy based metabonomic studies on the comparative biochemistry of the kidney and urine of the bank vole (Clethrionomys glareolus), wood mouse (Apodemus sylvaticus), white toothed shrew (Crocidura suaveolens) and the laboratory rat. Comparative biochemistry and physiology *127*, 357-367.

Gronwald, W., Klein, M.S., Zeltner, R., Schulze, B.D., Reinhold, S.W., Deutschmann, M., Immervoll, A.K., Boger, C.A., Banas, B., Eckardt, K.U., *et al.* (2011). Detection of autosomal dominant polycystic kidney disease by NMR spectroscopic fingerprinting of urine. Kidney international *79*, 1244-1253.

Hauet, T., Baumert, H., Amor, I.B., Gibelin, H., Tallineau, C., Eugene, M., Tillement, J.P., & Carretier, M. (2000a). Pharmacological limitation of damage to renal medulla after cold storage and transplantation by trimetazidine. The Journal of pharmacology and experimental therapeutics *292*, 254-260.

Hauet, T., Baumert, H., Gibelin, H., Hameury, F., Goujon, J.M., Carretier, M., & Eugene, M. (2000b). Noninvasive monitoring of citrate, acetate, lactate, and renal medullary osmolyte excretion in urine as biomarkers of exposure to ischemic reperfusion injury. Cryobiology *41*, 280-291.

Hauet, T., Gibelin, H., Godart, C., Eugene, M., & Carretier, M. (2000c). Kidney retrieval conditions influence damage to renal medulla: evaluation by proton nuclear magnetic resonance (NMR) pectroscopy. Clin Chem Lab Med *38*, 1085-1092.

Hauet, T., Gibelin, H., Richer, J.P., Godart, C., Eugene, M., & Carretier, M. (2000d). Influence of retrieval conditions on renal medulla injury: evaluation by proton NMR spectroscopy in an isolated perfused pig kidney model. The Journal of surgical research *93*, 1-8.

Hauet, T., Goujon, J.M., Tallineau, C., Carretier, M., & Eugene, M. (1999). Early evaluation of renal reperfusion injury after prolonged cold storage using proton nuclear magnetic resonance spectroscopy. The British journal of surgery *86*, 1401-1409.

Hauet, T., Mothes, D., Goujon, J.M., Caritez, J.C., Carretier, M., & Eugene, M. (1997a). Evaluation of injury preservation in pig kidney cold storage by proton nuclear magnetic resonance spectroscopy of urine. The Journal of urology *157*, 1155-1160.

Hauet, T., Mothes, D., Goujon, J.M., Caritez, J.C., Le Moyec, L., Carretier, M., & Eugene, M. (1997b). Evaluation of normothermic ischemia and simple cold preservation injury in pig kidney by proton nuclear magnetic resonance spectroscopy. The Journal of surgical research *68*, 116-125.

Heilmann, M., Neudecker, S., Wolf, I., Gubhaju, L., Sticht, C., Schock-Kusch, D., Kriz, W., Bertram, J.F., Schad, L.R., & Gretz, N. (2011). Quantification of glomerular number and size distribution in normal rat kidneys using magnetic resonance imaging. Nephrol Dial Transplant.

Hene, R.J., Van der Grond, J., Boer, W.H., Mali, W.P.T., & Koomans, H.A. (1994). Pre-transpiantation assessment of renal viability with 31P magnetic resonance spectroscopy. Kidney international *46*, 1694-1699.

Holmes, E., Nicholson, J.K., Nicholls, A.W., Lindon, J.C., Connor, S.C., Polley, S., & Connelly, J. (1998). The identification of novel biomarkers of renal toxicity using automatic data reduction techniques and PCA of proton NMR spectra of urine. Chemometrics and Intelligent Laboratory Systems *44*, 245-255.

Huhn, S.D., Szabo, C.M., Gass, J.H., & Manzi, A.E. (2004). Metabolic profiling of normal and hypertensive rat kidney tissues by hrMAS-NMR spectroscopy. Analytical and bioanalytical chemistry *378*, 1511-1519.

Klemm, A., Rzanny, R., FÃ¼nfstÃ¼ck, R., Werner, W., Schubert, J., Kaiser, W.A., & Stein, G. (1998). 31P-magnetic resonance spectroscopy (31P-MRS) of human allografts after renal transplantation. Nephrology, dialysis, transplantation : official publication of the European Dialysis and Transplant Association - European Renal Association *13*, 3147-3152.

Kwiatkowski, A., Wszola, M., Kosieradzki, M., Danielewicz, R., Ostrowski, K., Domagala, P., Lisik, W., Nosek, R., Fesolowicz, S., Trzebicki, J., *et al.* (2007). Machine perfusion preservation improves renal allograft survival. Am J Transplant *7*, 1942-1947.

Le Bihan, D., Breton, E., Lallemand, D., Aubin, M.L., Vignaud, J., & Laval-Jeantet, M. (1988). Separation of diffusuion and perfusion in intravoxel incoherent motion MR imaging. Radiology *168*, 497-505.

Lenz, E.M., Bright, J., Knight, R., Wilson, I.D., & Major, H. (2004). Cyclosporin A-induced changes in endogenous metabolites in rat urine: a metabonomic investigation using high field 1H NMR spectroscopy, HPLC-TOF/MS and chemometrics. Journal of pharmaceutical and biomedical analysis *35*, 599-608.

Liu, Q., Vekemans, K., van Pelt, J., Pirenne, J., Himmelreich, U., Heedfeld, V., Wylin, T., Brassil, J., Monbaliu, D., & Dresselaers, T. (2009). Discriminate Liver Warm Ischemic Injury During Hypothermic Machine Perfusion by Proton Magnetic Resonance Spectroscopy : A Study in a Porcine Model. Transplantation proceedings *41*, 3383-3386.

Malvezzi, P., Bricault, I., Terrier, N., & Bayle, F. (2009). Evaluation of Intrarenal Oxygenation by Blood Oxygen Level-Dependent Magnetic Resonance Imaging in Living Kidney Donors and Their Recipients : Preliminary Results. Transplantation proceedings *41*, 641-644.

Mills, P.H., Hitchens, T.K., Foley, L.M., Link, T., Ye, Q., Weiss, C.R., Thompson, J.D., Gilson, W.D., Arepally, A., Melick, J.A., *et al.* (2011). Automated detection and characterization of SPIO-labeled cells and capsules using magnetic field perturbations. Magn Reson Med.

Moers, C., Varnav, O.C., van Heurn, E., Jochmans, I., Kirste, G.R., Rahmel, A., Leuvenink, H.G., Squifflet, J.P., Paul, A., Pirenne, J., *et al.* (2010). The value of machine perfusion perfusate biomarkers for predicting kidney transplant outcome. Transplantation *90*, 966-973.

Montet, X., Ivancevic, M.K., Jorge-Costa, M., Pochon, S., PerchÃ¨re, A., & VallÃ©e, J.P. (2003). Noninvasive measurement of absolute renal perfusion by contrast medium-enhanced magnetic resonance imaging. Investigative radiology *38*, 584-592.

Niekisch, M.B., Von Elverfeldt, D., El Saman, A., Hennig, J., & Kirste, G. (2004). Improved pretransplant assessment of renal quality by means of phosphorus-31 magnetic resonance spectroscopy using chemical shift imaging. Transplantation *77*, 1041-1045.

Oostendorp, M., de Vries, E.E., Slenter, J.M., Peutz-Kootstra, C.J., Snoeijs, M.G., Post, M.J., van Heurn, L.W., & Backes, W.H. (2011). MRI of renal oxygenation and function after normothermic ischemia-reperfusion injury. NMR Biomed *24*, 194-200.

Palmucci, S., Mauro, L.A., Veroux, P., Failla, G., Milone, P., Ettorre, G.C., Sinagra, N., Giuffrida, G., Zerbo, D., & Veroux, M. (2011). Magnetic Resonance With Diffusion-Weighted Imaging in the Evaluation of Transplanted Kidneys : Preliminary Findings. Transplantation proceedings *43*, 960-966.

Pereira, R.S., Gonul, I.I., McLaughlin, K., Yilmaz, S., & Mahallati, H. (2011). Assessment of Chronic Renal Allograft Nephropathy Using Contrast-Enhanced MRI: A Pilot Study. American Journal of Roentgenology *194*, 407-413.

Sadowski, E.A., Djamali, A., Wentland, A.L., Muehrer, R., Becker, B.N., Grist, T.M., & Fain, S.B. (2010). Blood oxygen level-dependent and perfusion magnetic resonance imaging : detecting differences in oxygen bioavailability and blood flow in transplanted kidneys. Magnetic resonance imaging *28*, 56-64.

Serkova, N., Klawitter, J., & Niemann, C.U. (2003). Organ-specific response to inhibition of mitochondrial metabolism by cyclosporine in the rat. Transpl Int *16*, 748-755.

Seto, K., Ikehira, H., Obata, T., Sakamoto, K., Yamada, K., Kashiwabara, H., Yokoyama, T., & Tanada, S. (2001). Long-term assessment of posttransplant renal prognosis with 31 P magnetic resonance spectroscopy. Transplantation *72*, 627-630.

Siew, E.D., Ware, L.B., & Ikizler, T.A. (2011). Biological markers of acute kidney injury. J Am Soc Nephrol *22*, 810-820.

Thoeny, H.C., & De Keyzer, F. (2011). Diffusion-weighted MR Imaging of Native and Transplanted kidneys. *259*, 25-38.

Thoeny, H.C., Zumstein, D., Simon-zoula, S., Eisenberger, U., De Keyser, F., Hofmann, L., Vock, P., Boesch, C., Frey, F.J., & Vermathen, P. (2006). Functional Evaluation of Transplanted Kidneys with Diffusion-weighted and BOLD MR Imaging : Initial Experience. Radiology *241*, 812-821.

von Elverfeldt, D., Niekisch, M., Quaschning, T., El Saman, A., Kirste, G., Kramer-Guth, A., & Hennig, J. (2007). Kinetics of PME/Pi in pig kidneys during cold ischemia. NMR Biomed *20*, 652-657.

Vyhnanovska, P., Dezortova, M., Herynek, V., Taborsky, P., Viklicky, O., & Hajek, M. (2011). In Vivo (31)P MR Spectroscopy of Human Kidney Grafts Using the 2D-Chemical Shift Imaging Method. Transplantation proceedings *43*, 1570-1575.

Wang, Y., Bollard, M.E., Nicholson, J.K., & Holmes, E. (2006). Exploration of the direct metabolic effects of mercury II chloride on the kidney of Sprague-Dawley rats using high-resolution magic angle spinning 1H NMR spectroscopy of intact tissue and pattern recognition. Journal of pharmaceutical and biomedical analysis *40*, 375-381.

Waters, N.J., Waterfield, C.J., Farrant, R.D., Holmes, E., & Nicholson, J.K. (2005). Metabonomic deconvolution of embedded toxicity: application to thioacetamide hepato- and nephrotoxicity. Chemical research in toxicology *18*, 639-654.

Wight, J.P., Chilcott, J.B., Holmes, M.W., & Brewer, N. (2003). Pulsatile machine perfusion vs. cold storage of kidneys for transplantation: a rapid and systematic review. Clinical transplantation *17*, 293-307.

Wolff, S.D., & Balaban, R.S. (1988). NMR studies of renal phosphate metabolites in vivo: effects of hydration and dehydration. American journal of physiology *255*, 581-589.

Yamamoto, A., Zhang, J.L., Rusinek, H., Chandarana, H., Vivier, P.H., Babb, J.S., Diflo, T., John, D.G., Benstein, J.A., Barisoni, L., *et al.* (2011). Quantitative evaluation of acute renal transplant dysfunction with low-dose three dimensional MR renography. Radiology *260*, 781-789.

Zhao, L., Gao, H., Lian, F., Liu, X., Zhao, Y., & Lin, D. (2011). 1H NMR-based metabonomic analysis of metabolic profiling in diabetic nephropathy rats induced by streptozotocin. American journal of physiology *300*, F947-F956.

7

Acute Effects of Branched-Chain Amino Acid Ingestion on Muscle pH during Exercise in Patients with Chronic Obstructive Pulmonary Disease

Tomoko Kutsuzawa[1], Daisaku Kurita[2] and Munetaka Haida[3]
[1]*School of Health Sciences, Tokai University*
[2]*IT Education Center, Tokai University*
[3]*Tokai University Junior College of Nursing and Medical Technology*
Japan

1. Introduction

The use of ^{31}P-magnetic resonance (MR) spectroscopy (^{31}P-MRS) allows noninvasive measurement of high-energy phosphate compounds such as phosphocreatine (PCr) and adenosine triphosphate (ATP), and the low-energy breakdown product, inorganic phosphate (Pi), in exercising muscle. Ratios of measureable high- and low-energy phosphate metabolites (e.g., PCr/Pi or PCr/(PCr+Pi) have been utilized as indices of the overall bioenergetic state of the cell (Sapega et al., 1987). Extracellular Pi does not exist in sufficient quantities to significantly affect ^{31}P-MR spectra (Sapega et al., 1987). Intracellular pH (pHi) can also be measured noninvasively based on the pH-dependent chemical shift of cellular Pi that appears as PCr peaks on ^{31}P-MRS (Sapega et al., 1987; Taylor et al., 1983). A decrease in pHi during exercise suggests lactate accumulation in muscles (Sapega et al., 1987; Taylor et al., 1983).

We have previously found, using ^{31}P-MRS, that skeletal muscle metabolism in patients with chronic respiratory impairment undergoes specific changes (Kutsuzawa et al., 1992, 1995). Patients with chronic respiratory impairment display significant decreases in PCr and pHi during even mild exercise, suggesting that ATP production is reduced and that lactate levels accumulate rapidly in their muscles, suggesting reduced oxidative capacity. In addition, recent studies have demonstrated that reduced oxidative capacity in skeletal muscles correlates with an accelerated lactate response to exercise in patients with chronic obstructive pulmonary disease (COPD) (Maltais et al., 1996; Saey et al., 2005). Several factors such as inactivity, malnutrition and/or hypoxemia might contribute to altered muscle metabolism (Mannix et al., 1995; Payen et al., 1993; Sala et al., 1999).

Weight loss and muscle wasting are common features in patients with COPD (Bernard et al., 1998) and muscle wasting contributes to muscle weakness and exercise limitations in patients with COPD (Schols et al., 1993). Skeletal muscle is the major protein store that supplies amino acids to other tissues under specific conditions. Plasma concentrations of free amino acids indicate the balance between exogenous uptake and intercurrent metabolites in protein synthesis and breakdown (Wagenmakers, 1998). The branched-chain amino acids (BCAAs) leucine, isoleucine, and valine account for 35% of the essential amino acids contained in muscle proteins (Harper et al., 1984). Although essential amino acids other than BCAAs are mainly catabolized in the liver, BCAAs can be oxidized in skeletal muscle (Wagenmakers, 1998).

Several investigators have reported that the amino acid profile is altered in the plasma and skeletal muscle of patients with COPD (Engelen et al., 2000b; Hoffored et al., 1990; Pouw et al., 1998; Yoneda et al., 2001). Most of these studies have shown that plasma concentrations of the BCAAs leucine, isoleucine, and valine are reduced (Engelen et al., 2000b; Hoffored et al., 1990; Yoneda et al., 2001). Yoneda et al. (Yoneda et al., 2001) demonstrated that decreased concentrations of BCAAs in COPD are specifically related to weight loss and decreased muscle mass.

Energy expenditure greatly increases in skeletal muscle during exercise, and BCAA oxidization then maximally increases two- to three-fold (Knapik et al., 1991; Wolf et al., 1982). In addition, BCAAs might contribute to energy metabolism during exercise as substrates that expand the pool of tricarboxylic acid (TCA) cycle intermediates (Wagenmakers, 1998). Using ^{31}P-MRS, we have previously found that plasma concentrations of BCAAs correlate with muscle pH at the completion of exercise in patients with COPD (Kutsuzawa et al., 2009). Those findings were consistent with a role of BCAAs in muscle energy metabolism during exercise in patients with COPD.

Supplementation with amino acids, particularly BCAAs, should increase exercise capacity in COPD patients, who might be affected by altered muscle and plasma amino acid profiles. Several studies in healthy subjects have examined the effects of BCAA ingestion on lactate metabolism during long-term, exhaustive exercise (De Palo et al., 2001; MacLean et al., 1996; Vukovich et al., 1992). MacLean et al. (MacLean et al., 1996) examined the effects of a large oral dose (308 mg/kg) of BCAAs on muscle amino acid metabolism during 90 min of exercise. They found that lactate release and arterial lactate values were lower in the group given BCAAs compared to a control group. We have studied the effects of BCAA ingestion on muscle pH during repeated bouts of short-term (3-min) exercise in healthy subjects and have found that BCAA supplementation before exercise can cause the attenuation of acidosis in exercising muscle, probably due to a decrease in lactate production (Kutsuzawa et al., 2011). Another study (Doi et al., 2004) of muscle energy metabolism demonstrated that an infusion of glucose and BCAAs before exercise improved acidic pHi during exercise in patients with liver cirrhosis accompanied by a severe amino acid imbalance.

The effects of BCAA ingestion on muscle pH have been investigated in healthy young participants (Kutsuzawa et al., 2011), but whether such supplementation will benefit exercise capacity in patients with COPD remains unclear. We thus used ^{31}P-MRS to investigate the effects of BCAA ingestion on muscle pH during repeated bouts of short-term (3-min) exercise. Our hypothesis was that BCAA ingestion before a second bout of exercise could prevent metabolic acidosis in exercising muscle.

2. Methods

2.1 Subjects

Subjects comprised 10 ambulatory male outpatients with stable COPD (mean age, 70.4 ± 8.8 years) diagnosed according to spirometric findings from moderate to very severe airflow limitation (forced expiratory volume in 1 s (FEV_1)/forced vital capacity (FVC)<70% and FEV_1 <80% of the predicted value) (Global Initiative for Chronic Obstructive Lung Disease, 2010). None of the patients had ever received systemic corticosteroid therapy and two of them had been treated with oxygen inhalation at home. None of them had participated in pulmonary rehabilitation. Exclusion criteria were malignancy, cardiac failure, renal failure, liver cirrhosis, diabetes mellitus, and infection. The ethics committee at our institution approved the study protocol, and both the control individuals and patients provided written informed consent to participate. Tables 1 and 2 show the physical characteristics of the participants.

		Patients (n=10)		
Age	years	70.4	±	8.8
Height	cm	163.9	±	3.8
Weight	kg	55.6	±	10.0
BMI	kg/m^2	20.6	±	3.1
Forearm circumference	cm	22.9	±	1.7
TSF	cm	5.6	±	3.0
Grip power (left)	kg	36.7	±	5.5

Table 1. Anthropometric data from the patients. Values are given as mean ± SD. BMI, body mass index; TSF, triceps skinfold thickness.

		Patients (n=10)		
VC	L	2.75	±	0.77
VC (%of predicted)	%	84.1	±	21.8
FEV_1	L	1.02	±	0.40
FEV_1/FVC	%	40.3	±	9.4
FEV_1 (% of predicted)	%	41.5	±	15.4
pH		7.412	±	0.031
$PaCO_2$	Torr	41.3	±	4.8
PaO_2	Torr	79.8	±	7.6

Table 2. Spirometric and blood gas analysis data from the patients. Values are given as mean ± SD. VC, vital capacity; FEV_1, forced expiratory volume in 1 s; FVC, forced vital capacity; $PaCO_2$, partial pressure of CO_2; PaO_2, partial pressure of O_2.

2.2 Study design

All patients fasted overnight, then anthropometric parameters and grip strength were measured at our outpatient clinic. Maximal voluntary grip strength of the non-dominant arm was measured using a dynamometer (DM-100N; Yagami, Nagoya, Japan). Fasting venous blood was obtained from an antecubital vein. Arterial blood was taken from the brachial artery for blood gas analysis while breathing room air.

All patients then performed two consecutive, 3-min constant work-rate exercises (a control bout and a BCAA bout), using the non-dominant forearm. Differences in MRS variables among individuals might be smaller for the non-dominant arm because routine activities might not vary as much as those performed with the dominant arm. Ten minutes after the first bout (control bout) of exercise, the patients consumed 8.0 g of powdered BCAAs (2 packs of LIVACT®; Ajinomoto, Tokyo, Japan) with 100 ml of water. The second bout (BCAA bout) of exercise started at 60 min after BCAA ingestion. Patients remained seated during the interval between first and second bouts of exercise and were allowed water. Muscle metabolism was measured using ^{31}P-MRS during 1.5 min of rest, 3 min of exercise, and 4 min of recovery.

The exercise consisted of repetitively gripping a lever attached to a weight via a pulley system at a rate of 20 grips/min for 3 min while supine and breathing room air. The weight was lifted 5 cm by gripping the lever. To normalize the exercise intensity, the weight was adjusted to 7% of the maximum grip strength, which was suitable for this study because all patients could complete the exercise. Moreover, repetitive hand-gripping exercise in which the same weight (7% of maximal hang grip) is lifted 5 cm 20 times per min can differentiate healthy from altered muscle metabolism (as a decrease in pHi) (Kutsuzawa et al., 1992, 1995).

2.3 BCAA supplementation

LIVACT® is a BCAA powder that was developed to treat imbalances in amino acids among patients with liver cirrhosis. One pack of LIVACT (4.75 g) contains 4.0 g of BCAA (3808 mg of leucine, 1904 mg isoleucine and 2288 mg of valine). The composition ratio of leucine, isoleucine and valine at 2:1:1.2 effectively balances nitrogen as well as the plasma amino acid profile (Ohashi et al., 1989). The plasma BCAA level at 2 h after ingesting 8 g of BCAA increases 2-fold (Hamada et al., 2005).

2.4 Nutritional assessment

Nutritional status was evaluated by biochemical blood testing and anthropometric measurements including height, weight, non-dominant forearm circumference and triceps skin fold thickness (TSF). Body mass index (BMI) was calculated based on height and weight. The circumference of the non-dominant forearm was measured at the proximal third of the forearm, where the MRS surface coil was positioned. TSF of the non-dominant arm was measured using an EIYOKEN-TYPE skinfold caliper (Yagami).

Fasting blood samples from all patients were obtained by venipuncture before the control bout. In six of the 10 patients, second blood samples were obtained before the BCAA bout. Portions of samples were immediately cooled on ice and plasma obtained by centrifugation at 4°C was stored at -80°C for later amino acid analysis. Samples were deproteinized using 5% sulfosalicylic acid, then plasma levels of amino acids were measured by ion-exchange, high-pressure liquid chromatography with fluorometric detection (Model 8500; Hitachi, Tokyo, Japan) (Dyel et al., 1986). Total BCAAs comprised leucine + isoleucine + valine, and total amino acids included all measured amino acids. Serum albumin and prealbumin, as indices of nutritional status, were determined by routine methods in other portions of the samples.

2.5 ^{31}P-MRS

Unlocalized MR spectra were obtained using a 2.0-T, 31-cm-bore BEM 250/80 superconducting magnet (Otsuka Electronics Co., Osaka, Japan). The spectrometer was operated at 85 MHz for ^{1}H and at 34.5 MHz for ^{31}P. A 4-cm surface coil was placed on the proximal third of the non-dominant forearm. We accumulated ^{31}P-MR spectra every 3 s for 1 min using a single 90° pulse (50 µs) (Kutsuzawa et al., 1992). We then analyzed the ^{31}P-MR spectrum at rest (1 min before onset of exercise) and at the end of 3 min of exercise.

The signal area for Pi and PCr was determined from each spectrum by Gaussian curve fitting (Kutsuzawa et al., 1992). Relative concentrations of PCr and Pi were evaluated using normalized units of PCr/(PCr+Pi).

Muscle pH (i.e., pHi) was calculated as a difference in the chemical shift between Pi and the PCr peak (Stevens, 1987; Taylor et al., 1983). At physiological pH, Pi exists as HPO_4^{2-} and $H_2PO_4^-$ ions. The signal from HPO_4^{2-} is shifted downfield by 2.25 ppm from that of $H_2PO_4^-$. However, the two forms are in rapid exchange, so a single Pi peak is formed with a chemical shift reflecting the relative proportions of the two ions. The chemical shift in Pi can thus be used as a pH indicator, as follows:

$$pH = 6.75 + \log (\delta - 3.27)/(5.69 - \delta),$$

where δ is the difference of chemical shift in parts per million between the Pi and PCr signals (Taylor et al., 1983). The pH was determined from the weighted average of both Pi peaks if the peak was split.

We determined ΔpHi or ΔPCr/(PCr+Pi) as the difference between values just before and at the end of the exercise period.

2.6 Statistical analysis

All data are presented as means ± standard deviation (SD). MRS variables between the control and BCAA bouts of exercise and between resting and the end of exercise were compared using Student's paired *t*-test. The ΔpHi and ΔPCr/(PCr+Pi) between control and BCAA bouts were compared to determine the effects of BCAA supplementation using the paired Student's *t*-test. We used linear regression analysis to evaluate correlations between concentration of BCAA and BMI, between BCAA and spirometric data, and between BCAA and the MRS variable (ΔpHi of the first exercise bout) using the least-squares method. Goodness of fit was examined using the χ^2-test. A value of $p < 0.05$ was considered indicative of a significant difference.

3. Results

3.1 Physical characteristics and nutritional assessment

Table 1 shows the physical characteristics of the 10 patients. Mean body mass index of patients was 20.6 ± 3.1 kg/m^2 and 3 of the patients were considered malnourished (BMI <

20). Table 2 shows spirometric data from the patients with COPD. Mean FEV_1 was 1.02 ± 0.40 L. Based on the Global Initiative for Chronic Obstructive Lung Disease (GOLD) criteria (Global Initiative for Chronic Obstructive Lung Disease, 2010), 3 of the 10 patients were categorized as stage II, 4 as stage III and 3 as stage IV, but none showed severe hypoxemia (partial pressure of O_2 (PaO_2), 79.8 ± 7.6 Torr).

3.2 Nutritional assessment

Values of serum albumin did not decrease in the patients. Although the mean level of prealbumin was within normal range (22-40 mg/dl), two of the patients showed a prealbumin level below the lower limit of the normal range (Table 3).

		Patients (n=10)		
Albumin	g/dl	4.5	±	0.4
Prealbumin	mg/dl	25.9	±	6.5

Table 3. Albumin and prealbumin levels in fasting venous blood from patients. Values are given as mean ± SD.

Amino acid (nmol/L)	Range	Patients (n=10)		
Taurine	40 - 93	56.4	±	14.8
Threonine	67 - 190	101.5	±	21.0
Serine	72 - 190	92.1	±	20.8
Asparagine	45 - 97	43.1	±	8.5
Glutamic acid	12 - 63	38.1	±	12.0
Glutamine	420 - 700	699.5	±	146.1
Proline	78 - 270	132.2	±	35.1
Glycine	150 - 350	167.9	±	40.6
Alanine	210 - 520	339.5	±	55.0
Citrulline	17 - 43	36.5	±	14.7
Aminobutyric acid	7.9 - 27	13.2	±	4.1
Valine	150 - 310	199.9	±	34.6
Cystine	29 - 49	49.4	±	8.2
Methionine	19 - 40	23.7	±	5.2
Isoleucine	40 - 110	59.4	±	12.8
Leucine	48 - 180	103.2	±	21.6
Tyrosine	40 - 90	65.2	±	13.8
Phenylalanine	43 - 76	56.8	±	11.2
Histidine	59 - 92	70.7	±	12.7
Tryptophan	37 - 75	58.6	±	9.3
Ornithine	30 - 100	53.1	±	16.3
Lysine	110 - 240	191.5	±	47.8
Arginine	54 - 130	100.1	±	28.7
Total amino acids	2100 - 3500	2770.7	±	391.8
Total BCAAs	270 - 600	362.4	±	66.4

Table 4. Plasma amino acid concentrations before the first exercise bout. Values are given as mean ± SD. BCAA, branched-chain amino acid.

Table 4 shows values for individual plasma amino acids. Total amino acids and total BCAAs were not reduced from the normal range. The mean glutamine concentration was approximately at the upper limit of the normal range. Concentrations of total BCAAs tended to correlate with BMI ($r = 0.6099$, $p < 0.1$) in patients. Concentrations of total BCAAs did not correlate with FEV_1(%of the predicted value), which is an index of COPD severity.

Plasma amino acid profiles at 1 h after BCAA ingestion were examined in 6 of 10 patients (Table 5). Valine, leucine, and isoleucine significantly increased by more than 3- to 5-times after BCAA ingestion. Glutamine and arginine were also slightly but significantly increased.

Amino acid (nmol/L)	Fasting			After BCAA ingestion (n=6)		
Taurine	51.7	±	6.0	52.6	±	3.8
Threonine	112.4	±	15.6	110.8	±	19.4
Serine	101.7	±	18.1	104.7	±	20.5
Asparagine	45.5	±	8.6	43.5	±	7.3
Glutamic acid	32.6	±	11.5	31.3	±	14.2
Glutamine	749.2	±	165.0	889.4	±	167.4**
Proline	133.8	±	20.1	116.9	±	23.2*
Glycine	210.8	±	47.7	190.7	±	48.6*
Alanine	351.1	±	67.1	315.5	±	42.7
Citrulline	40.8	±	16.6	39.6	±	18.0
Aminobutyric acid	14.6	±	3.7	15.3	±	3.4
Valine	203.3	±	22.9	679.8	±	160.1**
Cystine	51.0	±	6.4	51.0	±	5.6
Methionine	25.1	±	4.6	22.9	±	4.2
Isoleucine	59.2	±	12.2	322.6	±	83.6**
Leucine	103.6	±	19.0	606.5	±	163.1**
Tyrosine	66.0	±	14.9	61.5	±	12.0
Phenylalanine	56.6	±	9.8	53.0	±	6.7
Histidine	74.2	±	10.8	77.7	±	10.4
Tryptophan	60.0	±	9.1	53.4	±	8.8**
Ornithine	59.0	±	17.1	59.3	±	17.7
Lysine	216.8	±	29.2	232.4	±	38.6
Arginine	111.1	±	29.7	128.1	±	36.3*
Total amino acids	2918.4	±	332.0	4246.0	±	320.3**
Total BCAAs	366.0	±	51.5	1609.0	±	386.9**

Table 5. Plasma amino acid concentration before and after ingestion of BCAAs. Valine, leucine, and isoleucine were increased more than 300% by 1 h after BCAA ingestion. Values are given as mean ± SD. *: $p < 0.05$ vs. before ingestion; **: $p < 0.01$ vs. before ingestion.

3.3 Muscle energy metabolism

Representative ^{31}P-MR spectra obtained from a 75-year-old patient with COPD at the end of exercise are shown in Figure 1. The peak for Pi was higher than that for PCr, and shifted toward that of PCr during the control bout of exercise (Fig. 1A). In contrast, the peak of Pi was lower than that of PCr, and the Pi peak went back toward the normal chemical shift (-4.9 ppm). The values of pHi were calculated as 6.39 (Fig. 1A) and 6.84 (Fig. 1B) during the control and BCAA bouts of exercise, respectively. Values of PCr/(PCr+Pi) during the control (Fig. 1A) and BCAA bout (Fig. 1B) of exercise were 0.467 (Fig. 1A) and 0.630 (Fig. 1B), respectively.

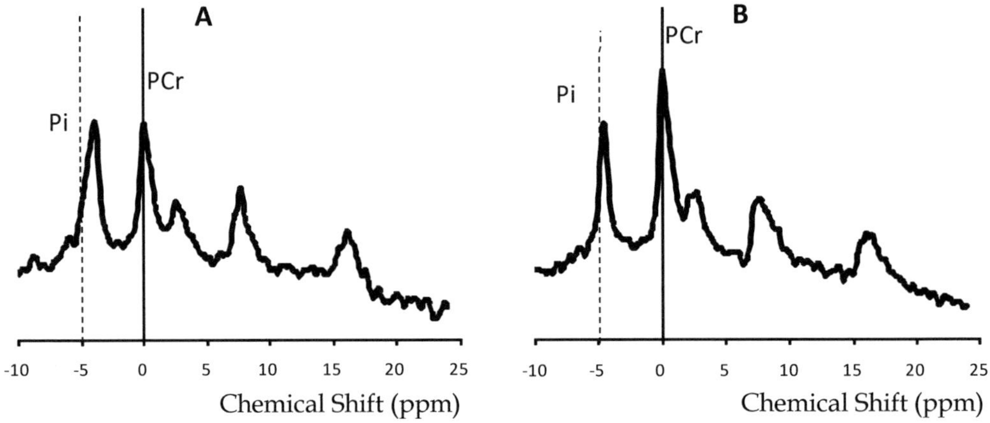

Fig. 1. ^{31}P-MR spectra after 3 min of exercise, obtained from a 75-year-old patient with COPD. A and B, First (control) and second (after BCAA ingestion) bouts of exercise, respectively; Pi, inorganic phosphate; PCr, phosphocreatine.

Calculated values of pHi and PCr/(PCr+Pi) in the control bout of exercise were 6.39 and 0.467, respectively, and those in the BCAA bout were 6.84 and 0.630, respectively.

Mean values of pHi and PCr/(PCr+Pi) at rest and at the end of each exercise are shown in Tables 6 and 7, respectively. Both pHi and PCr/(PCr+Pi) were significantly decreased at the end of each exercise bout. Mean values for pHi and PCr/(PCr+Pi) were significantly higher at the end of the BCAA bout than at the end of the control bout. Thus, ΔpHi and ΔPCr/(PCr+Pi) were significantly smaller in the BCAA bout. In addition, acidic changes in pHi were attenuated in 6 of the 10 patients in the BCAA bout (Fig. 2).

	Control bout			BCAA bout		
At rest	7.00	±	0.08	7.03	±	0.09
End of exercise	6.70	±	0.19 #	6.86	±	0.14 * †
ΔpH	-0.31	±	0.19	-0.17	±	0.17 *

Table 6. Changes in muscle pH. *, $p < 0.05$ vs. control bout; †, $p < 0.05$ vs. resting; #, $p < 0.01$ vs. resting. ΔpH, difference in pHi between resting and end of exercise.

	Control bout			BCAA bout		
At rest	0.870	±	0.023	0.876	±	0.032
End of exercise	0.423	±	0.056	0.502	±	0.103 * #
ΔPCr/(PCr+Pi)	-0.447	±	0.059 #	-0.373	±	0.094 *

Table 7. Changes in PCr/(PCr+Pi). *, $p < 0.05$ vs. control bout; #, $p < 0.01$ vs. resting. ΔPCr/(PCr+Pi), difference in PCr/(PCr+Pi) between resting and end of exercise.

The pHi of all participants in the control bout of exercise correlated with leucine concentration (r=0.6713) and tended to correlate with BCAA concentration (r=0.6015).

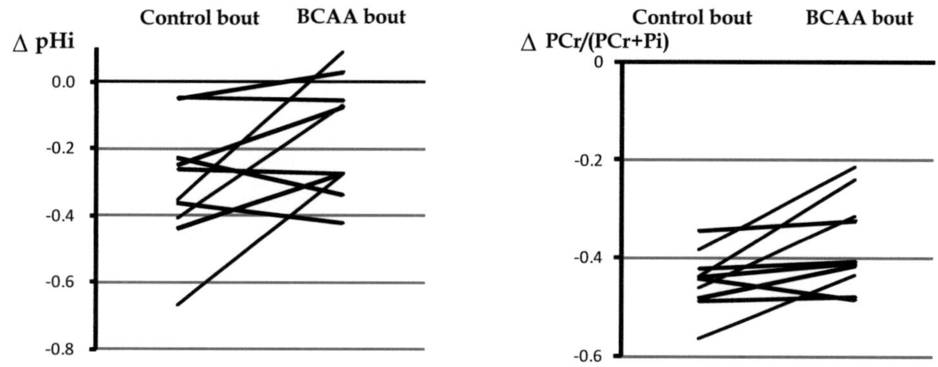

Fig. 2. Differences in pHi (ΔpHi) and PCr/(PCr+Pi) (ΔPCr/(PCr+Pi)) of each patient in control and BCAA bout. Six of 10 patients showed that ΔpHi and ΔPCr/(PCr+Pi) were reduced in the BCAA bout.

4. Discussion

We investigated the acute effects of a single BCAA ingestion on muscle energy metabolism during hand-grip exercise in patients with COPD and found a decrease in ΔpHi and ΔPCr/(PCr+Pi) for the BCAA bout. The finding suggests that BCAA supplementation before exercise can cause an attenuation of acidosis in exercising muscle among COPD patients, probably due to an increase in oxidative capacity and a decrease in lactate production.

4.1 Muscle pH

Values of pHi can be measured using ^{31}P-MRS as the pH-dependence of a chemical shift between cellular Pi and PCr peaks (Sapega et al., 1987; Taylor et al., 1983). In addition, pHi can be determined as the H^+ balance of consumption (PCr hydrolysis, buffering capacity and H^+ efflux) and lactate production processes (Kemp, 2004). A decrease in pHi during exercise suggests that lactic acid accumulates in exercising muscle cells due to anaerobic glycolysis (Kemp, 2004; Sapega et al., 1987; Taylor et al., 1983). The line width frequently increased and the Pi peak often split during exercise in patients, suggesting that the pH among muscle fibers is heterogeneous, and supporting the suggestion that this phenomenon reflects metabolic heterogeneity among muscle fiber types (Vandenborne et al., 1993).

The H^+ and lactate produced can either be buffered and removed intracellularly or released to the interstitium. Several transport systems as well as muscle buffering remove H^+ during intense skeletal muscle contraction. Buffers include free Pi, PCr and histidine residues in both proteins and some dipeptides, and the capacity of such buffers is decreased by high-intensity exercise via a decrease in protein buffering (Bishop et al., 2009). Supplementation with β-alanine, which increases muscle protein buffer capacity, attenuates the fall in blood pH during exercise (Baguet et al., 2010). Whether BCAA supplementation affects muscle buffer capacity remains unclear.

4.2 Plasma BCAA profile in COPD

Several studies have investigated plasma amino acid profiles in COPD patients (Engelen et al., 2000b; Hoffored et al., 1990; Pouw et al., 1998; Yoneda et al., 2001). No specific plasma amino acid profile has been identified, probably due to the heterogeneity of disease stages in COPD (for example, severity of airflow limitation, hypoxemia, and malnutrition). One study of Japanese patients with COPD (Yoneda et al., 2001) found that concentrations of glutamic acid and glutamine were elevated, whereas those of BCAAs were decreased except for leucine. We have previously investigated plasma amino acid levels in fasting venous blood among COPD patients and age-matched healthy subjects, revealing that plasma glutamine was elevated without overall changes in BCAAs (Kutsuzawa et al., 2009). The present study also showed that levels of plasma BCAA were within normal limits. One previous study (Yoneda et al., 2001) demonstrated that decreased concentrations of BCAAs in COPD are specifically related to weight loss and decreased muscle mass. Our previous (Kutsuzawa et al., 2009) and present studies have shown that the concentration of BCAAs correlated or tended to correlate with BMI ($r=0.54488$, $r=0.6099$), respectively, so nutritional status relates to a low BCAA concentration. However, severity of COPD did not correlate with the concentration of BCAAs, since no correlation was seen with FEV_1/FEV_1pred.

We measured BCAA levels immediately before the BCAA bout in 6 of 10 patients. Each BCAA concentration after BCAA ingestion increased significantly, by more than 3- to 5-fold compared to fasting values and to a consistent 2- to 3-fold more than the upper limit of the normal range. Another study demonstrated that plasma levels of BCAAs at 2 h after BCAA supplementation increase 2-fold after ingesting > 8 g of BCAAs (Hamada et al., 2005). Plasma levels of BCAA by the BCAA bout have thus been sufficiently increased. Increased plasma levels of BCAAs after administration subsequently enhance BCAA uptake by muscle during exercise (MacLean et al., 1996).

4.3 Plasma BCAAs and muscle energy metabolism

We have previously reported that plasma BCAA (leucine, isoleucine, valine) concentrations correlate with both intracellular pH and the PCr index during exercise (Kutsuzawa et al., 2009). The present study also showed the relationship between muscle pH and leucine ($r=0.6713$, $p<0.05$). Total BCAAs tended to correlate with muscle pH ($r=0.6015$, $p<0.1$). A previous study (Doi et al., 2004) investigated muscle energy metabolism in patients with liver cirrhosis accompanied by low plasma BCAA concentrations using ^{31}P-MRS and found an acidic pHi during exercise.

Low plasma BCAA concentrations might affect lactate metabolism through two mechanisms. Firstly, BCAAs expand the pool of TCA cycle intermediates (Rutten et al., 2005; Wagenmakers, 1998) and react with α-ketoglutarate to produce branched-chain α-keto acids and glutamic acid in the presence of BCAA aminotransferase (Vandenborne et al., 1993; Wagenmakers, 1998):

$$\text{BCAA} + \alpha\text{-ketoglutarate} \leftrightarrow \text{branched-chain } \alpha\text{-keto acids} + \text{glutamic acid}$$

BCAAs would therefore affect intracellular glutamic acid concentrations. During the first minutes of exercise, glutamic acid generates TCA cycle intermediates via the alanine aminotransferase reaction in skeletal muscle (Rutten et al., 2005):

pyruvate + glutamic acid → alanine + α-ketoglutarate

The accumulated pyruvate can generate alanine through this reaction instead of lactate during exercise. Engelen et al. discovered that glutamic acid concentrations in the quadriceps femoris muscles of COPD patients are reduced and might relate to a reduced lactic threshold (Engelen et al., 2000a).

Secondly, BCAAs can be oxidized during moderate to heavy exercise. Several studies have reported that endurance exercise activates the branched-chain α-keto acid dehydrogenase (BCKDH) complex, which catalyzes branched-chain α-keto acid to form coenzyme A compounds in human and rat skeletal muscle (Shimomura et al., 1995; Wagenmakers et al., 1989). Shimomura et al. (Shimomura et al., 1993) reported that activity of the BCKDH complex increases in rat hindlimb muscles after 5 min of electrically induced contraction. Rates of leucine oxidation were almost double from rest to moderate intensity in healthy individuals performing steady-state exercise (Lamont et al., 2001). The oxidation of BCAAs does not relate to glycolysis or produce lactate. This mechanism might also explain the correlation between pHi and total BCAA after exercise.

4.4 Effects of amino acid supplementation on patients with COPD

The effects of BCAA ingestion before and/or after exercise on muscle damage and on muscle metabolism have been investigated in athletes since the 1990s. Several studies have demonstrated that BCAA supplementation attenuates the increase in blood lactate dehydrogenase (Coombes et al., 2000; Koba et al., 2007) and creatine kinase (Coombes et al., 2000) after prolonged exercise. Another study has shown that supplementation with amino acids including BCAAs attenuates delayed-onset muscle soreness (Nosaka et al., 2006). These findings suggested that BCAAs attenuate the degree of exercise-induced muscle damage.

Intense muscle activity generates intracellular protons and lactate accumulation. Several investigators have studied the effects of BCAA supplementation on lactate accumulation during exercise (Blomstrand et al., 1996; De Palo et al., 2001; MacLean et al., 1996; Matsumoto et a., 2009; Vukovich et al., 1992) in healthy subjects and athletes. MacLean et al. (MacLean et al., 1996) examined the effects of a large oral dose (308 mg/kg) of BCAAs on muscle amino acid metabolism during 90 min of dynamic knee extensor exercise. They reported that long-term exercise after BCAA administration resulted in significantly greater muscle NH_3, alanine and glutamine levels, as well as lower lactate production. Matsumoto et al. (Matsumoto et al., 2009) studied the effects of BCAA supplementation on the lactate threshold during incremental exercise. They demonstrated that BCAA ingestion immediately before an incremental exercise test after 6 days of BCAA supplementation increased oxygen uptake and workload at the lactate threshold, the onset of blood lactate accumulation. Blomstrand et al. reported a smaller decrease in muscle glutamic acid levels in healthy volunteers who consumed BCAAs and then performed a prolonged submaximal exercise test when compared to a control group (Blomstrand et al., 1996).

Supplementation with amino acids, particularly BCAAs and/or glutamic acid, should increase exercise capacity in COPD patients, as this capacity may be affected by altered muscle and plasma amino acid profiles. A small number of studies have examined supplementation with BCAAs or glutamic acid during exercise in COPD patients. Menier et al. studied the effects of BCAA administration to COPD patients during rehabilitation and showed no effects of BCAA supplementation on maximal oxygen uptake or maximal work (Menier et al., 2001). Rutten et al. studied the metabolic and functional effects of glutamic acid intake in COPD patients. Oral glutamic acid ingestion (30 mg/kg body weight every 20 min for 80 min) did not increase muscle glutamic acid concentration or reduce plasma lactate levels in COPD patients or healthy controls (Rutten et al., 2008).

The effects of a single administration of BCAAs on muscle energy metabolism in COPD patients have not been investigated. The present study showed that BCAA ingestion attenuated ΔpHi and ΔPCr/(PCr+Pi) at the end of exercise compared with the control bout. The findings suggested that BCAA supplementation before exercise could increase oxidative phosphorylation and decrease lactate production, then attenuate acidosis in exercising muscle in COPD patients. We have previously investigated the effects of BCAA ingestion on muscle pH during similar repeated bouts of short-term (3-min) exercise in healthy young participants (Kutsuzawa et al., 2011). The pHi at the second exercise bout without BCAA ingestion was significantly decreased compared with the first bout. In contrast, neither pHi after 3 min of exercise nor ΔpHi differed significantly between the first and second exercise bouts after BCAA ingestion in healthy participants. Effects of BCAA ingestion on muscle pH may be intense in COPD patients, probably due to low BCAA concentrations. Muscle energy metabolism might be affected by BCAAs during exercise acting as an energy source and as substrates that expand the pool of TCA cycle intermediates.

Patients with COPD frequently develop hypoxemia at rest and/or during exercise, which can influence muscle energy metabolism. PaO_2 during exercise was not evaluated in the present study, although PaO_2 at rest ranged from 67 to 90 mmHg. Our previous study evaluated PaO_2 during the same hand-grip exercise in COPD patients, finding no significant decrease during exercise (Kutsuzawa et al., 1992). This suggests that reduced oxygen availability might not contribute to lactate accumulation in a control bout in COPD patients.

4.5 Limitations of study

The present study did not investigate muscle energy metabolism during two consecutive short-term bouts of exercise with a 1-h interval without BCAA supplementation. We previously studied the effects of a single administration of BCAAs on muscle pH during repeated short-term exercise (with or without BCAAs) in healthy young males (Kutsuzawa et al., 2011). In that study, healthy individuals performed repeated hand-grip exercises that consisted of the same weight, same distance, and double the frequency of the present study to induce low muscle pH. All participants who did not take BCAAs showed a pHi at completion of the second bout that was significantly decreased compared to that of the first bout. These findings suggested that the protocol resulted in decreased pHi at the end of the second bout of exercise as compared with the first bout. Therefore, pHi and PCr/(PCr+Pi) at the end of the second bout of hand-grip exercise in the present study might have been decreased.

This study did not measure concentrations of amino acids in muscle. Glutamic acid and BCAAs are taken up by skeletal muscle after consuming meals containing protein and the carbon skeletons are used for *de novo* glutamine synthesis (Wagenmakers, 1998). A few studies (Pouw et al., 1998; Engelen et al., 2000b) have measured concentrations of muscle amino acids in patients with COPD. Pouw et al. (Pouw et al., 1998) reported that levels of BCAAs in plasma and muscle do not differ between patients with COPD and healthy individuals. However, Engelen et al. (Engelen et al., 2000b) showed that plasma and muscle levels of leucine and isoleucine are significantly decreased in COPD subtypes with emphysema, indicating that leucine metabolism is altered in COPD patients. Both studies demonstrated a decrease in glutamic acid in muscles in such patients. Muscle concentrations of glutamic acid and BCAAs might thus be decreased in patients with COPD and low plasma BCAA concentrations.

Furthermore, we did not measure plasma concentrations of lactate, because the magnet in our MR equipment was too narrow to collect venous blood from the exercising forearm during exercise. We also did not determine whether attenuation of metabolic acidosis in muscle resulted in a decrease in plasma lactate levels. However, the present exercise model involved a small muscle mass, which produced only limited changes in arterial H^+ and lactate concentrations.

5. Conclusions

BCAA ingestion before a second bout of hand-grip exercise in patients with COPD resulted in a significant decrease in ΔpHi and ΔPCr/(PCr+Pi) at the end of the second bout of exercise. These findings suggest that BCAAs can help to prevent metabolic acidosis in exercising muscle among COPD patients, probably by increasing oxidative capacity and by decreasing lactate production. BCAA ingestion should thus improve exercise capacity in COPD patients.

6. Acknowledgments

This study was supported in part by a grant from the Department of Home Care Service, Tokai University School of Medicine.

7. References

Baguet, A., Koppo, K., Pottier, A., & Derave, W. (2010). β-Alanine supplementation reduces acidosis but not oxygen uptake response during high-intensity cycling exercise. *European Journal of Applied Physiology,* Vol. 108, No. 3, (February 2010), pp. 495-503, ISSN 14396319

Bernard, S., LeBlanc, P., Whittom, F., Carrier, G., Jobin, J., Belleau, R., & Maltais, F. (1998). Peripheral muscle weakness in patients with chronic obstructive pulmonary disease. *American Journal of Respiratory and Critical Care Medicine,* Vol. 158, No. 2, (August 1998), pp. 629-634, ISSN 1073449X

Bishop, D., Edge, J., Mendez-Villanueva, A., Thomas, C., & Schneiker, K. (2009) High-intensity exercise decreases muscle buffer capacity via a decrease in protein buffering in human skeletal muscle. *European Journal of Physiology,* Vol. 458, No. 5, (September 2009), pp. 929-936, ISSN 00316768

Blomstrand, E., Ek, S., & Newsholme, E. A. (1996). Influence of ingesting a solution of branched-chain amino acids on plasma and muscle concentrations of amino acids during prolonged submaximal exercise. *Nutrition,* Vol. 12, No. 7-8, (July 1996), pp. 485-490, ISSN 08999007

Coombes, J. S., & McNaughton, L. R. (2000). Effects of branched-chain amino acid supplementation on serum creatine kinase and lactate dehydrogenase after prolonged exercise. *Journal of Sports Medicine and Physical Fitness,* Vol. 40, No. 3, (September 2000), pp. 240-246, ISSN 00224707

De Palo, E. F., Gatti, R., Cappellin, E., Schiraldi, C., De Palo, C. B., & Spinella, P. (2001). Plasma lactate, GH and GH-binding protein levels in exercise following BCAA supplementation in athletes. *Amino Acids* Vol. 20, No. 1, (February 2001), pp. 1-11, ISSN 09394451

Deyl, Z., Hyanek, J., & Horakova, M. (1986). Profiling of amino acids in body fluids and tissues by means of liquid chromatography. *Journal of Chromatography* Vol. 379, (June 1986), pp. 177-250, ISSN 03784347

Doi, J., Shiraishi, K., Haida, M., & Matsuzaki, S. (2004). Abnormality of energy metabolism in the skeletal muscle of patients with liver cirrhosis and changes under administration of glucose and branched-chain amino acids. *Tokai Journal of Experimental and Clinical Medicine.* Vol. 29, No. 4, (December 2004), pp. 191-198, ISSN 03850005

Engelen, M. P. K. J., Schols, A. M. W. J., Does, J. D., Gosker, H. R., Deutz, N. E. P., Wouters, E. F. M. (2000a). Exercise-induced lactate increase in relation to muscle substrates in patients with chronic obstructive pulmonary disease. *American Journal of Respiratory and Critical Care Medicine,* Vol. 162, No. 5, (November 2000), pp. 1697-1704, ISSN 1073449X

Engelen, M. P. K. J., Wouters, E. F. M., Deutz, N. E. P., Menheere, P. P. C. A., & Schols, A. M. W. J. (2000b). Factors contribution to alterations in skeletal muscle and plasma amino acid profiles in patients with chronic obstructive pulmonary disease. *American Journal of Clinical Nutrition,* Vol. 72, No. 6, (December 2000), pp. 1480-1487, ISSN 00029165

Global Initiative for Chronic Obstructive Lung Disease. (2010). Definition, In: *Global strategy for the diagnosis, management, and prevention of chronic obstructive pulmonary disease,* August 10 2011, available from http://www.goldcopd.org/uploads/users/files/GOLDReport_April112011.pdf

Hamada, K., Koba, T., Sakurai, M., Matsumoto, K., Higuchi, T., Imaizumi, K., Hayase, H., & Ueno, H. (2005). Effective dose of branched-chain amino acids on blood response in healthy men. *Journal of Japanese Society of Clinical Nutrition,* Vol. 27, No. 1, (January 2005), pp. 1-10 (In Japanese), ISSN 02868202

Harper, A. E., Miller, R. H., & Block, K. P. (1984). Branched-chain amino acid metabolism. *Annual Review of Nutrition,* Vol. 4, (July 1984), pp. 409-454, ISSN 01999885

Hofford, J. M., Milakofsky, L., Vogel, W. H., Sacher, R. S., Savage, G. J., & Pell, S. (1990). The nutritional status in advanced emphysema associated with chronic bronchitis. A study of amino acid and catecholamine levels. *American Review of Respiratory Disease,* Vol. 141, No. 4 pt. 1, (April 1990), pp. 902-908, ISSN 00030805

Kemp, G. J. (2004). Mitochondrial dysfunction in chronic ischemia and peripheral vascular disease. *Mitochondrion* Vol. 4, No. 5-6, (September 2004), pp. 629-640, ISSN 15677249

Knapik, J., Meredith, C., Jones, B., Fieldry, R., Young, V., & Evans, W. (1991). Leucine metabolism during fasting and exercise. *Journal of Applied Physiology,* Vol. 70, No. 1, (January 1991), pp. 43-47, ISSN 87507587

Koba, T., Hamada, K., Sakurai, M., Matsumoto, K., Hayase, H., Imaizumi, K., Tsujimoto, H., & Mitsuzono, R. (2007). Branched-chain amino acids supplementation attenuates the accumulation of blood lactate dehydrogenase during distance running. *Journal of Sports Medicine and Physical Fitness,* Vol. 47, No. 3, (September 2007), pp. 316-322, ISSN 00224707

Kutsuzawa, T., Shioya, S., Kurita, D., Haida, M., Ohta, Y., & Yamabayashi, H. (1992). ^{31}P-NMR study of skeletal muscle metabolism in patients with chronic respiratory impairment. *American Review of Respiratory Disease,* Vol. 146, No. 4, (October 1992), pp. 1019-1024, ISSN 00030805

Kutsuzawa, T., Shioya, S., Kurita, D., Haida, M., Ohta, Y., & Yamabayashi, H. (1995). Muscle energy metabolism and nutritional status in patients with chronic obstructive pulmonary disease. A ^{31}P magnetic resonance study. *American Journal of Respiratory and Critical Care Medicine,* Vol. 152, No. 2, (August 1995), pp. 647-652, ISSN 1073449X

Kutsuzawa, T., Shioya, S., Kurita, D., & Haida, H. (2009). Plasma branched-chain amino acid levels and muscle energy metabolism in patients with chronic obstructive pulmonary disease. *Clinical Nutrition,* Vol. 28, No. 2, (April 2009), pp. 203-208, ISSN 02615614

Kutsuzawa, T., Kurita, D., & Haida, M. (2011). Acute effects of branched-chain amino acids on muscle pH during exercise. *Advances in Exercise and Sports Physiology,* Vol. 16, No. 4, (March 2011), pp. 101-107, ISSN 13403141

Lamont, L. S., McCullough, A. J., & Kalhan, S. (2001). Relationship between leucine oxidation and oxygen consumption during steady-state exercise. *Medicine and Science in Sports and Exercise,* Vol. 33, No. 2, (February 2001), pp. 237-241, ISSN 01959131

MacLean, D. A., Graham, T. E., & Saltin, B. (1996) Stimulation of muscle ammonia production during exercise following branched-chain amino acid supplementation in humans. *Journal of Physiology,* Vol. 493, No. 3, (June 1996), pp. 909-922, ISSN 00223751

Maltais, F., Simard, A., Simard, C., Jobin, J., Desgagnes, P., & LeBlanc, P. (1996). Oxidative capacity of the skeletal muscle and lactic acid kinetics during exercise in normal subjects and in patients with COPD. *American Journal of Respiratory and Critical Care Medicine,* Vol. 153, No. 1, (January 1996), pp. 288-293, ISSN 1073449X

Mannix, E. T., Boska, M. D., Galassetti, P., Burton, G., Manfredi, F., & Farber, M. O. (1995). Modulation of ATP production by oxygen in obstructive lung disease as assessed by ^{31}P-MRS. *Journal of Applied Physiology,* Vol. 78, No. 6, (June 1995), pp. 2218-2227, ISSN 87507587

Matsumoto, K., Koba, T., Hamada, K., Tsujimoto, H., & Mitsuzono, R. (2009). Branched-chain amino acid supplementation increases the lactate threshold during an incremental exercise test in trained individuals. *Journal of Nutritional Science and Vitaminology.* Vol. 55, No. 1, (April 2009), pp. 52-58, ISSN 03014800

Menier, R., Talmud, J., Laplaud, D., Bernard, M-P. (2001). Branched-chain aminoacids and retraining of patients with chronic obstructive lung disease. *Journal of Sports Medicine and Physical Fitness,* Vol. 41, No. 4, (December 2001), pp. 500-504, ISSN 00224707

Nosaka, K., Sacco, P., & Mawatari, K. (2006). Effects of amino acid supplementation on muscle soreness and damage. *International Journal of Sport Nutrition and Exercise Metabolism,* Vol. 16, No. 6, (December 2006), pp. 620-635, ISSN 1526484X

Ohashi, H., Sukegawa, E., Takami, T., Yoshida, T., & Muto, Y. (1989). Effects of supplementation with branched-chain amino acids on protein-nutritional status in rats treated by carbon tetrachloride. *Japanese Journal of Gastroenterology,* Vol. 86, No. 8, (August 1989), pp. 1645-1653 (In Japanese with English Abstract), ISSN 04466586

Payen, J. F., Wuyam, B., Reutenauer, P. L. H., Stiegliz, P., Paramelle, B., & Le Bas, J. F. (1993). Muscular metabolism during oxygen supplementation in patients with chronic hypoxemia. *American Review of Respiratory Disease,*Vol. 147, No. 3, (March 1993), pp. 592-598, ISSN 00030805

Pouw, M., Schols, A. M. W. J., Deutz, N. E. P., Wouters, E. F. M. (1998). Plasma and muscle amino acid levels in relation to resting energy expenditure and inflammation in stable chronic obstructive pulmonary disease. *American Journal of Respiratory and Critical Care Medicine* Vol. 157, No. 2, (February 1998), pp. 797-801, ISSN 1073449X

Rutten, E. P. A., Engelen, M. P. K. J., Schols, A. M. W. J., & Deutz, N. E. P. (2005). Skeletal muscle glutamate metabolism in health and disease: State of art. *Current Opinion in Clinical Nutrition and Metabolic Care,* Vol. 8, No. 1, (January 2005), pp. 41-51, ISSN 13631950

Rutten, E. P. A., Engelen, M. P. K. J., Gosker, H., Bast, A., Cosemans, K., Vissers, Y.L.J., Wouters, E. F. M., Deutz, N. E. P., & Schols, A. M. W. J. Metabolic and functional effects of glutamate intake in patients with chronic obstructive pulmonary disease (COPD). *Clinical Nutrition,* Vol. 27, No. 3, (June 2008), pp. 408-415, ISSN 02615614

Saey, D., Michaud, A., Couillard, A., Cote, C. H., Mador, M. J., LeBlanc, P., Jobin, J, & Maltais, F. (2005). Contractile fatigue, muscle morphometry, and blood lactate in chronic obstructive pulmonary disease. *American Journal of Respiratory and Critical Care Medicine,* Vol. 171, No. 10, (May 2005), pp. 1109-1115, ISSN 1073449X

Sala, E., Roca, J., Marrades, R. M., Alonso, J., Gonzales De Suso, J. M., Moreno, A., Barbera, J. A., Nadal, J., DeJover, L., Rodriguez-Roisin, R., & Wagner, P. D. (1999) Effects of endurance training on skeletal muscle bioenergetics in chronic obstructive pulmonary disease. *American Journal of Respiratory and Critical Care Medicine,* Vol. 159, No. 6, (June 1999), pp. 1726-1734, ISSN 1073449X

Sapega, A. A., Sokolow, D. P., Graham, T. J., & Chance, B. (1987). Phosphorus nuclear magnetic resonance: A non-invasive technique for the study of muscle bioenergetics during exercise. *Medicine and Science in Sports and Exercise,* Vol. 19, No. 4, (August 1987), pp. 410-420, ISSN 01959131

Schols, A. M. W. J., Soeters, P. B., Dingemans, A. M. C., Mostert, R., Franzen, P. J., & Wouters, E. F. M. (1993). Prevalence and characteristics of nutritional depletion in patients with stable COPD eligible for pulmonary rehabilitation. *American Review of Respiratory Disease,* Vol. 147, No. 5, (May 1993), pp. 1151-1156, ISSN 00030805

Shimomura, Y., Fujii, H., Suzuki, M., Fujitsuka, N., Naoi, M., Sugiyama, S., & Harris, R. A. (1993). Branched-chain 2-oxo acid dehydrogenase complex activation by tetanic contractions in rat skeletal muscle. *Biochimica et Biophysica Acta.* Vol. 1157, No. 3, (June 1993), pp. 290-296, ISSN 03044165

Shimomura, Y., Fujii, H., Suzuki, M., Murakami, T., Fujitsuka, N., & Nakai, N. (1995). Branched-chain α-keto acid dehydrogenase complex in rat skeletal muscle: Regulation of the activity and gene expression by nutrition and physical exercise *Journal of Nutrition,* Vol. 125, No. 6 SUPPL, (June 1995), pp. 1762S-1765S, ISSN 00223166

Stevens, A. N. (1987). NMR Spectroscopy: Application to metabolic research. In: *Functional studies using NMR,* McCready, V. R., Leach, M., & Ell, P. J., pp. 61-84, Springer-Verlag, ISBN 3-540-16213-5, Berlin Heidelberg

Taylor, D. J., Bore, P. J., Styles, P., Gadian, D. G., & Radda, G. K. (1983). Bioenergetics of intact human muscle. A ^{31}P nuclear magnetic resonance study. *Molecular Biology and Medicine,* Vol. 1, No. 1, (1983), pp. 77-94, ISSN 07351313

Vandenborne, K., Walter, G., Leigh, J. S., & Goelman, G. (1993). pH heterogeneity during exercise in localized spectra from single human muscles. *American Journal of Physiology,* Vol. 265, No. 5 (Cell Physiology 34), (November 1993), pp. C1332-1339, ISSN 00029513

Vukovich, M. D., Sharp, R. L., King, D. S., & Kershishnik, K. (1992). The effect of protein supplementation on lactate accumulation during submaximal and maximal exercise. *International Journal of Sport Nutrition,* Vol. 2, No. 4, (December, 1992), pp. 307-316, ISSN 10501606

Wagenmakers, A. J. M., Brookes, J. H., Coakley, J. H., Reilly, T., & Edwards, R. H. (1989). Exercise-induced activation of the branched-chain 2-oxo acid dehydrogenase in human muscle. *European Journal of Applied Physiology,* Vol. 59, No. 3, (October 1989), pp. 159-167, ISSN 14396319

Wagenmakers, A. J. M. (1998). Protein and amino acid metabolism in human muscle. *Advances in Experimental Medicine and Biology,* Vol. 441, (1998), pp. 307-319, ISSN 00652598

Wolfe, R. R., Goodenough, R. D., Wolfe, M. H., Royle, G. T., & Nodel, E. R. (1982). Isotopic analysis of leucine and urea metabolism in exercising humans. *Journal of Applied Physiology,* Vol. 52, No. 2, (February 1982), pp. 458-466, ISSN 87507587

Yoneda, T., Yoshikawa, M., Fu, A., Tsukaguchi, K., Okamoto, Y., & Takenaka, H. (2001). Plasma levels of amino acids and hypermetabolism in patients with chronic obstructive pulmonary disease. *Nutrition,* Vol. 17, No. 2, (February 2001), pp. 95-99, ISSN 08999007

Part 2

MRS Beyond the Clinic

8

NMR Spectroscopy as a Tool to Provide Mechanistic Clues About Protein Function and Disease Pathogenesis

Benjamin Bourgeois[1], Howard J. Worman[2] and Sophie Zinn-Justin[1]
[1]*Laboratoire de Biologie Structurale et Radiobiologie, CEA Saclay & URA CNRS 2096, Gif-sur-Yvette*
[2]*Department of Medicine and Department of Pathology and Cell Biology, College of Physicians and Surgeons, Columbia University, New-York*
[1]*France*
[2]*USA*

1. Introduction

Nuclear magnetic resonance (NMR) has become an important technique for determining the three-dimensional (3D) structure of biological macromolecules. Since 1985, it has been used to determine the structures of approximately 8,000 proteins, 1,000 DNA/RNA complexes and 180 protein/nucleic acid complexes (http://www.pdb.org/pdb/ statistics/holdings.do). At first, NMR was limited to relatively small and soluble proteins or protein domains. The study of large proteins was hindered by the presence of overlapping large peaks in the NMR spectra. This has been in part alleviated by the introduction of isotope (^{2}H, ^{15}N, ^{13}C) labeling and multidimensional (3D, 4D) experiments (Sattler et al., 1999). By using these techniques, it is now possible to study proteins up to 40 kDa. For instance, the 3D solution structure of the maltodextrin-binding protein (41kDa) has been recently solved using NMR (Madl et al., 2009; Figure 1A). Comprehensive NMR studies of integral membrane proteins in solution have long been impaired by substantial problems of sample preparation, including the inability to produce sufficient quantities of isotopically labelled protein as well as the difficulties associated with the limited thermal stability, sample heterogeneity and short lifetimes of such proteins. However, NMR allows investigation of the very conformational mobility that to a large extent interferes with the process of crystallization of membrane proteins. Thus, by focusing on proteins with a sufficient expression yield and screening sample and detergent conditions in a microtiter-plate format, it has been possible to determine 71 structures of integral membrane proteins corresponding to 49 unique proteins (http://www.drorlist.com/ nmr/MPNMR.html). The first NMR structure determination of a detergent-solubilized seven-helix transmembrane (7TM) protein, the phototaxis receptor sensory rhodopsin II (pSRII) from *Natronomonas pharaonis*, was recently reported to illustrate that NMR can provide structures of large membrane proteins (Gautier et al., 2010; Figure 1B). The challenge is now to apply similar techniques to the study of other 7TM proteins, including G-protein coupled receptors (GPCRs) that represent the most important class of targets for current therapeutic agents. These proteins can only be expressed in small quantities and are of limited stability, particularly in their unbound state. Samples must be conformationally and chemically homogeneous and stable at high concentrations. Despite these problems, there are encouraging indications suggesting that, in the near future, heterologous expression systems will provide labelled GPCRs in sufficient quantities for NMR analysis to characterize the details of the interactions between GPCRs and their ligands.

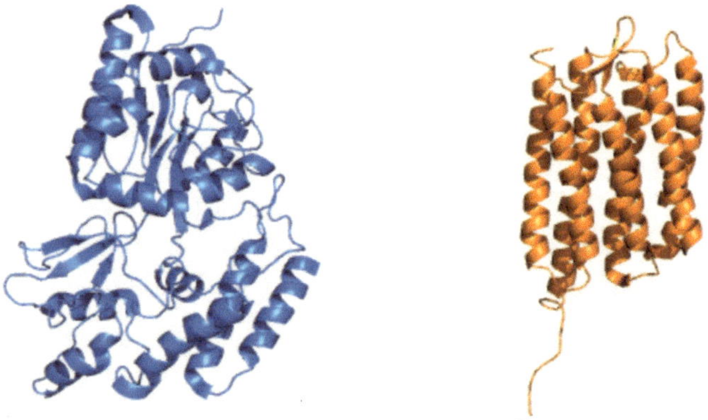

A B

Fig. 1. Ribbon representation of the solution NMR structures of **(A)** the maltodextrin-binding protein (PDB ID 2KLF; Madl et al., 2009) and **(B)** the phototaxis receptor sensory rhodopsin II (pSRII) from *Natronomonas pharaonis* (PDB ID 2KSY; Gautier et al., 2010).

Most NMR studies of biological macromolecules have been carried out in solution. Since about 10 years ago, developments in NMR technology, sample preparation, pulse-sequence methodology and structure calculation protocols have allowed the structure determination of several proteins by solid-state NMR spectroscopy. Thus, 17 structures corresponding to 11 unique proteins have been solved using oriented samples of protein/lipids mixture (http://www.drorlist.com/ nmr/SPNMR.html). In particular, the M2 protein, a small membrane protein that enables hydrogen ions to enter the influenza A viral particle, was characterized by NMR to better understand its 3D structure and its interaction with drugs used against flu (Hu et al., 2010; Sharma et al., 2010; Figure 2A). Solid-state NMR was also used to solve 18 structures corresponding to 5 proteins forming fibrils (Van Melckebeke et al., 2010; Figure 2B) and 8 proteins yielding microcrystalline samples (Jehle et al., 2010; Figure 2C). Like liquid-state NMR, solid-state NMR is based on local structure information. As a consequence, large amounts of data on several differently labelled samples are typically required to obtain sufficient long-range information. However, NMR is particularly useful to study fibrils and microcrystals because these preparations are highly ordered on a local scale and consequently show narrow resonance lines. In recent years, considerable progress has been made in using solid-state NMR spectroscopy to determine atomic-resolution structures of amyloid fibrils associated with serious disorders such as Alzheimer disease, Parkinson disease, prion diseases and type 2 diabetes mellitus (for review: Tycko, 2011). Although the architecture of fibrils is considered to be a continuous stack of β-sheet ladders termed a cross-β structure, there may be significant variations in the supramolecular organization of the peptides within the fibrils. NMR provides detailed insight on the structural organization of these fibrils, highlighting their assembly process and inspiring the design of fibril-binding compounds and inhibitors.

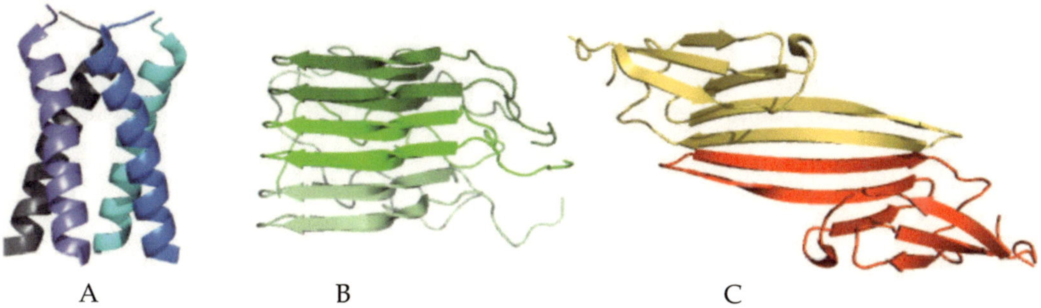

Fig. 2. Ribbon representation of the solid-state NMR structures of **(A)** the M2 transmembrane peptide of the influenza A virus in DMPC lipid bilayers (PDB ID 2KQT; Cady et al., 2010), (B) the HET-s(218-289) prion in its amyloid form (PDB ID 2KJ2; Van Melckebeke et al., 2010) and (C) the α-crystallin domain in αB-crystallin oligomers (PDB ID 2KLR; Jehle et al., 2010).

NMR can be used to study a large panel of molecular complexes, including those characterized by a low affinity binding interaction. At the present time, NMR has been used to solve about 1,500 3D structures of protein complexes. The majority of these structural studies have been performed on complexes characterized by submicromolar affinities. In cases of weak binding, characterized by a millimolar to micromolar affinity, it is possible to map and characterize details of the interface. The simplest and most popular approach is the so-called "chemical shift mapping" technique wherein changes in backbone chemical shifts of one molecule are monitored during titration with another molecule by recording a series of heteronuclear single-quantum correlation (HSQC) spectra (Figure 3). Upon addition of a ligand, chemical shift, line width and intensity changes of specific HSQC peaks indicate that the corresponding residues experience a modification of their chemical environment. This modification is due to the complex formation, and may result either from the proximity between the observed residue and the ligand or from binding-induced conformational changes in the first molecule close to the observed residue. The exact effects of the complex formation on the HSQC spectrum depend on the relative values of the NMR time scale and the exchange rate of the complex. The NMR time scale refers to the chemical shift scale: differences in chemical shifts between species in exchange. If this difference is larger than the exchange rate, then the exchange is classified as SLOW. If this difference is equal to the exchange rate, then the exchange is INTERMEDIATE. If this difference is smaller than the exchange rate, the exchange is FAST. Protein-protein interactions with Kd < 1μM (tight binding) are generally in slow exchange. In this case, two NMR signals are seen for the free and bound forms. During the titration, the free form signal gradually disappears and the bound form signal appears. Protein-protein interactions with Kd > 1mM (weak binding) are generally in fast exchange. In such cases, only one averaged signal is seen with a chemical shift fractionally weighted according to the populations and chemical shifts of the free and bound forms. Protein-protein interactions with a Kd between 1 μM and 1 mM are generally in intermediate exchange. This gives rise to broadened signals from both the free and bound forms. During addition of a ligand, identification of the NMR peak changes and mapping of these changes onto the protein structure provides information on the binding interface and the conformational changes of the protein due to the interaction (Figure 3). Analysis of these data opens up great opportunities for understanding the dynamics of interaction networks

(Mackereth et al., 2011). Which molecules are in competition for binding to the studied protein? Which molecules bind simultaneously? Is a conformational change necessary for the complex formation? Is this conformation change involved in the regulation of other interactions? How multiple domain proteins exploit their flexibility in order to recognize their targets?

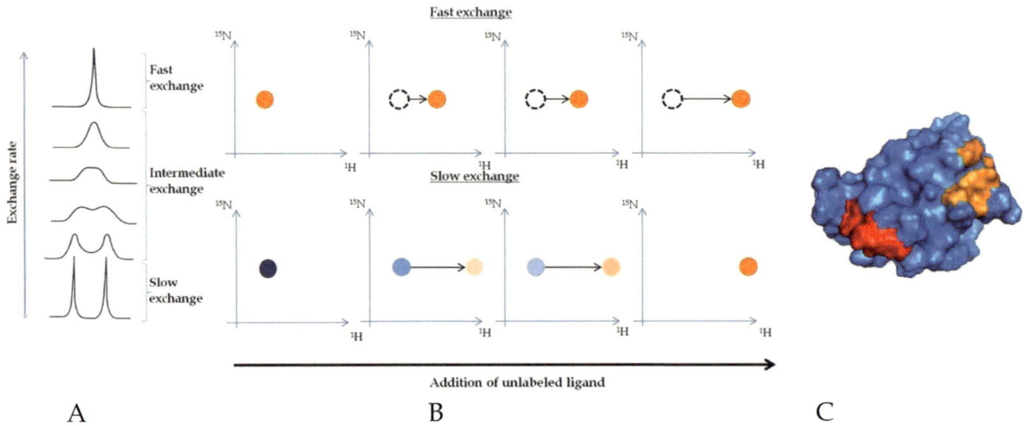

Fig. 3. Mapping of binding sites by NMR. **(A)** In the presence of free and ligand-bound proteins, the NMR signal varies as a function of the exchange rate. Its chemical shifts and linewidths evolve from a FAST exchange to a SLOW exchange condition. When the exchange is FAST, only one averaged chemical shift is observed. When it is SLOW, the chemical shifts corresponding to the free and bound forms are observed. **(B)** The chemical shift changes measured during the titration of a labelled protein with its binding partner are displayed in the case of FAST exchange (upper panel) and SLOW exchange (lower panel). **(C)** Residues whose NMR chemical shifts and/or linewidths change during the titration with ligands A and B are colored in red and orange, respectively, on the surface representation of the 3D structure of the labelled protein. This "chemical shift mapping" study shows that the labelled protein recognizes its two ligands by different surfaces.

NMR allows for direct observations of NMR-active nuclei (^{1}H, ^{15}N, ^{13}C, ^{31}P) within any NMR-inactive environment and can therefore be employed to investigate the structures of appropriately labelled biomolecules either in cell extracts or inside live cells. It has been used to structurally characterize biomolecules in the presence of cell extracts, in order to investigate post-translational modifications, conformational changes and binding events at the residue level within macromolecules in conditions mimicking the cellular environment (Liotakis et al., 2010). To accomplish this, NMR-active labelled recombinant proteins are injected into cell extracts and their chemical shift evolution is followed in the extracts after addition of specific enzyme co-factors or binding partners. These experiments are particularly powerful at describing the molecular binding events regulated by post-translational modifications. Furthermore, NMR has been applied to the observation of protein-protein interactions and the determination of protein structures in *E. coli*. The so-called STINT-NMR approach entails sequentially expressing two (or more) proteins within a single bacterial cell in a time-controlled manner and monitoring the protein interactions using in-cell NMR spectroscopy (Burz et al., 2006). NMR has also been used to follow the behavior of intrinsically disordered proteins in the crowded environment of bacterial cells

(Dedmon et al., 2002). The 3D structure of the putative heavy-metal binding protein TTHA1718 from *Thermus thermophilus HB8* was solved from data acquired on living *E. coli* samples (Sakakibara et al., 2009). In eukaryotic cells, the first in-cell NMR studies were performed by injecting proteins into *Xenopus laevis* oocytes (Selenko et al., 2006). Cell-penetrating peptides have also been used to deliver labelled proteins that can be observed in living cells (Inomata et al., 2009). However, the low sensitivity of the method and the short lifetime of the samples have so far prevented the acquisition of structural data in most of these eukaryotic systems. Development of ultra-fast methods for multidimensional experiments has already contributed to the first successes of in-cell NMR and should be further exploited to follow biological events.

Solid-state and liquid-state NMR techniques are now essential tools for understanding biological processes from a mechanistic point of view at the atomic level. They can describe critical steps of a disease mechanism, highlight the mechanism of action of a particular drug and inspire the design of binding compounds and complex assembly inhibitors. We will now focus on the use of NMR for the elucidation of the molecular mechanisms of specific genetic diseases caused by either missense mutations or amino acid deletions/insertions in several proteins located at the nuclear envelope.

2. NMR and genetic diseases involving the nuclear envelope

We have used NMR to study the molecular mechanisms of genetic diseases caused by mutations in genes encoding inner nuclear membrane proteins (see for examples Krimm et al., 2002 and Caputo et al., 2006). These proteins play critical roles in nuclear structure and positioning (Figure 4). They also influence genome spatial and temporal organization and genome functional properties. Because of their many biological functions, the pathological mechanisms resulting from mutations are complex and not well understood (Dauer & Worman, 2009). A wide range of diseases affecting different organs system have been linked to mutations in the *LMNA* gene, encoding the A-type nuclear lamins, which are intermediate filament proteins mainly located at the inner nuclear membrane of differentiated somatic cells. These diseases include dilated cardiomyopathy with variable muscular dystrophy, Dunnigan-type familial partial lipodystrophy, a Charcot-Marie-Tooth type 2 disease, mandibuloacral dysplasia and Hutchinson-Gilford progeria syndrome. Adult-onset autosomal dominant leukodystrophy is caused by duplication of the gene encoding lamin B1, which is an intermediate filament protein located at the inner nuclear membrane of all nucleated somatic mammalian cells. In addition, several diseases are linked to mutations in genes encoding integral proteins of the inner nuclear membrane that are associated with nuclear lamins, such as emerin, LBR and MAN1. Structural studies of the proteins involved in these so-called "laminopathies" or "nuclear envelopathies" have provided mechanistic clues about the functions of the nuclear envelope and insights into the disease pathogenesis.

Some mutations causing laminopathies are frameshifts or premature termination codons resulting in truncated protein. In these cases, the protein is generally rapidly degraded and its function is lost. NMR can however be used to structurally characterize the native protein, thus providing molecular details on its lost function (Caputo et al., 2006). Others mutations generate amino acid substitutions that can destabilize the protein leading to its premature degradation, interfere with its degradation pathway or modify its interaction with other proteins or nucleic acids. In these cases, NMR can provide information on the structural consequences of the mutation (Krimm et al., 2002). Does the mutation affect a hydrophobic residue in the core of the protein and thus destabilize its 3D structure? Does it affect a residue at the surface of the protein that is critical for a specific interaction with a biological partner? Structural studies utilizing NMR, by identifying the structural consequences of the missense mutations, can point out specific disease mechanisms. Such information could be used to develop therapies targeted to the defects.

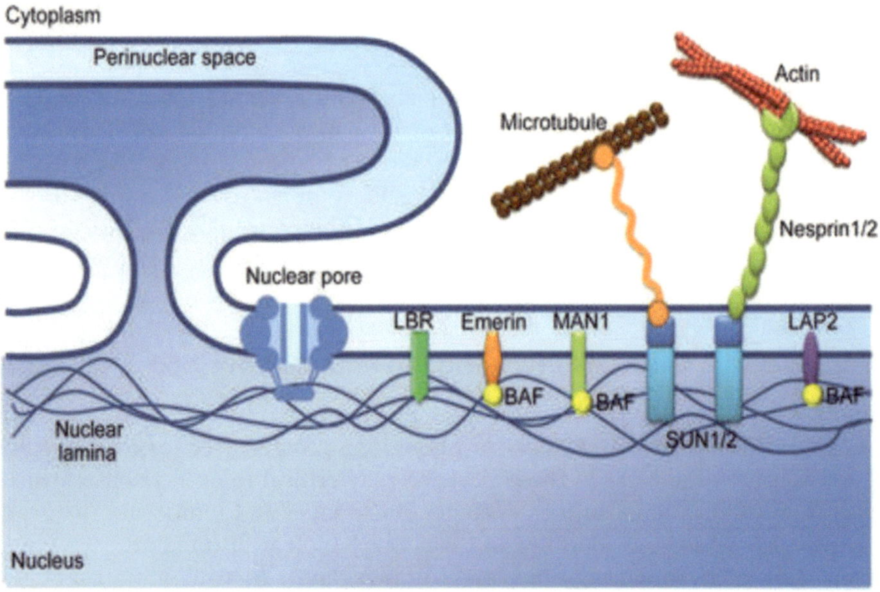

Fig. 4. Architecture of the nuclear envelope (reproduced with permission from Chi et al., 2009). The nuclear lamina, comprising the A- and B-type lamins, interacts with several proteins anchored at the inner nuclear membrane such as LBR, emerin, MAN1 and SUN1/2. SUN1/2 proteins also interact with outer nuclear membrane proteins that in turn bind to microtubules and actin. This network of protein-protein interactions is essential for cell structural organization.

We have used NMR to study A-type lamins, showing how different types of mutations that cause different diseases affect protein structure, hence providing clues about pathogenesis. We have also used NMR to study LEM domain proteins, which mediate interactions between the inner nuclear membrane and DNA and are involved in bone and muscle diseases. We have further analysed in detail MAN1, a LEM domain protein that regulates a key signal transduction pathway and whose heterozygous loss of function causes sclerosing bone dysplasias.

Many proteins associated with cellular control and signalling mechanisms such as A-type lamins and LEM domain proteins are modular in structure in that they contain both well-folded domains and poorly-structured regions (Wright & Dyson, 2009). The presence of poorly-folded regions facilitates protein accessibility to modifying enzymes and interaction with a wide variety of targets. However, this also hinders protein structural characterization, as the poorly-structured regions can adopt a large number of conformations and fold into different structures on binding to different target proteins. The pathological consequences of mutations located in the poorly-folded regions would then not be observed on the 3D structure of the mutated protein but instead linked to modifications of its binding properties. To tackle the structural description of these proteins, we chose to (1) solve the 3D solution structures of their globular domains and (2) characterize the relative positioning of domains within sub-regions. This "divide-and-conquer" approach is based on the combination of NMR spectroscopy and small-angle X-ray scattering (SAXS) and is a powerful method to characterize the structural ensemble of partially disordered proteins (Madl et al., 2011). From the description of the three-dimensional structures of sub-regions of A-type lamins and LEM domain proteins, we then (1) determined the impact of disease-linked mutations on the structure and stability of the proteins, (2) mapped interaction surfaces of proteins with their biological partners, (3) positioned the mutations relatively to these functionally important surfaces and (4) characterized the 3D structure of complexes involving these proteins.

3. How do mutations in A-type lamins cause different diseases?

3.1 Architecture of the lamin intermediate filaments

Nuclear lamins are classified as either A-type or B-type according to homology in sequence, biochemical properties and localization during the cell cycle. In humans, the *LMNB1* and *LMNB2* genes encode lamin B1 and B2, respectively, which are expressed in most or all nucleated somatic cells. The *LMNA* gene encodes the A-type lamins and the major isoforms, lamin A and lamin C, are expressed in most differentiated somatic cells. Lamins A and C are produced by alternative RNA splicing. They share a common region from amino acids 1-566 and differ at their C-terminus, from amino acids 567-664 for prelamin A, the lamin A precursor that is processed to lamin A, and from amino acids 567-572 for lamin C.

Like all intermediate filament proteins, lamins are fibrous in nature and share a tripartite structural organization. A non-α-helical N-terminal region (head) and a C-terminal region (tail) flank a central α-helical coiled-coil domain (rod). Lamins differ from the cytoplasmic intermediate filament proteins in that they have an extended rod domain (42 amino acid longer), that they have a nuclear localization signal (NLS) between their rod and tail regions and that they display a typical tertiary structure in this tail region (Herrmann et al., 2009; Figure 5). In contrast to most cytoplasmic intermediate filament proteins, lamins also contain sites for phosphorylation by mitotic kinases and most contain carboxy-terminal CAAX motifs that signal posttranslational modification by farnesylation. The lamin α-helical central rod domain is divided into three coiled regions (termed 1A, 1B and 2), which mediate lamin assembly into filaments. *In vitro* experiments have revealed that elementary lamin dimers first assemble through longitudinal N–C interactions and then these assemblies associate through lateral interactions to form intermediate filaments.

X-ray crystallography has been used to determine the atomic structure of various fragments of the lamin intermediate filament rod domain (Herrmann et al., 2009). In particular, it has been used to solve the crystal structure of a human lamin A fragment comprising residues 305 - 387, which corresponds to the second half of coil2 (PDB ID 1X8Y; Strelkov et al., 2004). This structure revealed a left-handed parallel coiled-coil extending to the predicted end of the rod domain (Figure 5). Essentially the same fragment of lamin B1 has also been resolved and a similar structure was observed (PDB ID 3MOV). Interestingly, the crystal structure of another human lamin A fragment (residues 328–398), which is largely overlapping with fragment 305–387 but harbours a short segment of the tail domain, was also solved. Unexpectedly, there is no parallel coiled-coil form within the crystal. Instead, the α-helices are arranged such that two antiparallel coiled-coil interfaces are formed (PDB ID 2XV5). The most significant interface has a right-handed geometry, which results from a characteristic 15-residue repeat pattern that overlays the canonical heptad repeat pattern (Figure 5). Analysis of these different modes of coil association gives some clues about the mechanisms of lamin polymerization in cells (Kapinos et al., 2011). Several polymerization mechanisms have been proposed that could co-exist and be modulated by specific chaperone-type molecules as well as post-translational modifications.

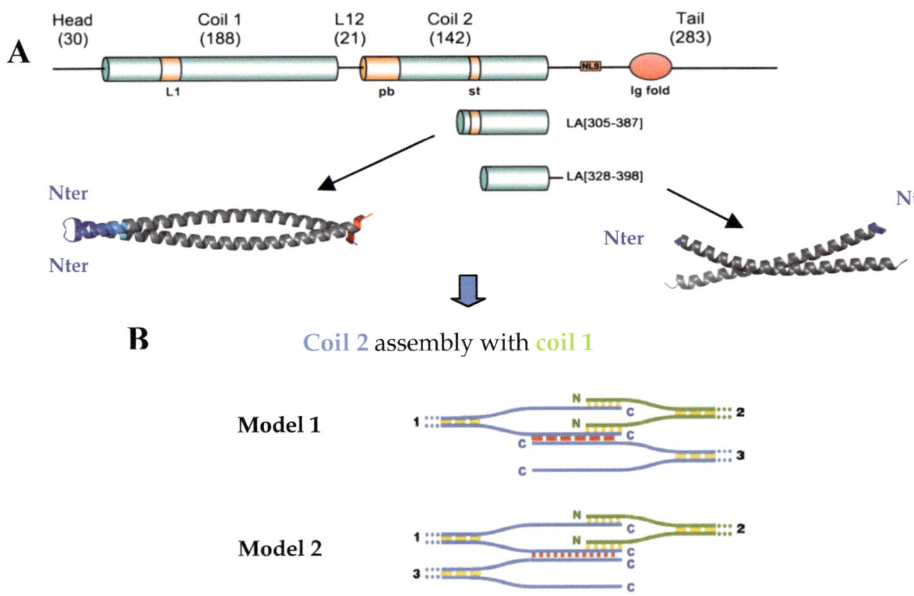

Fig. 5. Architecture of lamins, adapted with permission from Kapinos et al., 2011. **(A)** General structural organization of lamin monomers. Two A-type lamin coil 2 fragments were studied at atomic resolution (PDB IDs 1X8Y and 2XV5). Their X-ray structures are displayed in the cartoon, in which the sequence of amino acids 328-382, common to both fragments, is colored in gray and the remaining residues colored blue (N-terminus) or red (C-terminus). **(B)** Two models of lamin filament structural organization proposed from the analysis of the rod fragment X-ray structures. The C-terminal rod sections of two dimers labelled 1 and 3 are colored blue and the N-terminal rod section of dimer 2 is colored green. Broken lines represent coiled-coil interfaces that have been observed in crystal structures and dotted lines indicate other theoretically possible coiled coil interactions.

We have solved the 3D solution structure of the C-terminal globular domain of A-type lamins, which participates to the recognition of various lamin binding proteins (PDB ID 1IVT; Krimm et al., 2002). Determination of this structure was made from experimental measured values of short inter-proton distances (<6 Å) obtained by ^{1}H, ^{15}N and ^{13}C NMR on a ^{13}C and ^{15}N labelled sample of the domain. Figure 6A shows the well-dispersed ^{1}H-^{15}N HSQC spectrum of the C-terminal globular domain of A-type lamins. The labeling was essential to assign the inter-proton distances obtained by ^{1}H NMR to specific proton pairs. Molecular modeling calculations were used to calculate a family of 3D structures, all very close one to the other, compatible with the distances measured by NMR (Figure 6B). These structures, which reflect the structure of the domain in solution, have an immunoglobulin fold between residues 430 and 545. Crystal structures of this C-terminal domain of A-type lamins have also been solved and show similar structural organization (Dhe-Paganon et al., 2002; PDB IDs 1IFR and 1UFG).

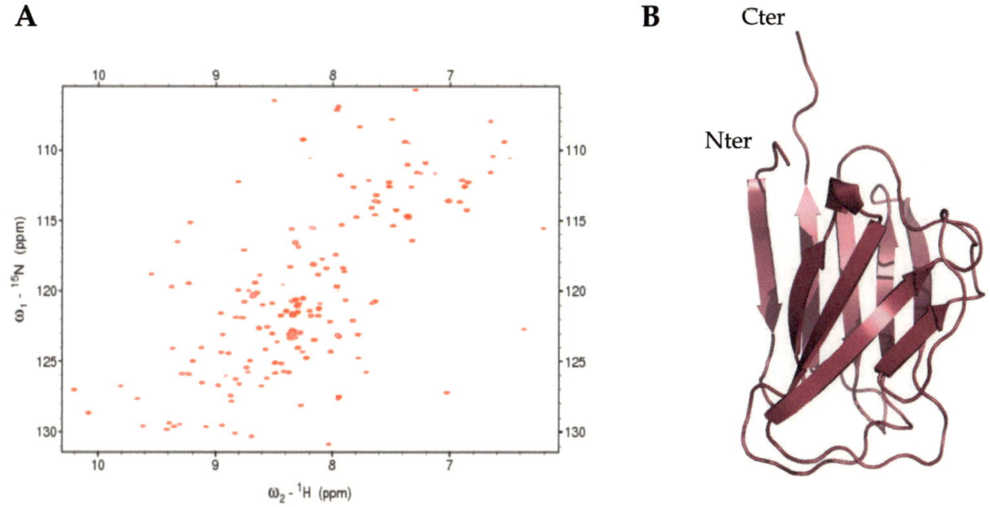

Fig. 6. Structural characterization of the globular domain found in the tail region of lamins. (A) ^{1}H-^{15}N HSQC spectrum of the domain from human A-type lamin. This spectrum was acquired on a 40 µM protein sample in 250 µl phosphate buffer pH 7.4 over 1 hour using a 700 MHz Bruker spectrometer. Each residue of the domain is revealed by a peak whose position depends on the residue chemical environment. Well-folded domains exhibit well-dispersed peaks, as shown for the lamin tail domain. (B) Cartoon representation of the 3D structure of the fragment of amino acids 428-549 from human A-type lamin, as calculated from NMR experimental data.

3.2 Post-translational modification of A-type lamins

Lamins undergo post-translational modifications that alter their localization, assembly and binding properties. Prelamin A is converted into lamin A by four enzymatic post-translational processing steps: farnesylation of a cysteine in a CAAX motif at the carboxyl terminus of the protein, endoproteolytic cleavage of the last three amino acids of the protein, carboxyl methylation of the newly exposed farnesylcysteine and subsequent endoproteolytic release of the last 15 amino acids, including the farnesylcysteine methyl ester. B-type lamins also contain a CAAX motif and undergo the first three of these enzymatic reactions but not the last. A-type and B-type lamins are also phosphorylated by cyclin dependent kinases, which regulate nuclear lamina assembly and disassembly during mitosis. Other phosphorylation, acetylation and sumoylation events have also been reported whose physiological importance is largely unknown. According to the PhosphoSite database, more than 60 phosphorylation sites are present in human A-type lamins. Most of these are located in unstructured regions of the proteins (Figure 7). These phosphoresidues could be important for lamin functions by regulating interactions with other nuclear proteins.

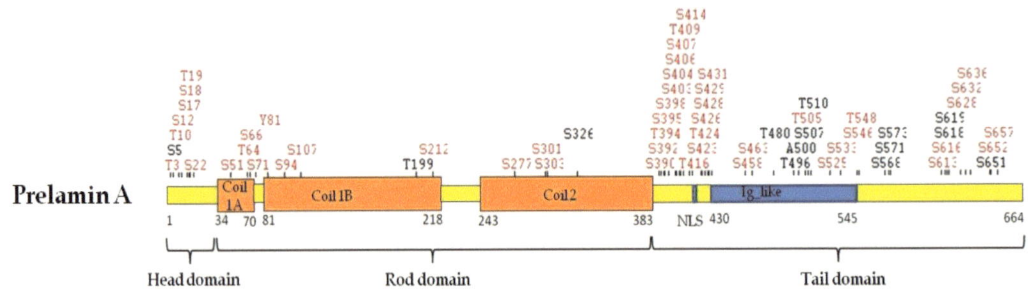

Fig. 7. Phosphorylation sites in human A-type lamins that have been reported in the PhosphoSite database (http://www.phosphosite.org/).

Post-translational modifications can be followed by NMR, either by adding the appropriate enzyme to the labelled protein sample or by diluting the labelled protein into cell extracts and adding the appropriate co-factor (Liotakis et al., JACS 2010). Series of NMR spectra are then recorded to follow the protein chemical shift evolution with time. Residues whose chemical shifts are modified because of the presence of enzymes in the sample are identified. These residues are either the targets of the enzyme or are close to the modified residues. NMR is particularly efficient in dissecting the modification kinetics of protein regions rich in inter-dependant modification sites.

3.3 Localization and structural impact of disease-linked missense mutations identified in A-type lamins

Several different diseases are caused by mutations in the *LMNA* gene encoding lamin A and C (Worman et al., 2010). More than 1,500 mutations have been identified within this gene. Amino acid substitutions in various regions of A-type lamins cause striated muscle diseases, partial lipodystrophy or progeroid disorders but in most cases a correlation between the localization of the mutation and the disease phenotype is not readily apparent. We searched for a correlation between the localization of the mutated residue in the lamin 3D structure and the disease phenotype. We focused on the lamin tail globular domain, because amino acid substitutions in this region cause either striated muscle diseases, lipodystrophy or progeroid disorders. Analysis of the position of the mutated residues in the NMR structure of the immunoglobulin-like domain and experimental measurement of the impact of several selected mutations on this structure were carried out (Krimm et al., 2002). We observed that most dominantly inherited mutations causing diseases of striated muscle affect residues of the hydrophobic core of the immunoglobulin-like domain (Figure 8A). These mutations probably destabilize the 3D structure of this domain, leading to an overall loss of protein function. Such destabilization has been experimentally verified for the Arg453Trp mutant. In contrast, dominantly inherited mutations causing Dunnigan-type familial partial lipodystrophy, a disease affecting adipose tissues, affect residues located at the surface of the immunoglobulin-like domain and cluster at a specific positively charged site (Figure 8B). This site is conserved in A-type and B-type lamins. This suggests that mutations causing adipose tissue diseases do not destabilize the domain structure but may hinder the interaction of A-type lamin with a binding partner that plays a critical role in adipose tissue. Recessive mutations in the immunoglobulin-like domain of A-type lamins causing progeroid disorders also affect residues located at the surface of this domain and cluster at a specific site (Figure 8C; Verstraeten et al., 2006). This hot spot is distinct from the surface affected in partial lipodystrophy and is conserved in A-type lamins. It may correspond to another protein binding site specific to A-type lamins, with mutations causing progeroid disorders hindering this putative interaction. Experiments to identify the proteins interacting with A-type lamins at the different identified hot spots are now underway.

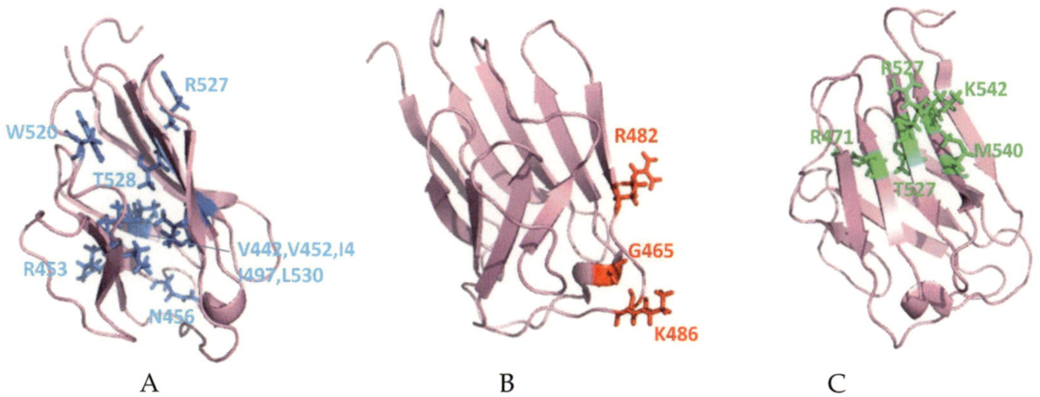

Fig. 8. Localization of the residues identified as mutated in laminopathies in the 3D structure of the tail globular domain of A-type lamins (PDB ID 1IVT; Krimm et al., 2002; Verstraeten et al., 2006). In **(A)**, residues mutated in striated muscle diseases are displayed in blue sticks. In **(B)**, residues mutated in adipose tissue diseases are displayed in red sticks. In **(C)**, residues mutated in progeria-like diseases are displayed in green sticks.

3.4 Perspectives: NMR study of how lamin post-translational modifications affect protein structure and interactions

Several studies have shown that the lamin tail globular domain and the flexible lamin regions are involved in binding to other proteins. We know that flexible regions of lamins are highly modified in cells (Figure 7). This suggests that post-translational modifications could be involved in regulating lamin recognition. In fact, post-translational modification of partners has already been shown to be involved in regulating lamin binding. For example, lamin A is involved in the sequestration of c-Fos, a member of the dimeric activator protein 1 (AP-1) transcription factor family that regulates different cellular pathways including cell proliferation, death survival differentiation and oncogenic transformation. Phosphorylation of c-Fos by ERK1/2 protein kinase reduces lamin A/c-Fos interaction, thus activating AP1 complexes (Gonzales et al., 2008).

In-cell NMR is a useful way to analyse these regulation pathways involving post-translational modifications of lamins or lamin partners. Using NMR chemical shift mapping as presented in part 1, modified residues can be identified onto the lamin tail or onto its binding partners. Next, interaction between modified or unmodified lamins and their binding partners, and conversely between lamins and modified or unmodified partners, can be tested. Our strategy is to produce recombinant lamins and partners and inject them into human cell extracts with or without addition of cofactors that are essential for post-translational-modifications. Figure 9 shows our first ^{1}H-^{15}N HSQC spectra of the tail region of lamin C incubated into 293T cell extracts during 1 to 24 hours. This experiment shows that it is possible to follow the fate of a partially unfolded protein in cell extracts during one day.

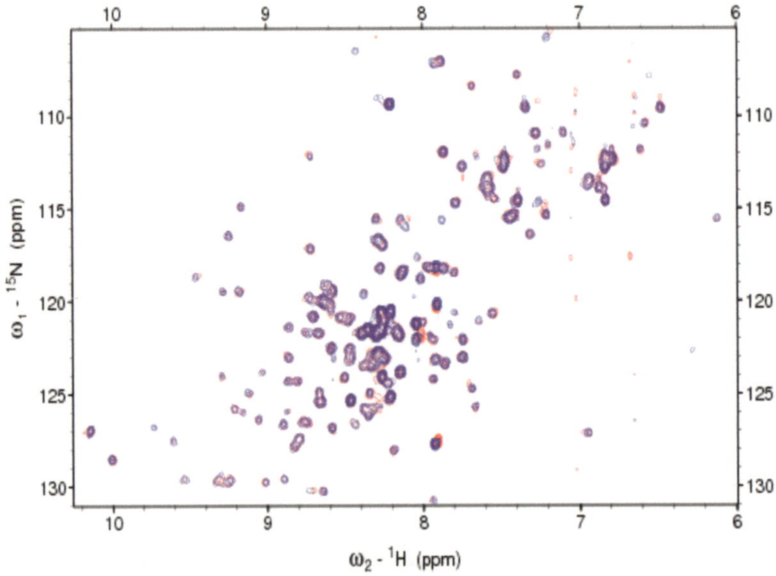

Fig. 9. Following modification and binding events involving the lamin C tail in 293T cell extracts: feasibility experiments. ^{1}H-^{15}N HSQC spectra were recorded on a Bruker 700 MHz spectrometer after 1 hour (red) and 24 hours (blue) of incubation of a 50 μM sample of labelled protein in 250 μl of cell extracts at 5mg/ml. The protein is stable in these conditions. Co-factors should then be added in order to allow modification of the labelled protein.

4. How do mutations in LEM domain proteins affect interactions between the nuclear envelope and chromatin?

4.1 Architecture of LEM domain proteins

LAP2 isoform β (LAP2 β), emerin and MAN1 are human nuclear proteins that share a highly conserved structural motif called the LEM domain (Lin et al., 2000). The LEM domain contains approximately 50 amino acids. It is located at the N-terminus of these proteins and is often separated from the rest of the protein by predicted unstructured regions (Figure 10). Both MAN1 and emerin possess one copy of the LEM domain in their N-terminal nucleoplasmic region whereas LAP2 β contains a LEM-like domain and a LEM domain connected by a predicted unstructured linker.

The 3D solution structures of emerin and LAP2 β LEM domains and LAP2 β LEM-like domain have been solved using NMR (Wolff et al., 2001; Laguri et al., 2001; Cai et al., 2001). These LEM and LEM-like domains share a similar 3D structure, mainly composed of a short N-terminal helix and two large α-helices interacting through a set of conserved amino acids residues (Figure 10). NMR characterization of the fragment from amino acids 1-168 of LAP2 β containing both the LEM-like and LEM domains has shown that the two domains are structurally independent, non-interacting domains connected by an approximately 60-residue flexible linker (Cai et al., 2001).

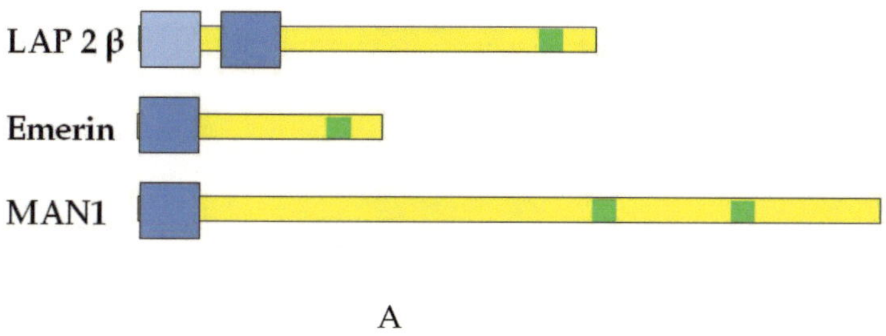

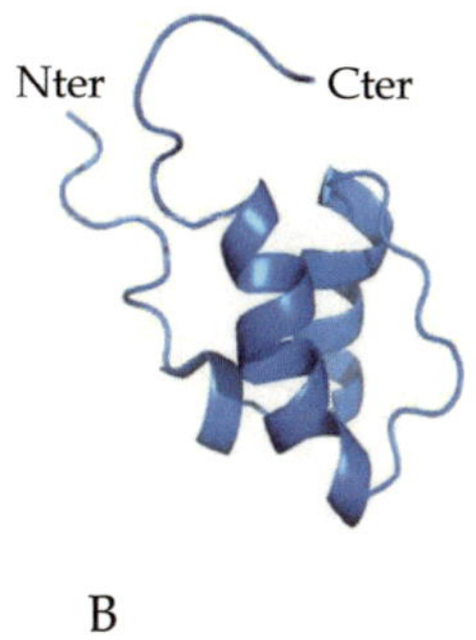

Fig. 10. Schematic organization of nuclear envelope proteins containing a LEM domain. **(A)** Three human inner nuclear membrane proteins are displayed: LAP2 β, MAN1 and emerin. Dark blue boxes represent LEM domains, the light blue box represents a LEM-like domain, green rectangles represent transmembrane segments. **(B)** Ribbon representation of the average solution structure of the LEM domain of LAP2 β (PDB ID 1H9F; Laguri et al., 2001).

4.2 LEM domains recognize the DNA binding BAF protein

Barrier-to-autointegration factor (BAF) is a highly conserved metazoan protein, which functions in nuclear assembly, chromatin organization and gene transcription. BAF dimers bind to double-stranded DNA non-specifically and thereby bridge DNA molecules to form a large, discrete nucleoprotein complex. BAF is able to interact simultaneously with both LAP2 and DNA *in vitro* (Shumaker et al., 2001). This suggested that LEM proteins and BAF mediate chromatin attachment to the nuclear envelope during nuclear assembly or interphase, or both.

The interaction between the fragment containing amino acids 1-168 of LAP2 β and the BAF-DNA complex was characterized by NMR (Cai et al., 2001). It was proposed on the basis of chemical shift mapping experiments that the LEM-like domain recognizes DNA (Figure 11A) while the LEM domain recognizes the DNA binding protein BAF (Figure 11B). However, when the whole BAF-DNA complex was added to the labelled LAP2 β fragment, only the peaks corresponding to the LEM domain shifted, indicating that only the LEM domain interacts with the BAF–DNA nucleoprotein complex (Figure 11C).

Subsequently, the solution structure of the BAF-emerin LEM domain complex was solved on the basis of NMR data (Cai et al., 2007). This structure revealed that one BAF dimer interacts with one emerin LEM domain (Figure 12A). The stoechiometry of the complex prevents association between one molecule of BAF dimer and multiple LEM domain proteins. Moreover, the interaction surface between BAF and emerin does not overlap with the two symmetry related DNA binding sites on the BAF dimer (Figure 12B). Thus, BAF can simultaneously interact with emerin and DNA.

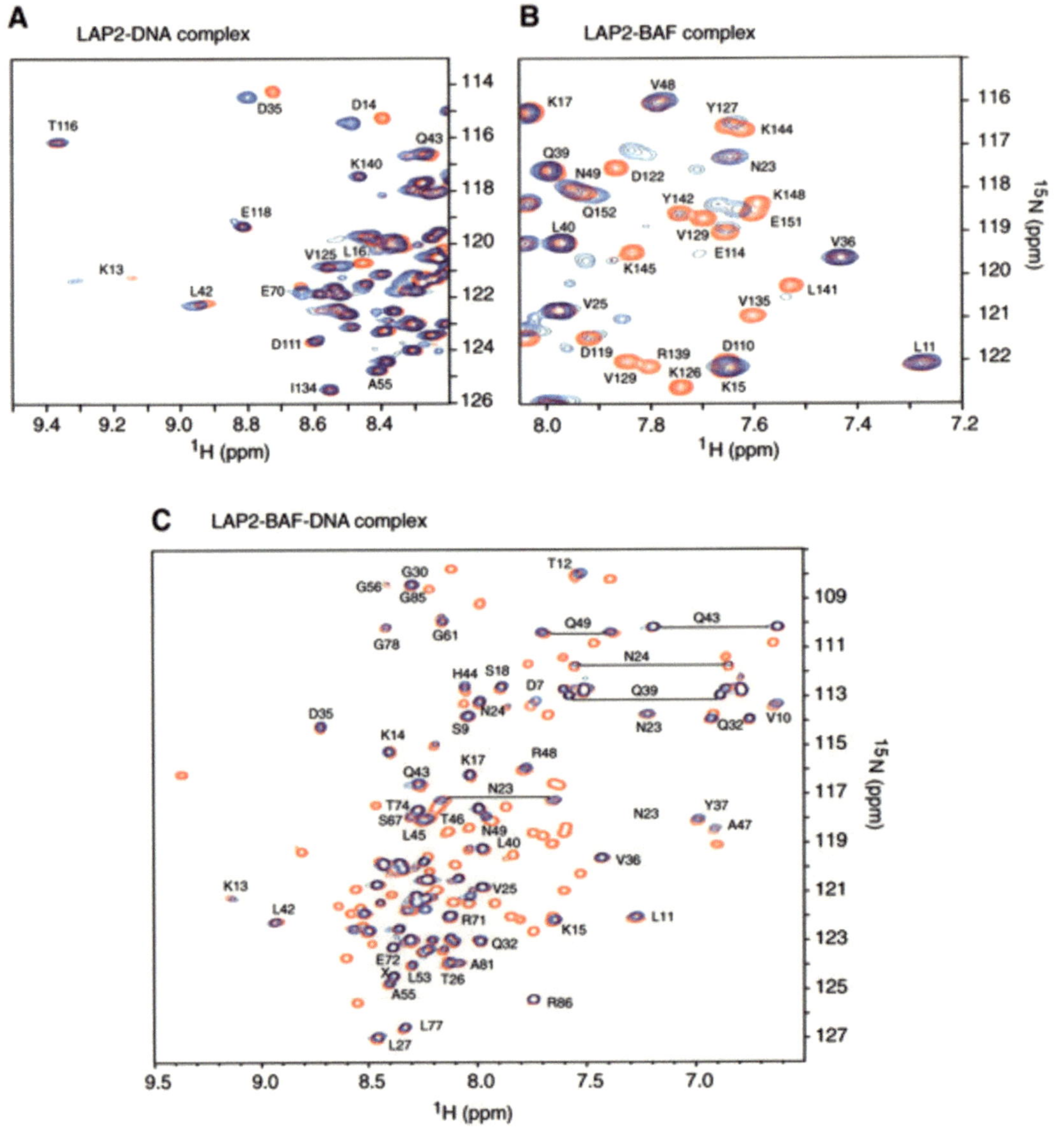

Fig. 11. Mapping the LAP2 β residues involved in BAF–DNA nucleoprotein recognition (reproduced with permission from Cai et al., 2001). (**A**) Comparison of the ^{1}H-^{15}N HSQC spectra of LAP2 β region containing amino acids 1-168 in the absence (red) and presence of 1.5 equivalents (blue) of a duplex DNA dodecamer. Only cross-peaks of the LEM-like domain shift upon DNA binding. (**B**) Comparison of ^{1}H-^{15}N HSQC spectra of LAP2 β region 1-168 in the absence (red) and presence (blue) of one equivalent of BAF. Only the cross-peaks in the LEM domain change significantly upon binding to BAF. (**C**) Comparison of the ^{1}H-^{15}N HSQC spectra of LAP2 β region containing amino acids 1-168 in the absence (red) and presence (blue) of the BAF–DNA nucleoprotein complex. Only the peaks originating from the LEM domain disappear upon binding the BAF–DNA nucleoprotein complex.

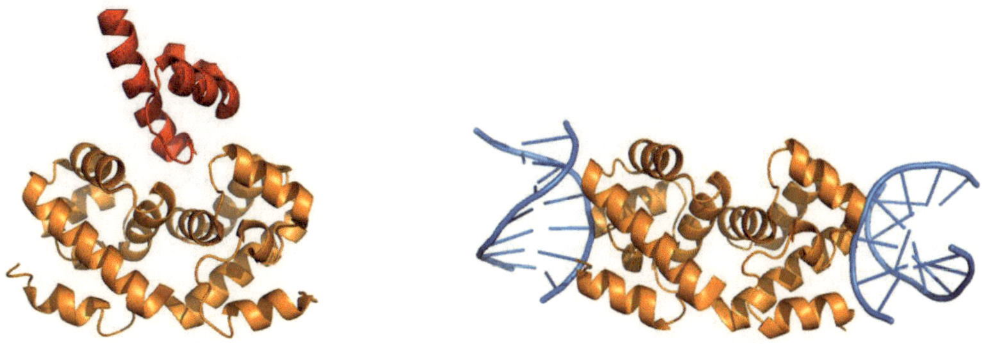

A B

Fig. 12. Ribbon representation of **(A)** the solution structure of the BAF_2 dimer (orange) bound to the emerin LEM domain (red) (PDB ID 2ODG; Cai et al., 2007) and **(B)** the X-ray structure of the BAF_2 dimer (orange) bound to DNA (blue) (PDB ID 2BZF; Bradley et al., 2005).

4.3 Localization and structural impact of disease-linked mutations identified in emerin and BAF

X-linked Emery-Dreyfus muscular dystrophy (EDMD) is characterized by early contractures of the spine, Achilles tendon and elbows, muscle wasting in a humerperoneal distribution and dilated cardiomyopathy with conduction system abnormalities (Muchir & Worman, 2007). It is caused by mutations in the *EMD* gene encoding emerin (Bione et al., 1994), an integral protein of the inner nuclear membrane. At present, 130 mutations homogeneously distributed along the *EMD* gene have been reported (Brown et al., 2011). Approximately 90% of these mutations result in the complete absence of protein as characterized by immunohistochemical staining. The few mutations allowing modified emerin protein expression yield protein that is expressed in reduced amounts and is frequently mislocalized. The majority of patients with residual emerin expression display clinical phenotypes indistinguishable from their null counterparts. However, it is difficult to argue that there is no discernable genotype-phenotype correlation, as clinical data collection on EDMD patients is often incomplete. Moreover, the relationship between emerin absence or decreased expression and muscle abnormalities is poorly understood. As emerin has been hypothesized to regulate muscle specific gene expression and nuclear architecture, some have suggested that absence or reduced levels affect cellular susceptibility to mechanical stress, cellular proliferation and differentiation (Fidziańska & Hausmanowa-Petrusewicz, 2003; Frock el al., 2006).

Recently, a mutation (A12T) in the *BANF1* gene encoding BAF has been shown to induce a progeroid syndrome that shares physiopathological characteristics with Hutchinson-Gilford progeria syndrome (HGPS) (Puente et al., 2011). HPGS has received considerable attention because of its striking premature aging phenotype, including alopecia, diminished subcutaneous fat, premature atherosclerosis, and skeletal abnormalities. The vast majority of HGPS cases are associated with a de novo nucleotide substitution at position 1824 (C->T) in the *LMNA* gene encoding A-type lamins (Eriksson et al., 2003; De Sandre-Giovannoli et al., 2003). This mutation does not affect the coded amino acid (and is thus generally referred to as G608G), but partially activates a cryptic splice donor site in exon 11 of *LMNA*, leading to the production of a prelamin A mRNA that contains an internal deletion of 150 base pairs. This transcript is then translated into a protein known as progerin, which lacks 50 amino acids near the C terminus. The new progeroid syndrome caused by a mutation in BAF differs from HGPS by the fact that affected patients have not cardiovascular deficiencies and live longer. A 3D model of BAF shows that the mutated residue is located on the surface of the protein (Figure 13). Nevertheless, the A12T mutation is not predicted to affect BAF dimerization or binding to either DNA or emerin, raising the possibility that this amino acid substitution could impair the interaction with other proteins, its subcellular localization or its stability. Examination of the effect of the BAF A12T mutation in the fibroblasts of affected patients showed a reduction in protein levels, indicating that this mutation affects the stability of BAF. Surprisingly, the decrease in BAF appears to be linked to a delocalization of emerin in the endoplasmic reticulum and abnormalities in the nuclear lamina. In HeLa cells that overexpressed a phosphomimetic BAF missense mutant S4E, but not S4A, emerin also mislocalized from the nuclear envelope (Bengtsson & Wilson, 2005). Furthermore, phosphorylation of serine 4 inhibited BAF binding to emerin and lamin A in blot overlay assays. These results suggest that the N-terminal region of BAF is normally involved in emerin localization at the nuclear envelope and that the A12T mutation could destabilize a lamin-emerin-BAF complex. Structural data on this complex are lacking so further structural analysis of the consequences of the BAF A12T mutation is not currently possible.

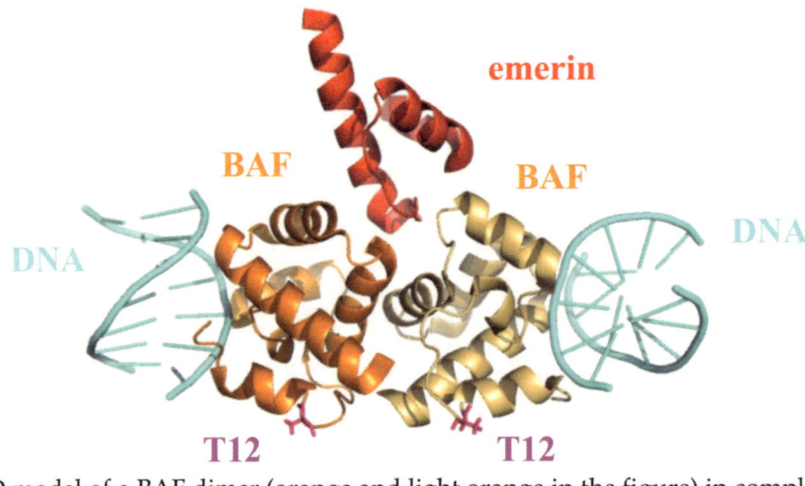

Fig. 13. 3D model of a BAF dimer (orange and light orange in the figure) in complex with emerin (red) and DNA (cyan) built from the PDB files 2ODG and 2BZF. The position of the T12 residue in mutant BAF is indicated in pink sticks (Puente et al., 2011).

5. How do mutations in the inner nuclear envelope MAN1 deregulate TGFβ signaling?

5.1 Architecture of MAN1, a LEM domain protein with an R-Smad binding C-terminal region

The *LEMD3* gene encodes MAN1, an integral protein of the inner nuclear membrane (Lin et al., 2000). MAN1 consists of 911 amino acids and exhibits two transmembrane domains

(Figure 14A). Its N-terminal and the C-terminal regions are located on the nucleoplasmic side of the membrane. The N-terminal nucleoplasmic region of MAN1 (amino acids 1-471) contains an N-terminal LEM (Figure 14B). This domain is essential for emerin, lamin and BAF binding (Liu et al., 2003; Mansharamani & Wilson, 2005). We have used ^{1}H, ^{15}N and ^{13}C NMR and SAXS to study the structural organization of the C-terminal nucleoplasmic region of MAN1 (Caputo et al., 2006; Kondé et al., 2010). This region is composed of a globular winged helix (WH) domain (Figure 14C), a linker region, a globular U2AF Homology Motif (UHM) domain (Figure 14D) and a C-terminal unstructured region. The WH domain presents a fold found in several transcription factors and it recognizes DNA (Caputo et al., 2006). The UHM domain is essential for MAN1 binding to Smad2 and Smad3 that are transcriptional regulators of the TGFβ pathway (Lin et al., 2005; Pan et al., 2005). The C-terminal region also recognizes other transcription regulators as the death-promoting transcriptional repressor Btf and the transcriptional repressor germ-cell-less GCL (Mansharamani & Wilson, 2005).

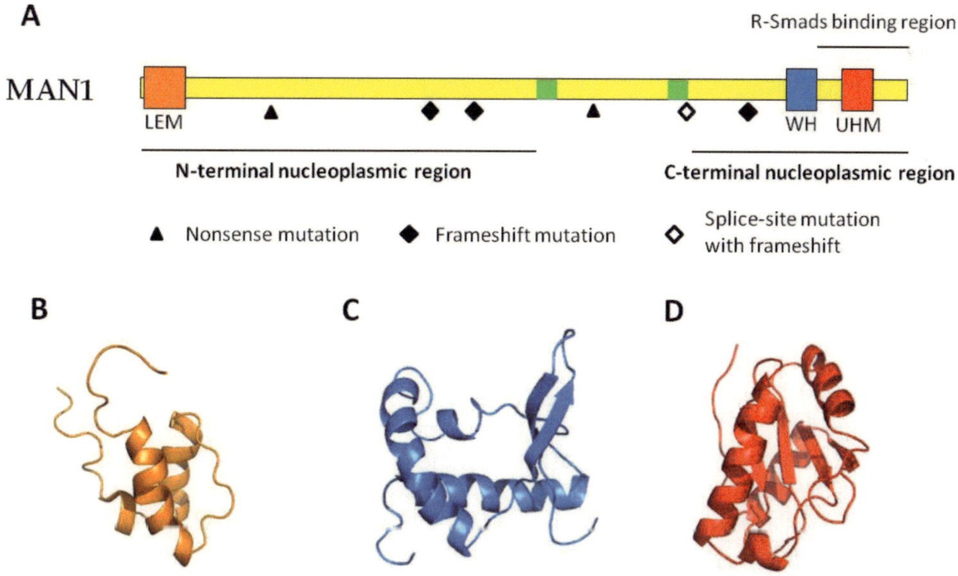

Fig. 14. Structural organization of the MAN1 protein. **(A)** Domain composition of MAN1 (the two transmembrane regions are colored in green) and localization of the mutations causing bone genetics diseases (Hellemans et al., 2004). **(B)** Model of the LEM domain of MAN1, built by homology on the basis of the LAP2 β LEM domain structure (PDB ID 1H9F; Laguri et al., 2001). **(C)** NMR structure of the WH domain (PDB ID 1CH0; Caputo et al., 2006). **(D)** Model calculated for the UHM domain on the basis of the secondary structure information deduced from the NMR chemical shift analysis and the 3D structure of the UHM domain of U2AF65 (PDB ID 1O0P; Kondé et al., 2010).

To understand the mechanisms of regulation of the TGFβ pathway by MAN1, we characterized the molecular determinants of its interaction with Smad2 and Smad3. We showed that the first WH domain is not essential for Smad2 binding. However, the linker region as well as the UHM domain and the C-terminus are all involved in Smad2 binding. NMR and SAXS data were used to reconstitute the fluctuating 3D structure of the Smad2 binding region of MAN1 (Kondé et al., 2010).

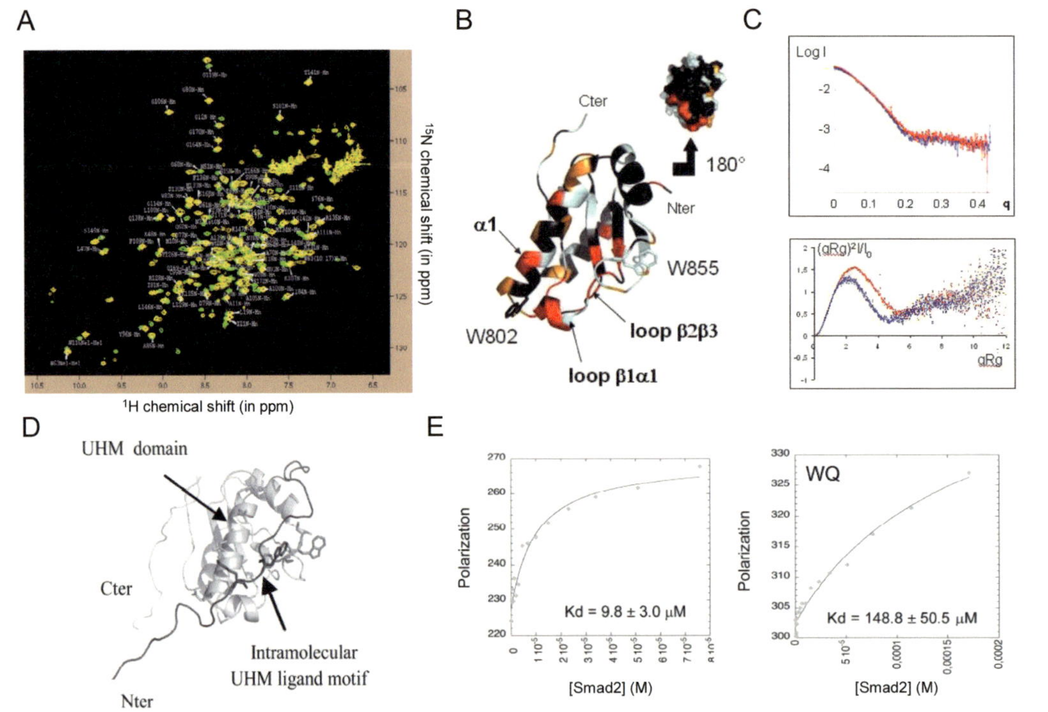

Fig. 15. Structural organization of the Smad2 binding motif of MAN1 (adapted with permission from Kondé et al., 2010). **(A)** NMR ^{1}H-^{15}N HSQC spectra of the wild-type (yellow) and mutated (W765A-Q766A, green) Smad2 binding motif of MAN1, representing the NMR finger print of the fold adopted by these protein fragments. Each NMR peak is assigned to the backbone NH bond of a specific amino acid in MAN1 sequence, and its position in the spectrum reflects its chemical environment in the protein domain. **(B)** NMR chemical shift mapping of the UHM region interacting with the linker. On the black ribbon representation of the MAN1 UHM model, residues whose ^{1}H-^{15}N HSQC peak is largely shifted and could not be assigned due to the mutations W765A and Q766A are colored in red, residues whose HSQC peak is shifted by more than 1.5 times the root mean square deviation of the chemical shift difference distribution but could still be assigned are coloured in orange, and residues whose HSQC peak could not be assigned in the MAN1LuhmWQ spectra are colored in cyan. The surface of the opposite face of the UHM domain is showed as an additional view. **(C)** Comparison of the SAXS data recorded on the wild-type (blue) and mutated (W765A-Q766A, red) Smad2 binding motif of MAN1. The upper view displays the superposition of the logarithm of the SAXS intensities as a function of the amplitude of the diffusion vector $q = 4*\pi*\sin(\theta)/\lambda$. The lower view corresponds to the superposition of the Kratky plots: the diffusion vector amplitude multiplied by the gyration radius is plotted on the abscissa and the square of the abscissa multiplied by the SAXS intensity divided by the intensity at 0 is plotted on the ordinate. This representation reveals the type of structure: compact, partially folded or unfolded. **(D)** Model of the Smad2 binding domain of MAN1 consistent with the NMR and SAXS data. The backbone is represented as a ribbon; the side chains of W765 and Q766, in the linker, and of several residues lining the hydrophobic cavity of the UHM domain are displayed as sticks. **(E)** Fluorescence polarization curves of the labelled wild-type (left) and mutated (W765A-Q766A, right) Smad2 binding fragment of MAN1 as a function of the concentration in Smad2.

We mutated the highly conserved W765 and Q766 of the linker region and observed the consequences of these mutations on the NMR ^{1}H-^{15}N spectrum of the Smad2 binding region (Figure 15A). Residues with NMR signals modified by the mutations were mapped onto the UHM domain (Figure 15B). They all clustered on one face of the domain and delineated a hydrophobic pocket in which the tryptophane residue binds. We performed SAXS experiments on samples of wild type and mutated Smad2 binding region. SAXS provides accurate information on folding and conformation in solution for both rigid and flexible macromolecules and the indirect Fourier transform of the SAXS intensity gives access to the real space electron pair distance distribution of molecules in solution. Figure 15C (upper panel) shows that the SAXS curves of the wild type and mutated protein fragments are similar, reflecting their common global fold. Calculation of the electron pair distance distributions using GNOM gave access to the radius of gyration Rg, the maximal distance and the I0 value that cannot be measured experimentally and is proportional to the mass. From these values, a Kratky representation was displayed (Figure 15C, lower panel) that highlighted structural differences between wild-type and mutated proteins: the maximum of the curve corresponding to (SRg)2 I/Io is shifted towards higher SRg values, reflecting the more elongated/less structured state of the mutant. Moreover, the wild type protein shows a gyration radius between 20 and 21 Å and a maximal distance between 68 and 72 Å, whereas the mutant shows a gyration radius between 23.3 and 24 Å and a maximal distance is close to 90 Å. This result validates our previous NMR based analysis that strongly suggests a role of W765 and Q766 in anchoring the linker onto the UHM domain. In contrast, the C-terminus of the Smad2 binding region of MAN1 is partially unfolded. From these observations, the positions of the linker and C-terminus regions relatively to the UHM domain were calculated, yielding to a model of the whole Smad2 binding region of MAN1 (Figure 15D). The functional importance of the positioning of the linker region onto the UHM domain was shown using fluorescence binding experiments: mutations of the W765 and Q766 residues into alanine yielded a 15-fold decrease of the affinity of MAN1 for Smad2 (Figure 15E).

5.2 Mechanism of bone diseases caused by the absence of the C-terminal region of MAN1

Heterozygous loss-of-function mutations in *LEMD3* encoding MAN1 cause the sclerosing bone dysplasias osteopoikilosis, Buschke-Ollendorff syndrome and non-sporadic melorheostosis (Hellemans et al., 2004). Several arguments suggest that the bone diseases result from enhanced TGF-ß signalling in cells.

First, all the disease-causing mutations including nonsense or frameshift mutations induce loss of the C-terminal nucleoplasmic fragment of MAN1, which is essential for Smad2 recognition (Figure 14A). Second, the TGF-β pathway is enhanced in cells from patients (Hellemans et al., 2004). Loss of the MAN1-Smad2 interaction may lead to the release of activated Smad2 and Smad3, thus causing an increase of Smad2 dependant transcription (Lin et al., 2005; Pan et al., 2005). It has been proposed that MAN1-Smad2 interaction not only sequestrates Smad2 and Smad3 at the inner nuclear envelope, but also favours their nuclear export (Pan et al., 2005; Figure 16). However, the mechanism by which the nucleoplasmic MAN1 C-terminal region would stimulate this nuclear export remains unclear. MAN1 could simply act as a "nuclear envelope sink" for activated nuclear Smad proteins, sequestering them at the inner nuclear membrane (Figure 16-1) and competitively inhibiting interactions with other nuclear factors involved in gene regulation (Figure 16-2).

Another hypothesis, also proposed for the MAN1 paralog NET25 (Huber et al., 2009), is that MAN1 functions as a scaffold protein recruiting Smad2, Smad3 and kinases/phosphatases to the inner nuclear membrane. Phosphorylation of Smad linker residues by kinases such as MAPKs or dephosphorylation of Smad C-terminal residues by phosphatases would then lead to enhanced nuclear export (Figure 16-3).

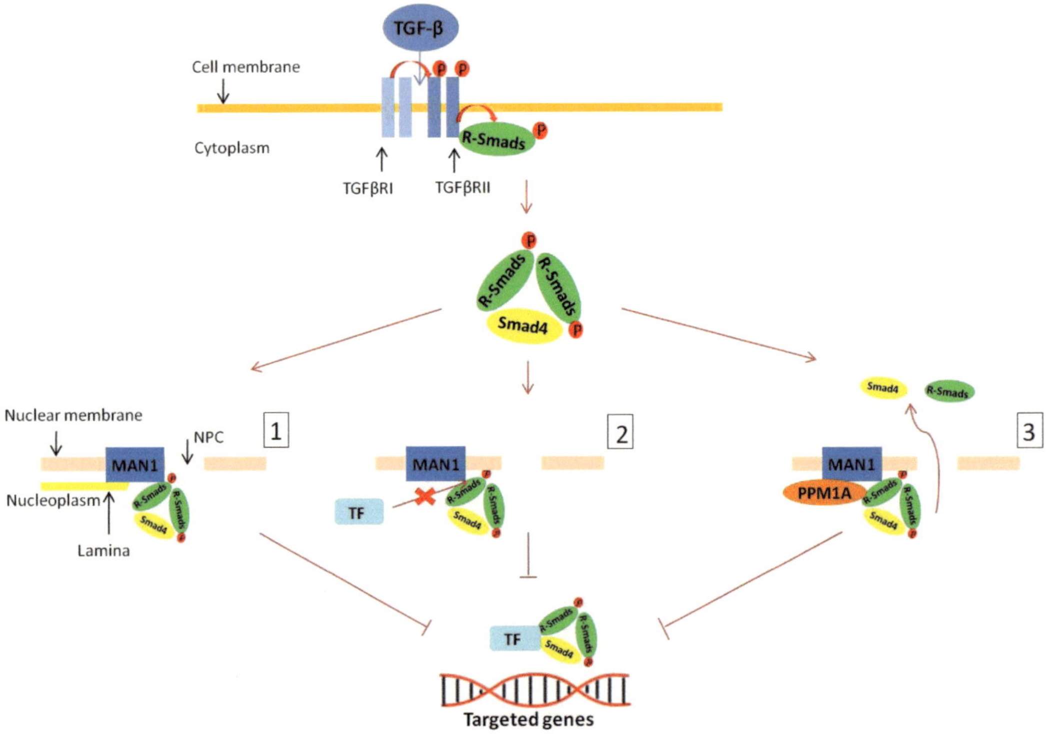

Fig. 16. The role of MAN1 in the TGF-β signaling pathway. The TGF-ß family of cytokines comprises key regulators of metazoan embryonic development and adult tissue homeostasis. In the canonical pathway, ligands of both the TGF-ß and the bone morphogenetic protein members of this family bind to heteromeric serine/threonine kinase receptor complexes, which in turn phosphorylate R-Smad transcription factors at their C-terminal tails. Upon phosphorylation, the R-Smads trimerize. This trimerization allows the R-Smads to interact with the common mediator Smad4. Then, these complexes translocate to the nucleus where they interact with various transcription factors, bind to DNA, and regulate transcription of targeted genes. MAN1 is able to influence the TGF-ß signalling by directly interacting with Smad2 and Smad3 (Hellemans et al., 2004; Lin et al., 2005). This leads to an inhibition of the TGF-ß signalling pathway (Pan et al., 2005). We suggest several putative mechanisms for the TGF-β pathway regulation by MAN1. **(1)** MAN1 could sequestrate the activated complexes R-Smads-Smad4 at the inner nuclear membrane, thus decreasing R-Smads accessibility to its targeted genes. **(2)** MAN1 could also compete with transcription factors for R-Smads binding resulting in a decrease of the transcriptional activity of R-Smads proteins. **(3)** MAN1 could recruit enzymes that modify R-Smads resulting in dissociation of active R-Smads-Smad4 complexes and nuclear export of R-Smads.

We used protein binding assays and isothermal calorimetry experiments to map the Smad2 binding site onto the MAN1 structure (Kondé et al., 2010). These experiments suggested that MAN1 recognizes Smad2 through a motif similar to the Smad Interaction Motif found in transcription factors. MAN1 could thus compete with transcription factors for Smad2 and Smad3 binding. Further experiments are needed to characterize the fate of Smads after MAN1 binding.

6. Conclusion

^{1}H, ^{15}N and ^{13}C NMR spectroscopy provide structural data which, when combined to SAXS data, allow the determination of the 3D structures of partially unfolded proteins. It is now possible to describe not only the structural consequences of disease-linked mutations located in well-folded domains but also their impact on the structural organisation of modular proteins (Mackereth et al., 2011). Such results provide mechanistic clues about how partially folded proteins use conformational switches in order to regulate their functions and highlight the connection between conformational variability, interaction and disease pathogenesis. Regulation of the function of modular proteins is also based on protein modifications. Recent studies propose that NMR characterization of a ^{15}N labelled protein in cell extracts can be a unique tool to examine changes in protein structure and interaction properties upon modification (Liokatis et al., 2010).

Characterization of interaction properties of disease-linked proteins is critical to understanding pathogenic mechanisms and may identify other genes to be screened in similar pathologies. NMR is a powerful tool to map low affinity (mM to μM) interaction surfaces and determine high affinity (nM to pM) complex structures, and must be used in conjunction with other methods such as isothermal calorimetry or fluorescence to deduce the nature, affinity and stochiometry of the interaction. Analysis of these parameters aims at highlighting the competitive or synergic role of the studied interaction within the large cellular protein-protein interaction network, and at identifying how disease-linked mutations perturb this functional network.

All theses different approaches highlight NMR spectroscopy as a technique adapted to the description of the consequences of disease-linked mutations in partially unfolded and multi-partner proteins, as those associated with cellular control and signalling mechanisms. It has become an essential tool for understanding such biological processes from a mechanistic point of view at the atomic level. It can describe critical steps of disease mechanisms, highlight the mechanism of action of a particular drug and inspire the design of binding compounds and complex assembly inhibitors. NMR could be used in the future to develop therapies targeted to the defects.

7. References

Bengtsson L & Wilson KL (2005). Barrier-to-autointegration factor phosphorylation on Ser-4 regulates emerin binding to lamin A in vitro and emerin localization in vivo. *Mol Cell Biol*, Vol. 17, No.3, pp. 1154-63

Bione S, Maestrini E, Rivella S, Mancini M, Regis S, Romeo G & Toniolo D (1994). Identification of a novel X-linked gene responsible for Emery-Dreifuss muscular dystrophy. *Nat Genet*, Vol. 8, No.4, pp. 323-7

Bradley CM, Ronning DR, Ghirlando R, Craigie R & Dyda F (2005). Structural basis for DNA bridging by barrier-to-autointegration factor. *Nat Struct Mol Biol*, Vol.12, No.10, pp.935-6

Burz DS, Dutta K, Cowburn D & Shekhtman A (2006). Mapping structural interactions using in-cell NMR spectroscopy (STINT-NMR). *Nature Methods*, Vol.3, pp. 91-93

Cady SD, Schmidt-Rohr K, Wang J, Soto CS, Degrado WF & Hong M (2010). Structure of the amantadine binding site of influenza M2 proton channels in lipid bilayers. *Nature*, Vol.443, No.7281, pp. 689-92

Cai M, Huang Y, Ghirlando R, Wilson KL, Craigie R & Clore GM (2001). Solution structure of the constant region of nuclear envelope protein LAP2 reveals two LEM-domain structures: one binds BAF and the other binds DNA. *EMBO J*, Vol.20, No.16, pp. 4399-407

Cai M, Huang Y, Suh JY, Louis JM, Ghirlando R, Craigie R & Clore GM (2007). Solution NMR structure of the barrier-to-autointegration factor-Emerin complex. *J Biol Chem*, Vol.282, No.19, pp. 14525-35

Caputo S, Couprie J, Duband-Goulet I, Kondé E, Lin F, Braud S, Gondry M, Gilquin B, Worman HJ & Zinn-Justin S (2006). The carboxyl-terminal nucleoplasmic region of MAN1 exhibits a DNA binding winged helix domain. *J Biol Chem*, Vol.281, No.26, pp. 18208-15

Chi YH, Chen ZJ & Jeang KT (2009). The nuclear envelopathies and human diseases. *J Biomed Sci*, Vol.16, pp. 96

Dauer WT & Worman HJ (2009). The nuclear envelope as a signaling node in development and disease. *Dev Cell*, Vol.17, No.5, pp. 626-38

Dedmon MM, Patel CN, Young GB & Pielak GJ (2002). FlgM gains structure in living cells. *Proc. Natl Acad. Sci. USA*, Vol.99, pp. 12681-12684

De Sandre-Giovannoli A, Bernard R, Cau P, Navarro C, Amiel J, Boccaccio I, Lyonnet S, Stewart CL, Munnich A, Le Merrer M & Lévy N. (2003). Lamin a truncation in Hutchinson-Gilford progeria. *Science*, Vol. 300, No. 5628, pp. 2055.

Dhe-paganon S, Werner ED, Chi YI & Shoelson SE (2002). Structure of the globular tail of nuclear lamin. *J Biol Chem*, Vol.277, No.20, pp. 17381-4

Eriksson M, Brown WT, Gordon LB, Glynn MW, Singer J, Scott L, Erdos MR, Robbins CM, Moses TY, Berglund P, Dutra A, Pak E, Durkin S, Csoka AB, Boehnke M, Glover TW & Collins FS (2003). Recurrent de novo point mutations in lamin A cause Hutchinson-Gilford progeria syndrome. *Nature*, Vol.423, No.6937, pp. 293-8

Fidziańska A & Hausmanowa-Petrusewicz I (2003). Architectural abnormalities in muscle nuclei. Ultrastructural differences between X-linked and autosomal dominant forms of EDMD. *J Neurol Sci*, Vol.210, No.1-2, pp. 47-51

Frock RL, Kudlow BA, Evans AM, Jameson SA, Hauschka SD & Kennedy BK (2006). Lamin A/C and emerin are critical for skeletal muscle satellite cell differentiation. *Genes Dev*, Vol.20, No.4, pp. 486-500

Gautier A, Mott HR, Bostock MJ, Kirkpatrick JP & Nietlispach D (2010). Structure determination of the seven-helix transmembrane receptor sensory rhodopsin II by solution NMR spectroscopy. *Nat Struct Mol Biol*, Vol.17, No.6, pp. 768–774

Gonzáles JM, Navarro-Puche A, Casar B, Crespo P & Andrés V (2008). Fast regulation of AP-1 activity throught interaction of lamin A/C, ERK1/2, and c-Fos at the nuclear envelope. *J Cell Biol*, Vol.183, No.4, pp. 653-66

Hellemans J, Preobrazhenska O, Willaert A, Debeer P, Verdonk PC, Costa T, Janssens K, Menten B, Van Roy N, Vermeulen SJ, Savarirayan R, Van Hul W, Vanhoenacker F, Huylebroeck D, De Paepe A, Naeyaert JM, Vandesompele J, Speleman F, Verschueren K, Coucke PJ & Mortier GR (2004). Loss-of-function mutations in LEMD3 result in osteopoikilosis, Buschke-Ollendorff syndrome and melorheostosis. *Nat Genet*, Vol.36, No.11, pp. 1213-8

Herrmann H, Strelkov SV, Burkhard P & Aebi U (2009). Intermediate filaments: primary determinants of cell architecture and plasticity. *J Clin Invest*, Vol.119, No.7, pp. 1772-83

Hu F, Luo W & Hong M (2010). Mechanisms of Proton Conduction and Gating in Influenza M2 Proton Channels from Solid-State NMR. *Science*, Vol.330, No.6003, pp. 505-508.

Huber MD, Guan T & Gerace L (2009). Overlapping functions of nuclear envelope proteins NET25 (Lem2) and emerin in regulation of extracellular signal-regulated kinase signalling in myoblast differentiation. *Mol Cell Biol*, Vol.29, No.21, pp. 5715-28

Inomata K, Ohno A, Tochio H, Isogai S, Tenno T, Nakase I, Takeuchi T, Futaki S, Ito Y, Hiroaki H & Shirakawa M (2009). High resolution multi-dimensional NMR spectroscopy of proteins in human cells. *Nature*, Vol.458, pp. 106-109

Jehle S, Rajagopal P, Bardiaux B, Markovic S, Kühne R, Stout JR, Higman VA, Klevit RE, van Rossum BJ & Oschkinat H (2010). Solid-state NMR and SAXS studies provide a structural basis for the activation of alphaB-crystallin oligomers. *Nat Struct Mol Biol*, Vol.17, No.9, pp. 1037-42

Kapinos LE, Burkhard P, Herrmann H, Aebi U & Strelkov SV (2011). Simultaneous formation of right- and left-handed anti-parallel coiled-coil interfaces by a coil2 fragment of human lamin A. *J Mol Biol*, Vol.408, No.1, pp. 135-46

Kondé E, Bourgeois B, Tellier-Lebegue C, Wu W, Pérez J, Caputo S, Attanda W, Gasparini S, Charbonnier JB, Gilquin B, Worman HJ & Zinn-Justin S (2010). Structural analysis of the Smad2-MAN1 interaction that regulates transforming growth factor-β signaling at the inner nuclear membrane. *Biochemistry*, Vol.49, No.37, pp. 8020-32

Krimm I, Ostlund C, Gilquin B, Couprie J, Hossenlopp P, Mornon JP, Bonne G, Courvalin JC, Worman HJ & Zinn-Justin S (2002). The Ig-like structure of the C-terminal domain of lamin A/C, mutated in muscular dystrophies, cardiomyopathy, and partial lipodystrophy. *Structure*, Vol.10, No.6, pp. 811-23

Laguri C, Gilquin B, Wolff N, Romi-Lebrun R, Courchay K, Callebault I, Worman HJ & Zinn-Justin S (2001). Structural characterization of the LEM motif common to three human inner nuclear membrane proteins. *Structure*, Vol.9, No.6, pp. 503-11

Lin F, Blake DL, Callebault I, Skerjanc IS, Holmer L, McBurney MW, Paulin-Levasseur M & Worman HJ (2000). MAN1, an inner nuclear membrane protein that shares the LEM domain with lamina-associated polypeptide 2 and emerin. *J Biol Chem*, Vol.275, No.7, pp. 4840-7

Lin F, Morrison JM, Wu W & Worman HJ (2005). MAN1, an integral protein of the inner nuclear membrane, binds Smad2 and Smad3 and antagonizes transforming growth factor-beta signaling. *Hum Mol Genet*, Vol.14, No.3, pp. 437-45

Liotakis S, Dose A, Schwarzer D & Selenko P (2010). Simultaneous detection of protein phosphorylation and acetylation by high-resolution NMR spectroscopy. *J Am Chem Soc*, Vol.132, No.42, pp. 14704-5

Liu J, Lee KK, Segura-Totten M, Neufeld E, Wilson KL & Gruenbaum Y (2003). MAN1 and emerin have overlapping function(s) essential for chromosome segregation and cell division in Caenorhabditis elegans. *Proc Natl Acad Sci U S A*, Vol.100, No.8, pp. 4598-603

Mackereth C, Madl T, Bonnal S, Simon B, Zanier K, Gasch A, Rybin V, Valcarcel J & Sattler M (2011). Multi-domain conformational selection underlies pre-mRNA splicing regulation by U2AF. *Nature*, Vol.475, pp. 408-411

Madl T, Bermel W & Zangger K (2009). Use of relaxation enhancements in a paramagnetic environment for the structure determination of proteins using NMR spectroscopy. *Angew Chem Int Ed Engl*, Vol.48, No.44, pp. 8259-8262

Madl T, Gabel F & Sattler M (2011). NMR and small-angle scattering-based structural analysis of protein complexes in solution. *J Struct Biol*, Vol.173, No.3, pp. 472-82

Mansharamani M & Wilson KL (2005). Direct binding of nuclear membrane protein MAN1 to emerin in vitro and two modes of binding to barrier-to-autointegration factor. *J Biol Chem*, Vol.280, No.14, pp. 13863-70

Muchir A & Worman HJ (2007). Emery-Dreifuss muscular dystrophy. *Curr Neurol Neurosci Rep*, Vol.7, No.1, pp. 78-83

Pan D, Estévez-Salmerón LD, Stroschein SL, Zhu X, He J, Zhou S & Luo K (2005). The inner nuclear membrane protein MAN1 physically interacts with R-Smad proteins to repress signaling by the transforming growth factor-{beta} superfamily of cytokines. *J Biol Chem*, Vol.280, No.16, pp. 15992-6001

Puente XS, Quesada V, Osorio FG, Cabanillas R, Cadiñanos J, Fraile JM, Ordóñez GR, Puente DA, Gutiérrez-Fernández A, Fanjul- Fernández M, Lévy N, Freije JM & López-Otín C (2011). Exome sequencing and functional analysis identifies BANF1 mutation as the cause of a hereditary progeroid syndrome. *Am J Hum Genet*, Vol.88, No.5, pp. 650-6

Sakakibara D, Sasaki A, Ikeya T, Hamatsu J, Hanashima T, Mishima M, Yoshimasu M, Hayashi N, Mikawa T, Wälchli M, Smith BO, Shirakawa M, Güntert P & Ito Y (2009). Protein structure determination in living cells by in-cell NMR spectroscopy. *Nature*, Vol.458, pp. 102-105

Sattler M, Schleucher J & Griesinger C (1999). Heteronuclear multidimensional NMR experiments for the structure determination of proteins in solution employing pulsed field gradients *Progr Magn Res Spect*, Vol.34, pp. 93-158

Selenko P, Serber Z, Gade B, Ruderman J & Wagner G (2006). Quantitative NMR analysis of the protein G B1 domain in Xenopus laevis egg extracts and intact oocytes. Proc. Natl Acad. Sci. USA, Vol.103, pp. 11904-11909

Sharma M, Yi M, Dong H, Qin H, Peterson E, Busath DD, Zhou HX & Cross TA (2010). Insight into the mechanism of the influenza A proton channel from a structure in a lipid bilayer. *Science*, Vol.330, No.6003, pp. 509-12

Shumaker DK, Lee KK, Tanhehco YC, Craigie R & Wilson KL (2001). LAP2 binds to BAF.DNA complexes: requirement for the LEM domain and modulation by variable regions. *EMBO J*, Vol.20, No.7, pp. 1754-64

Strelkov SV, Schumacher J, Burkhard P, Aebi U & Herrmann H (2004). Crystal structure of the human lamin A coil 2B dimer: implications for the head-to-tail association of nuclear lamins. *J Mol Biol*, Vol.343, No.4, pp. 1067-80

Tycko R (2011). Solid-State NMR studies of amyloid fibril structure. *Annu Rev Phys Chem*, Vol.62, pp. 279-299

Van Melckebeke H, Wasmer C, Lange A, Ab E, Loquet A, Böckmann A & Meier BH (2010). Atomic-resolution three-dimensional structure of HET-s(218-289) amyloid fibrils by solid-state NMR spectroscopy. *J Am Chem Soc*, Vol.132, No.39, pp. 13765-75

Verstraeten VL, Broers JL, van Steensel MA, Zinn-Justin S, Ramaekers FC, Steijlen PM, Kamps M, Kuijpers HJ, Merckx D, Smeets HJ, Hennekam RC, Marcelis CL & Van den Wijngaard A (2006). Compound heterozygosity for mutations in LMNA causes a progeria syndrome without prelamin A accumulation. *Hum Mol Genet*, Vol.15, No.16, pp. 2509-22

Wolff N, Gilquin B, Courchay K, Callebault I, Worman HJ & Zinn-Justin S (2001). Structural analysis of emerin, an inner nuclear membrane protein mutated in X-linked Emery-Dreifuss muscular dystrophy. *FEBS let*, Vol.501, No.2-3, pp. 171-6

Worman HJ, Ostlund C & Wang Y (2010). Diseases of the nuclear envelope. *Cold Spring Harb Perspect Biol*, Vol.2, No.2

Wright PE & Dyson HJ (2009). Linking folding and binding. *Curr Opin Struct Biol*, Vol.19, No.1, pp. 31-8

9

Structural and Vibrational Properties and NMR Characterization of (2'-furyl)-Imidazole Compounds

Ana E. Ledesma[1], Juan Zinczuk[2], Juan J. López González[3] and Silvia A. Brandán[4*]

[1]*INQUINOA-UNSE, Facultad de Agronomía y Agroindustrias, Universidad Nacional de Santiago del Estero, Santiago del Estero*
[2]*Instituto de Química Rosario (CONICET-UNR), Facultad de Ciencias Bioquímicas y Farmacéuticas, Rosario, Santa Fé*
[3]*Departamento de Química Física y Analítica, Facultad de Ciencias Experimentales, Universidad de Jaén, Jaén*
[4]*Cátedra de Química general, Instituto de Química Inorgánica, Facultad de Bioquímica, Química y Farmacia, Universidad Nacional de Tucumán, San Miguel de Tucumán, Tucumán, República*
[1,2,4]*Argentina*
[3]*Spain*

1. Introduction

The furylimidazoles compounds have a great importance in biochemistry and pharmacology because many of them present interesting properties[1,2]. They are also found in artificial compounds[3], such as agrochemicals,[4] pharmaceuticals[5], dyes[6], plastics, solvents, photographic chemicals, electronics, corrosion inhibitors,[7] preservatives, and polymers[8]. They can be used in synthetic organic chemistry as building blocks, due to their presence as key structural units in many natural products and in important pharmaceuticals. For example, the nature of the N- atoms in the imidazole molecule makes possible an extraordinary variety of reactions and this is the main reason for the great biological importance of the amino acid, histidine.

---

* Corresponding Author

[1] Salerno & Perillo, 2005
[2] Szabo, 2002.
[3] Gould et. al., 2006.
[4] Higashio & Shoji, 2004.
[5] Monterrey et al., 2004.
[6] Ooyama et al., 2007.
[7] Rohwerder & Michalik, 2007.
[8] Stroganova, et al., 2000.

Polymers of these compounds, which have potential as semi-conducting material are of great importance, because of their good thermal and chemical stability and relative ease of functionalization, which potentially permit the fine tuning of their physical and electronic properties[9]

In fact, these compounds provide one of the best studied examples of annular tautomerism, such as the 4(5)-substituted imidazoles[10,11,12]. Recently, the theoretical and experimental studies on structure, electronic and vibrational properties for the (2′-furyl)-imidazole series were reported by us[13,14,15,16,17].

Examination of the spectroscopic data for the each furanics molecules indicated that Nuclear Magnetic resonance spectroscopy, coupled with IR spectroscopy, was potentially the best analytical technique to provide confirmatory structural evidence for their formation. On the other hand, in general, the chemical shifts for the substituted imidazole ring, relative to the unsubstituted rings, suggest that the mesomeric effect of the five-membered rings contributes less to the interaction between two rings than does their inductive effects. It would indicate which rings is more electron-withdrawing in its overall electronic effect than the furan ring, as well as observed in the pyridine-thiophenes and furans[18]. The downfield shifts of the ^{13}C NMR signals for the carbon atom at the point of substitution on the imidazole ring would be explicate of the significant inductive electron-withdrawing effects of the 2-heteroaryl rings.

For this, reason for predicting the reactivity of this molecules due to the different position of the substituent, in this chapter, a comparison of the structural and vibrational properties of the four molecules belong to the (2′-furyl)-imidazole series was performed in order to evaluate the experimental and theoretical results based on B3LYP calculations by using 6-31G* and 6-311++G** basis sets. The optimized geometries and frequencies for the normal modes of vibration were calculated using both theory levels. For a complete assignment of the compounds, the DFT (Density functional Theory) calculations were combined with the scaled quantum mechanical force field (SQMFF) methodology[19,20,21] in order to fit the theoretical wavenumbers to the experimental ones. In all molecules of this series, the changes in the chemical shifts of the hydrogen and carbon atoms were also studied. In addition, the electronic properties of those molecules were evaluated by means of natural bond orbital (NBO) and atoms in molecules (AIM) studies in order to analyze the nature and magnitude of the intramolecular interactions. In this chapter, the experimental and theoretical studies of

---

[9] Nevin et al., 2008.
[10] Bellina et al., 2007.
[11] Popov et al., 2004.
[12] Sztanke et al., 2005.
[13] Ledesma et al., 2008.
[14] Ledesma et al., 2010.
[15] Ledesma et al., 2009a.
[16] Ledesma et al., 2009b.
[17] Zinczuk et al., 2009.
[18] Jones & Civcir, 1997.
[19] Rauhut & Pulay,1995a.
[20] Rauhut & Pulay, 1995b.
[21] Kalincsak & Pongor, 2002.

structures and vibrational properties of 2-(2′-furyl)-imidazole, 4-(2′-furyl)-imidazole, 5-(2′-furyl)-imidazole and N-(2′-furyl)-imidazole are compared and analyzed.

2. Structure and properties of the (2'-furyl)-imidazole series

2.1 Structural analysis

All compounds of this series are present in two different stable conformations according to the syn and anti position of the oxygen atom with respect to the N—H bond, named syn and anti conformers, respectively, as show in Figure 1.

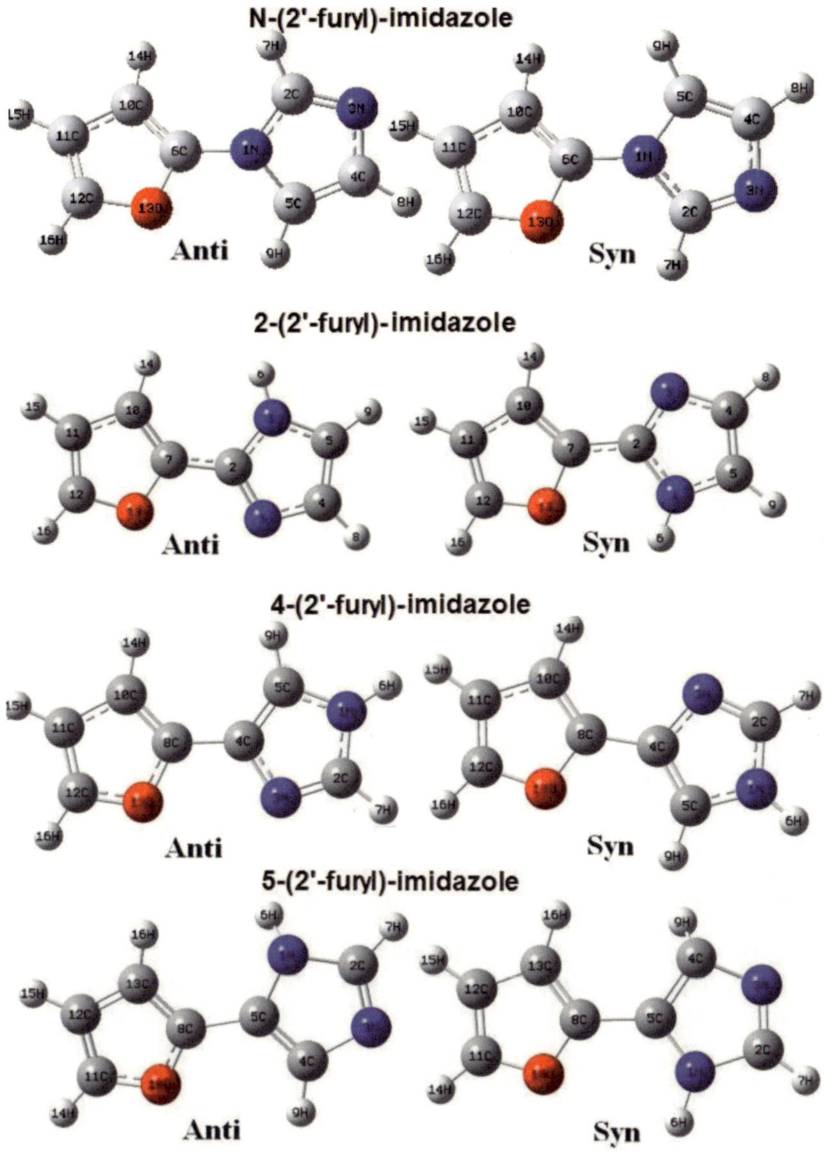

Fig. 1. Molecular structures of the (2′-furyl)-imidazole series

Experimentally, all molecules of this series have different characteristics or they are solid of different nature. Thus, the first series's member, N-(2′-furyl)-imidazole, is a liquid at room temperature and probably the two conformers are present in it. For the second series's member, 2-(2′-furyl)-imidazole, the crystallography analysis shows that both conformers are present in the crystalline lattice with equal occupancy and alternated arrangement in the N-H---N bonded polymeric chains along the crystal [101] direction. Only three units of the polymeric structure are shown in Figure 2. Finally, the 4-(2′-furyl)-imidazole and 5-(2′-furyl)-imidazole compounds are present in a tautomeric mixture in the solid state as a white power.

The calculation indicates that both conformers of N-(2′-furyl)-imidazole have C_1 symmetries, in the 2-(2′-furyl)-imidazole they have C_1 and C_s symmetries, while in the remaining molecules all conformers present C_s symmetries.

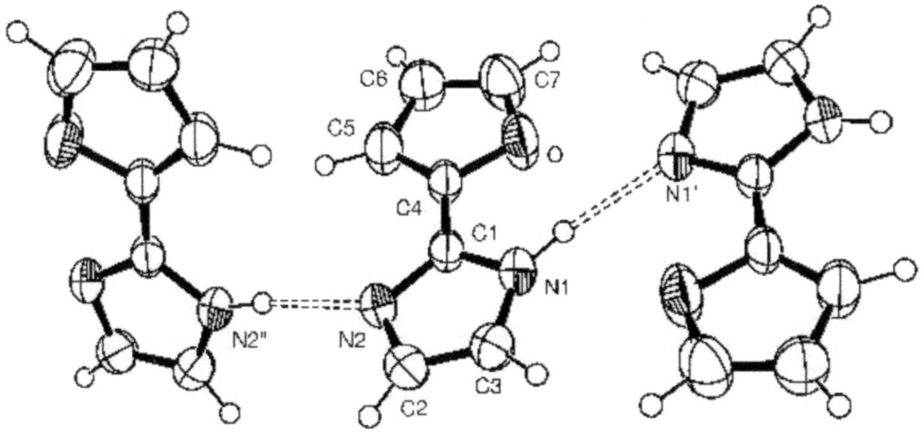

Unit 2 Unit 1 Unit 3

Fig. 2. View of a N—H---N bonded polymer chain in solid 2-(2′-furyl)-imidazole. The central monomer is related with the right and left side monomers through a crystallographic inversion center and a two fold axis rotation, respectively. The H-bonding is indicated by dashed lines

Table 1 shows a comparison of the total energy and dipole moment values for all molecules by using the 6-31 and 6-311++G** basis sets at B3LYP theory level. Note that all predicts values are similar between them and, only for the N-(2′-furyl)-imidazole, the calculation predicts that the anti conformation is the most stable, while that for the remaining compounds the syn conformation is the most stable.

The comparison between the experimental geometrical parameters (obtained for 2-(2′-furyl)-imidazole) with the corresponding theoretical values are shown in Table 2. The analysis shows that the length of C=C bond of the furan ring, does not change for all molecules, while the length of C=C bond of the imidazole ring varies according the following order: (4)5-(2′-furyl)-imidazole > N-(2′-furyl)-imidazole > 2-(2′-furyl)-imidazole. This trend is explained taking into account the next of this bond respect to the furan ring, since in the first molecule that bond is in alpha position respect to C=C bond corresponding to the furan ring, favoring the electronic delocalization, while in the remaining structures those bonds are in beta and gamma positions, respectively. This effect also explains the observed tendency for the C-N bond next to furan ring.

Conf.	*E* (B3LYP/6-31G*) (Hartrees)	*ΔE* kJ/mol	*μ*	E (B3LYP/6-311++G**) (Hartrees)	*ΔE* kJ/mol	*μ*
			N-(2′-furyl)-imidazole			
anti	-455.03903057	0	3.63	-455.16243953	0	3.82
syn	-455.03834901	1.8	3.80	-455.16160715	2.2	3.99
			2-(2′-furyl)-imidazole			
anti	-455.04955562	15.30	3.90	-455.17597057	15.42	4.08
syn	-455.05531501	0.0	2.97	-455.18185872	0.0	2.92
			4-(2′-furyl)-imidazole			
anti	-455.0490477	12.25	3.94	-455.1754201	12.54	4.10
syn	-455.0537122	0.0	3.23	-455.1802136	0.0	3.24
			5-(2′-furyl)-imidazole			
anti	-455.0512980	5.73	3.90	- 455.1772971	5.68	4.17
syn	-455.0534867	0.0	3.37	- 455.1794579	0.0	3.42

[a] In Debyes

Table 1. Total Energies (*E*) and relatives (*ΔE*) calculates (in Hartree), dipolar moments (*μ*) for all structures

Another very important difference between all series members is related to the dihedral angles. Thus, the angles values are 180° and 0° for the 2 and 4(5) isomers, while for the first isomer those values are between 30-40° and 160-170° respectively.

The stability of the different conformers were investigated using the Electrostatic Surface Potential, ESP maps[22,23] because these surfaces are important for describing overall molecular charge distributions as well as anticipating sites of electrophilic addition[23]. The molecular ESP values for the anti and syn conformers of each member's series by using 6-31G* basis set are given in Table 3 while Figure 3 shows the ESP maps for all conformers of this series. The red color represents negatively charged areas of the surface (i.e., those areas where accepting an electrophile is most favorable). The atomic charges derived from the ESPs (MK) and natural atomic charges were also analyzed and the corresponding values are given in Table 4. Note that the most important differences in all cases are observed on the imidazole ring. The important factor responsible for the lesser stability of same conformer is

[22] Sadlej-Sosnowska, 2007.
[23] Vektariene at al., 2007.

the electrostatic repulsion between the two lone pairs on N and O. Hence, a strong red color on both atoms is observed in the corresponding Figure 3.

Parameters	2-(2′-furyl)-Imidazole#	4-(2′-furyl)-Imidazole*		5-(2′-furyl)-Imidazole*		N-(2′-furyl)-Imidazole*	
Distances (Å)		*anti*	*syn*	*anti*	*syn*	*anti*	*syn*
$C{=}C_{furan}$	1.343 1.319	1.369 1.359	1.365 1.358	1.369 1.358	1.369 1.357	1.360 1.356	1.360 1.356
$C{=}C_{imidazole}$	1.345	1.379	1.377	1.380	1.380	1.367	1.367
C-N	1.374 1.369 1.342	1.382 1.377 1.366	1.383 1.378 1.366	1.385 1.373 1.367	1.385 1.372 1.366	1.380 1.379 1.390	1.380 1.379 1.392
C-C	1.413	1.429	1.432	1.431	1.431	1.435	1.435
C-O	1.362	1.361 1.364	1.365 1.370	1.365 1.367	1.364 1.367	1.370 1.359	1.372 1.360
C, $N{-}C_{inter\text{-}ring}$	1.438	1.450	1.445	1.439	1.439	1.392	1.389
Ángles (Degrees)							
N1-C2-N3	111.6 (2)	111.8	111.8	111.6	105.3	111.8	111.7
C2-N3-C4	105.6 (2)	105.5	105.3	105.6	111.8	105.6	105.7
N3-C4-C5	108.7 (2)	110.2	110.0	110.7	107.3	110.7	110.7
C4-C5-N1	108.4 (2)	105.1	110.8	104.6	104.4	105.3	105.4
C5-N1-C2	105.6 (2)	107.2	107.3	107.3	111.0	106.3	106.3
C6-C10-C11	107.1 (2)	106.6	106.4	106.4	106.5	105.6	105.5
C10-C11-C12	106.6(24)	106.0	106.0	106.2	106.2	106.5	106.6
C11-C12-O13	110.6(4)	110.5	110.6	110.3	110.4	110.0	111.1
C12-O13-C6	106.6(6)	107.3	106.9	107.3	107.2	106.5	106.6
O13-C6-C10	109.2 (2)	109.5	109.8	109.5	109.5	110.2	110.0

obtained by Ray X diffraction
* Theoretical parameters calculated at B3LYP/6-311++G** level of theory

Table 2. Geometrical parameters for all compounds of the series

Átom	N-(2′-furyl)-imidazole		2-(2′-furyl)-imidazole		4-(2′-furyl)-imidazole		5-(2′-furyl)-imidazole	
	anti	*syn*	*anti*	*syn*	*anti*	*syn*	*anti*	*syn*
N 1	-18.27	-18.26	-18.28	-18.28	-18.28	-18.28	-18.28	-18.28
C 2	-14.68	-14.68	-14.68	-14.67	-14.68	-14.68	-14.68	-14.68
N 3	-18.37	-18.37	-18.38	-18.38	-18.38	-18.37	-18.37	-18.37
C 4	-14.72	-14.72	-14.71	-14.72	-14.71	-14.71	-14.72	-14.72
C 5	-14.70	-14.70	-14.70	-14.71	-14.70	-14.70	-14.69	-14.69
H 6	-1.10	-1.10	-0.97	-0.98	-0.97	-0.97	-0.97	-0.98
C 7	-1.07	-1.08	-1.07	-1.10	-1.07	-1.07	-1.10	-1.10
H 8	-14.63	-14.63	-14.69	-14.68	-14.69	-14.69	-14.67	-14.67
H 9	-1.07	-1.07	-1.07	-1.07	-1.07	-1.07	-1.07	-1.07
C 10	-14.72	-14.72	-14.75	-14.74	-14.75	-14.75	-14.73	-14.73
C 11	-14.72	-14.72	-14.75	-14.73	-14.75	-14.75	-14.73	-14.73
C 12	-14.67	-14.67	-14.70	-14.68	-14.70	-14.70	-14.68	-14.68
O 13	-22.22	-22.22	-22.26	-22.24	-22.26	-22.25	-22.24	-22.23
H 14	-1.07	-1.07	-1.10	-1.09	-1.10	-1.11	-1.08	-1.08
H 15	-1.07	-1.07	-1.10	-1.09	-1.10	-1.10	-1.08	-1.08
H 16	-1.06	-1.06	-1.09	-1.07	-1.09	-1.08	-1.08	-1.07

Table 3. Molecular electrostatic potentials for all members of the series calculated at B3LYP/6-31G* level of theory

For the N-(2′-furyl)-imidazole a region can be observed where the delocalization of charge decrease (blue region between two rings) due to the breaking-off planarity of the both rings, while the remain molecules show π-electron delocalizated surfaces that evidence stables aromatic systems, being smaller for the N-(2′-furyl)-imidazole compound.

These results can be related with the energies of the HOMO and LUMO for all molecules. Table 4 shows the comparison of the HOMO and LUMO orbitals energies values as well as the GAP energies values of them.

The corresponding values for the N-(2′-furyl)-imidazole show that this compound is the most stable of the series, as expected, because it presents the longer GAP values. On the other hand, the calculated energy HOMO orbital value for 4-(2′-furyl)-imidazole is higher than the other ones due to the fact that it is the most reactive compound of this series.

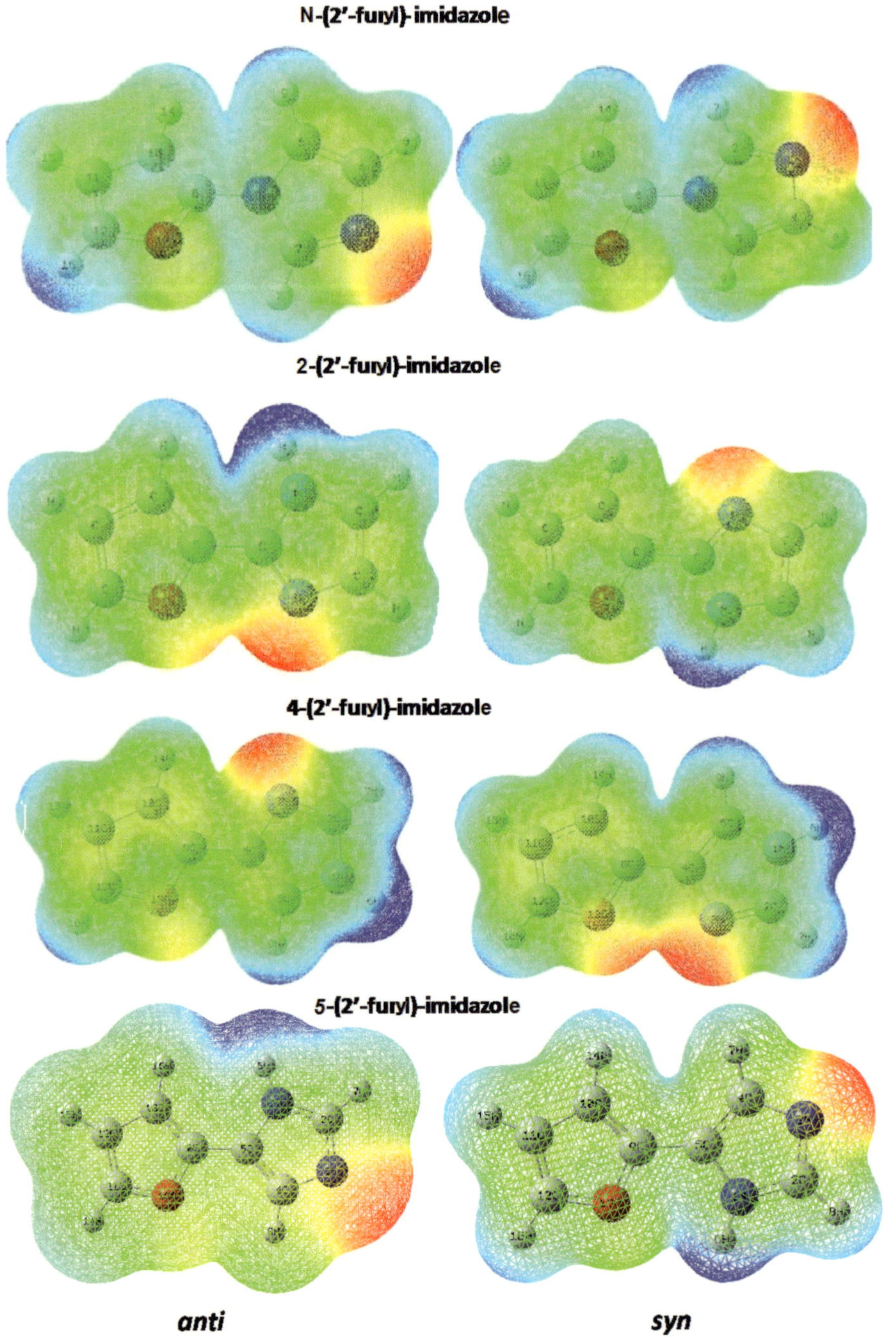

Fig. 3. Electrostatic Surface Potential calculated on the molecular surface of the conformers for all compounds of the series. Color, in u.a.: from red -0.103 to blue 0.103.

Orbital	N-(2′-furyl)-Imidazole		2-(2′-furyl)-Imidazole		4-(2′-furyl)-Imidazole		5-(2′-furyl)-Imidazole	
	syn	*anti*	*syn*	*anti*	*syn*	*anti*	*syn*	*anti*
HOMO	-0.21	-0.22	-0.19	-0.19	-0.18	-0.18	-0.19	-0.19
LUMO	-0.01	-0.01	-0.01	-0.01	0.00	0.00	-0-01	-0-01
GAP	0.20	0.20	0.17	0.17	0.18	0.18	0.17	0.17
GAP (kJ/mol)	535.0	542.9	464.2	464.2	495.4	495.4	466.8	466.8

Table 4. HOMO and LUMO orbitals Energíes (u.a.) and gap of energy (u.a.) for all members of the series

2.2 Nuclear magnetic resonance characterization

All nuclear magnetic resonance spectra were recorded for diluted solutions in DMSD-d_6 and the calculated chemical shifts of the ^1H NMR and ^{13}C NMR for the two conformers of each compound were obtained by GIAO method[24] using the B3LYP/6-311++G** theory level, as it is usually used for chemical shift NMR calculations on reasonably large molecules[25,26]. The calculations have been performed using the geometries optimized for this theory level and by using TMS as reference. A comparison of the results is present in Table 5 and it shows that for 2-(2′-furyl)-imidazole the calculated ^{13}C chemical shifts from CSGT method are in accordance with the experimental values, while the closest values were obtained with the GIAO method and the 6-311++G** basis set. Furthermore, the calculated shifts with both methods for the C(2), C(7), and C(1) atoms are higher than the experimental values. One important observation is that the results obtained from the conformational average have better agreement with data experimental, as expected, due to the presence of the two conformers in the solution. On the other hand, a comparison is present in Table 6 and it shows the calculated shifts with the two methods used where, for the H atom show significant differences with the experimental results. The addition of the polarization and diffuses functions at the basis set improves the results; however, the CSGT method predicts shifts practically different than the GIAO method for this atom. This disparity would be attributed to the fact that the GIAO method uses basis functions which depend on the field while the CSGT method achieves gauge invariance by performing a continuous set of gauge transformations, for each point, obtaining an accurately description of the current density[17,18].

The peak belonging to H atom of the N–H bond appears at 11.37 ppm. A small shift of these peaks towards lower fields implies the existence of some intermolecular interaction between nonbonding electrons.

Table 7 shows the experimental and calculated chemical shifts for 4(5)-(2′-furyl)-imidazole. These chemical shift values indicate that in the H atom is weakly held by two imidazole rings. At an intermediate rate of exchange, the H atom is partially decoupled, and a broad

[24] Ditchfield, 1974.

[25] Cheeseman et al., 1996.

[26] Keith & Bader, 1993.

N-H peak results. The most intense peak of this spectrum belongs to the C atom of the reference, while the following four peaks belong to the C atoms of the furyl group. The calculated chemical shifts are in agreement with the experimental ones, with RMSD values of 2.53 and 0.32 ppm for the ^{13}C and ^{1}H atoms, respectively. The agreement with our experimental data in these solvents is good, except for the H atom of the H-N bond in chloroform. This is because the calculations are for the gas phase, while the experimental values are for the $CDCl_3$ solution, where the molecular interactions are important. It is important to mention that the registered NMR spectra at room temperature and low temperature were not sufficient to identify the tautomeric mixture of 1, because the speed of exchange of protons is higher than the response time of NMR.

Chem. Shift	C(10)	C(11)	C(5)	C(12)	C(2)	C(4)	C(7)
Exp.[a]	106.4	111.6	122.5	122.5	138.0	142.5	146.2
syn [b]	93.9	100.7	102.8	119.7	126.4	129.6	135.5
[c]	99.2	104.1	107.9	123.6	132.0	135.3	141.3
[d]	103.8	111.4	113.4	132.6	141.0	143.8	135.9
anti [b]	97.5	102.5	102.6	119.6	126.7	127.9	136.4
[c]	102.3	105.7	107.9	123.7	132.3	134.1	142.4
[d]	107.8	113.6	113.5	132.9	141.3	142.1	151.5
AVERAGE[b]	98.7	101.6	102.7	119.7	126.6	128.7	135.9
[c]	100.8	104.9	107.9	123.9	132.1	134.7	141.8
[d]	105.8	112.5	113.5	138.8	141.1	142.9	151.0

[#] In DMSO-d_6; [##]Related to TMS; [a] Experimental; [b] GIAO 6-31G**; [c] CSGT 6-31G**; [d] GIAO 6-311++G**

Table 5. Experimental[#] and calculated[##] ^{13}C chemical shifts in ppm

Chem. shifts	H C(10)	H C(11)	H C(12)	H C(4)	H C(5)
Exp.[a]	6.57	6.82	6.82	7.10	7.71
syn [b]	6.02	6.09	7.16	6.50	6.87
[c]	3.60	3.79	4.74	4.10	4.38
[d]	6.26	6.70	7.37	6.70	7.05
anti [b]	6.70	6.16	7.05	6.47	6.85
[c]	3.88	4.30	4.66	4.12	4.33
[d]	3.92	6.38	7.25	6.70	7.03
AVERAGE[B]	6.36	6.12	7.10	6.49	6.86
[c]	3.74	4.04	7.70	4.11	4.35
[d]	5.09	6.32	7.31	6.70	7.04

[#] In DMSO-d_6; [##]Related to TMS; [a] Experimental; [b] GIAO 6-31G**; [c] CSGT 6-31G**; [d] GIAO 6-311++G**

Table 6. The experimental and calculated ^{1}H chemical shifts in ppm

Position	δ C		δ H, multiplicidad in ppm	
	Exp.[b]	Theor[c]	Exp.[b]	Theor[c]
10	104.3	103.55	6.54 (d, J=3.3 Hz, 1H)	6.29
11	111.3	108.82	6.43 (dd, J=1.8, J=3.3 Hz, 1H)	6.17
5	114.7	111.03	7.33 (d, J=0.9 Hz, 1H)	6.98
4	131.6	132.40		
12	135.6	138.1	7.71 (d, J=0.9 Hz, 1H)	7.26
2	141.2	141.35	7.39 (dd, J=0.9, J=1.5 Hz, 1H)	7.16
8	149.0	153.20		
N-H			11.37 (bs,1H)	7.86

[a] B3LYP/6-311++G**, average values; [b] In $CDCl_3$; [c] Related to TMS

Table 7. Experimental and calculated Chemical shifts (in ppm) for 4(5)-(2'-furyl)-imidazole

A comparison between the experimental and calculated chemical shifts for the C and H atoms for N-(2'-furyl)-imidazole are given in Tables 8 and 9, respectively. The calculation results show that the GIAO method reproduces quite well the ^{13}C and ^{1}H experimental chemical shifts values as shown by the calculated root mean square deviations (RMSD) values for each conformer. Furthermore, the shifts of the H atoms for both structures are similar in both conformers and practically equal to the average values. As expected, the latter values have a better agreement with the experimental data, probably because both conformers are present in the solution.

Chem. Shifts	C10	C11	C5	C4	C12	C2	C6	RMSD
Exp.[a]	96.2	111.6	117.5	130.0	135.4	138.9	144.5	
anti [b]	96.5	112.7	117.7	133.2	135.4	140.4	149.5	*0.9*
syn [b]	93.6	112.7	116.1	132.9	134.7	139.1	149.7	*0.9*
AVERAGE[B]	95.0	112.7	116.9	133.1	135.0	139.7	149.6	*0.9*

[a] Related to $DCCl_3$; [b] GIAO, B3LYP/6-311++G*

Table 8. ^{13}C Experimental and calculated Chemical shifts (in ppm) for N-(2'-furyl)-imidazole

Chem. Shifts	H14	H15	H8	H9	H16	H7	RMSD
Exp.[a]	**6.14**	**6.44**	**7.13**	**7.22**	**7.26**	**7.81**	
anti [b]	5.87	6.29	7.05	7.05	7.16	7.30	*0.10*
syn [b]	5.73	6.28	6.81	7.01	7.08	7.62	*0.10*
AVERAGE[B]	5.80	6.29	6.93	7.03	7.12	7.46	*0.09*

[a] Related to $DCCl_3$; [b] GIAO, B3LYP/6-311++G*

Table 9. ^{1}H Experimental and calculated Chemical shifts (in ppm) for N-(2'-furyl)-imidazole

3. Vibrational analysis

For this analysis the vibrational frequencies were separated in two groups, the first group corresponds to the skeletal vibrations ring and the second ones to those vibrations related to the C-H groups, both are show in Tables 10 and 11, respectively. The analysis shows that the frequencies values for the C=C stretching of the imidazole ring is according to the respective length bonds. Furthermore, the frequencies values for the C=N stretching mode are longer for the N-(2′-furyl)-Imidazole, due to the highest p character of bound, which impedes the resonance effects between two rings. Changes in the frequencies values related to the C-O stretching modes are not observed, in accordance with the corresponding length bonds, where the variations were only observed for the imidazole ring. The vibrational ring modes are practically observed in the same region for all series molecules, while the corresponding torsions are in agreement with the imidazole ring in all series members and they are next to the reported values for the imidazole compound.

Description	N-(2′-furyl)-Imidazole	2-(2′-furyl)-Imidazole	4-(2′-furyl)-Imidazole	5-(2′-furyl)-Imidazole
	anti, syn	*anti, syn*		
ν $(C=C)_{furano}$	1625 1511	1625 1504	1638 1467	1638 1491
ν $(C=C)_{imidazol}$	1521	1547, 1538	1516	1518
ν (C=N)	1493	1462,1453	1484	1484
ν (C-N)	1305, 1285 1224 1104	1428, 1393 1365, 1358 1159, 1133	1304 1275 1120	1307 1342 1119
ν (C-C)	1374	1380	1378	1342
ν (C-O)	1162 1065	1181 1075	1162 1067	1162 1067
βR_f	904 892	897 894	885 868	885 868
βR_i	984 910	965,952 927,911	942 916	964 918
τR_i	656 650	665 650	685 655	655 634
τR_f	615 594	624,622 593,591	621 591	624 591
ν $(C, N\text{-}C)_{int}$	409	402	404	404

Table 10. Experimental Vibrational Frequencies for all modes of imidazole and furan rings of the series.

A notable difference between the frequencies of the C-H stretching modes is observed. The rotating of the imidazole ring with the furan ring increase or decrease the frequencies assigned to the alilic hydrogen.

Description	N-(2′-furyl)-imidazole	2-(2′-furyl)-imidazole	4-(2′-furyl)-imidazole	5-(2′-furyl)-imidazole
	anti, syn	*anti, syn*		
ν C-H	3155			
	3151	3149	3137	3137
	3126	3118	3122	3120
	3122	3109	3101	3101
	3120	3088	3081	3081
	3104	3011	3037	3037
Β C-H	1410			
	1348	1300,1260	1225	1251
	1245	1229,1222	1204	1235
	1112	1106,1102	1081	1204
	1059	1084	1050	1081
	1014	1010	1006	1006
γ C-H	882			
	871	883,862	830	865
	816	843,835	813	813
	793	810,797	800	800
	737	748,733	750	776
	733	719	715	725

Table 11. Experimental vibrational frequencies for C-H groups

4. Conclusions

All compounds studied in this chapter were synthesized and only, the 2-(2'-furyl)-1H-imidazole compound was isolated as a crystalline solid, which allowed the molecular structure's determination by means of the ray X diffraction. In all cases, the theoretical method that better reproduces the experimental data is the B3LYP/6-311++G** combination, for this, the calculated molecular geometries and vibrational spectra were performed at this theory level. Each molecule presents two stable conformations, anti and syn, according to the orientations of the furan and imidazole rings. The calculations predicted that the conformation syn is the most stable, with exception of the isomer one, for which the anti conformer was the most stable. The distances among both rings only present appreciable changes for the isomer one which because the union in this case is by means of the C-N instead C-C like in the remaining ones. In the 4(5)-(2'-Furyl) Imidazole isomers, the infrared spectra at low temperature allowed the complete assignment of the both member's series. The PEM analysis shows that when the π-electron delocalizated surface is longer, the hydrogen atoms are less retained by the carbon atoms and, for this reason, an increasing in the respective length bonds is observed. Due to this, the H atom is very labile in consequence can be easily substituted. The later behavior is observed when the frequencies of the C-H groups in the N-(2'-Furyl)-imidazole are analyzed in reference to the other compounds of this series. Finally, the N-(2'-Furyl)-imidazole compound is the most stable member of the series.

5. References

[1] Salerno, A. ; Perillo, I. A., ^{1}H- and ^{13}C-NMR Analysis of a Series of 1,2-Diaryl-1H-4,5-dihydroimidazoles, 2005, *Molecules*, Vol 10, N° 2 (Febrary 2005), pp 435–443, ISSN: 1420-3049

[2] Szabo, B., Imidazoline antihypertensive drugs: a critical review on their mechanism of action, 2002, *Pharmacol. Therapeut.* Vol 93, N° 1 (January 2002) , pp. 1-35(35). ISSN: 0163 -7258

[3] Gould, S. L.; Kodis, G.; Liddell, P. A.; Palacios, R. E.; Brune, A.; Gust, D.; Moore, T. A; Moore, A. L., Artificial photosynthetic reaction centers with carotenoid antennas, *Tetrahedron* 2006, Vol 62, N° 9 (February 2006), pp 2074-2096. ISSN: 0040-4020

[4] Higashio, Y.; Shoji, T.; Erratum to "Heterocyclic compounds such as pyrrole, pyridines, piperidine, indole, imidazol and pyrazines" [Appl. Catal. A: Gen. 221 (2001) 197–207], *Applied Catalysis A: General* 2004, Vol 260, N° 2 (March 2004), pp 249-251. ISSN: 0926-860X

[5] Monterrey I. G.; Campiglia, P.; Lama, T.; La Colla, P.; Diurno, M. V.; Grieco, P.; Novellino, Synthesis of new pyrido [4,3- g and 3,4- g]quinoline-9,10-dione and dihydrothieno [2,3-g and 3,2-g]quinoline-4,9-dione derivatives and preliminary evaluation of cytotoxic activity, *E. Arkivoc* 2004 (v) 85 (February 2004), pp 85 - 96. ISSN: 1551-7004

[6] Ooyama, Y.; Mamura, T.; Yoshida, K., A facile synthesis of solid-emissive fluorescent dyes: dialkylbenzo[b]naphtho[2,1-d]furan-6-one-type fluorophores with strong blue and green fluorescence emission properties, *Tetrahedron Lett.* 2007, Vol 48 (June 2007), pp 5791-5793. ISSN: 0040-4039

[7] Rohwerder, M.; Michalik, A., Conducting polymers for corrosion protection: What makes the difference between failure and success?, *Electrochimica Acta.* 2007, Vol 53, N°20 (December 2007), pp 1300-1313. ISSN: 0013-4686

[8] Stroganova, T. A.; Butin, A. V.; Sorotskaya, J. N.; Kul'nevich, V. G., (Aryl)(2-furyl)alkanes and their derivatives, 20. Synthesis of symmetric bis- and tris(2-furyl)methanes, *E. Arkivoc 2000* (iv), 1, (September 2000), pp 641 - 659. ISSN 1551-7012.

[9] Nevin K.; Dilek E.; Pervin U. C., Synthesis and characterization of novel heterosubstituted pyrroles, thiophenes, and furans, *E. Arkivoc 2008* (xii) (March 2008), pp 17-29. ISSN 1551-7012.

[10] Bellina, F.; Cauteruccio, S.; Rossi, R., Efficient and Practical Synthesis of 4(5)-Aryl-1H-imidazoles and 2,4(5)-Diaryl-1H-imidazoles via Highly Selective Palladium-Catalyzed Arylation Reactions, 2007, *J. Org. Chem.*, Vol 72, N° 22 (October 2007), pp 8543–8546. ISSN: 0022- 3263

[11] Popov, S. A.; Andreev, R. V.; Romanenko, G. V.; Ovcharenko, V. I.; Reznikov, V. A., Aminonitrone-N-hydroxyaminoimine Tautomeric Equilibrium in the Series of 1-

Hydroxy-2-imidazolines, 2004, *J.Mol. Struct.*, Vol 697, N° 1–3 (April 2004), pp 49-60. ISSN: 0022-2860

[12] Sztanke, K.; Fidecka, S.; dzierska, E. K; Karczmarzyk, Z.; Pihlaja, K.; Matosiuk, D., 2005, *Eur. J.Med. Chem., Vol* 40, N° 2, pp 127. ISSN: 0223- 5234

[13] Ledesma, A. E.; Brandán, S. A.; Zinczuk, J.; Piro, O. E.; López González, J. J.; Ben Altabef, A., 2008, Structural and vibrational study of 2-(2'-furyl)-1H- imidazole, *J. Phys. Org. Chem.*, Vol 21, N° 12 (December 2008), pp 1086–1097, ISSN: 1099-1395

[14] Ledesma, A. E.; Zinczuk, J.; López González, J. J.; Ben Altabef, A.; Brandán, S. A., Structural, vibrational spectra and normal coordinate analysis for two tautomers of 4(5)-(2'-furyl)-imidazole, *J. Raman Spectrosc.*, 2010, Vol 41, N°5 (Mayo 2010), pp 587–597, ISSN: 1097-4555

[15] Ledesma A. E.; Zinczuk, J.; López González, J. J.; Ben Altabef, A.; Brandán, S. A., Synthesis and vibrational analysis of N-(2'-Furyl)-Imidazole, *J. Raman Spectrosc.*, 2009, Vol 40, N°8 (August 2009), pp. 1004–1010, ISSN: 1097-4555

[16] Ledesma, A. E.; Zinczuk, J.; López González, J. J. ; Ben Altabef, A.; Brandán, S. A., Structural and vibrational study of 4-(2'-furyl)-1-methylimidazole *J. of Molecular Structure*, 2009, Vol 924–926 (April 2009), pp 322–331, ISSN: 0022-2860

[17] Zinczuk, J.; Ledesma, A. E.; Brandán, S. A.; Piro, O. E.; López-González, J. J.; Ben Altabef, A., Structural and vibrational study of 2-(2'- furyl)-4,5-1H-dihydroimidazole, *J. Phys. Org. Chem.*, 2009, Vol 21 (April 2010), pp 1–12, ISSN: 1099-1395.

[18] Jones, R. A.; Civcir, P. U. Extended Heterocyclic Systems 2. The Synthesis and Characterisation of (2-Furyl)pyridines, (2-Thienyl)pyridines, and Furan-Pyridine and Thiophene-Pyridine Oligomers, Tetrahedron 1997, Vol 53, N° 34 (August 1997), pp 11529- 11540. ISSN: 0040- 4020

[19] Rauhut, G.; Pulay, P., Transferable Scaling Factors for Density Functional Derived Vibrational Force Fields, *J. Phys. Chem.* 1995, Vol 99, N°10 (March 1995), pp 3093-31100. ISSN: 1089-5639

[20] Rauhut, G.; Pulay, P., Transferable Scaling Factors for Density Functional Derived Vibrational Force Fields. [Erratum to document cited in CA122:199802], *J. Phys. Chem.* 1995, Vol 99, N° 39 (September 1995), pp 14572. ISSN: 1089-5639

[21] Kalincsak, F.; Pongor, G., Extension of the density functional derived scaled quantum mechanical force field procedure, *Spectrochim. Acta A* 2002, Vol 58, N° 5 (March 2002), pp 999- 1011(13), ISSN: 1386-1425

[22] Sadlej-Sosnowska, N., Molecular Similarity Based on Atomic Electrostatic Potential, *J. Phys. Chem. A*, 2007, Vol 111, N° 43 (October 2007), pp 11134–11140. ISSN: 1089-5639

[23] Vektariene, A. ; Vektaris, G.; Svoboda, J., 11th *International Electronic Conference on Synthetic Organic Chemistry* (ECSOC-11), 2007.

[24] Ditchfield, R., Self-consistent perturbation theory of diamagnetism, *Mol. Phys.*, 1974, Vol 27, N°4 pp 789- 807. ISSN: 00268976

[25] Cheeseman, J.; Trucks, G. ; Keith, T.; Frisch, M., A comparison of models for calculating nuclear magnetic resonance shielding tensors, *J. Chem. Phys.*, 1996, Vol 104, N°14 (April 1996), pp 5497–5509. ISSN: 1089-5639

[26] Keith, T. A.; Bader, R. F. W., Calculation of magnetic response properties using a continuous set of gauge transformations, *Chem. Phys.*, 1993, Vol 210, N°1-3 (May 1993), pp 223–231. ISSN: 0301-0104

10

NMR Spectroscopy: A Useful Tool in the Determination of the Electrophilic Character of Benzofuroxans - Case Examples of the Reactions of Nitrobenzofuroxans with Dienes and Nucleophiles

M. Sebban, P. Sepulcri, C. Jovene, D. Vichard, F. Terrier and R. Goumont*

University of Versailles, ILV (Institut lavoisier de Versailles)

France

1. Introduction

2,1,3-Benzoxadiazoles **1** and related 1-oxides **2**, commonly referred to as benzofurazans and benzofuroxans, respectively are heteroaromatic 10π-electron ring systems whose carbocyclic ring is intrinsically very susceptible to nucleophilic attack.[1-9] Most importantly, the introduction of a NO_2 group at C-4 enhances the electrophilic reactivity of this ring by several orders of magnitude, making it comparable to that of a trinitro substituted benzene ring. This property has raised considerable interest in the 1970-1980's, mostly in connection with the recognition that the ease of covalent nucleophilic addition to the carbocyclic ring is responsible for the inhibitory effect exerted by some mononitrobenzofurazans and -benzofuroxans on the biosynthesis of nucleic acid and protein in leucocytes, and the observed activity against leukaemia. Also much attention was directed to the S_NAr reactivity of compounds like 4-chloro- and 4-fluoro-7-nitrobenzofurazans (**3-4**) which have become commonly used as fluorogenic reagents for detection and quantification of amino and thiol residues on proteins, drugs and biologically active molecules.

In the last decades, we have been engaged in an effort to investigate the reactivity of strongly electrophilic aromatic and heteroaromatic substitutions and related σ-complex processes. In this context, we discovered that some appropriate substitutions of the carbocyclic ring of benzofurazan and benzofuroxan structures enhance so much the electron-deficiency of this ring that the resulting compounds can be reasonably ranked as superelectrophilic heteroaromatics. Referring meanly to the readily accessible prototype substrates, namely 4,6-dinitrobenzofuroxan (DNBF, **A**), this review will highlight this behaviour which has proved to be very useful to assess the nucleophilic reactivity of extremely weak carbon base. In the same context, some remarkable reactivity sequences deriving from an aza substitution of the carbocyclic ring or a change in the nature of the annelated ring will be also emphasized with a particular focus on the behaviour of this extremely electrophilic substrates, namely 6-nitro [2,1,3] oxadiazolo [4, 5-b] pyridine 1-oxide,

* Corresponding Author

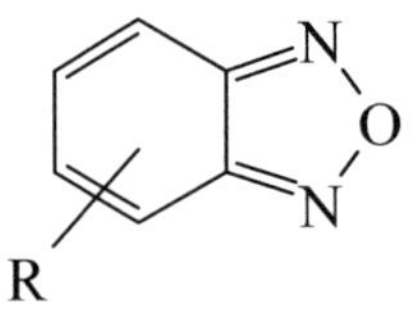

1

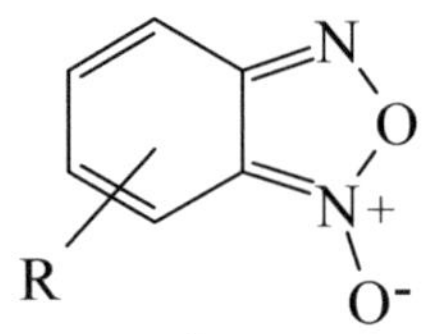

2

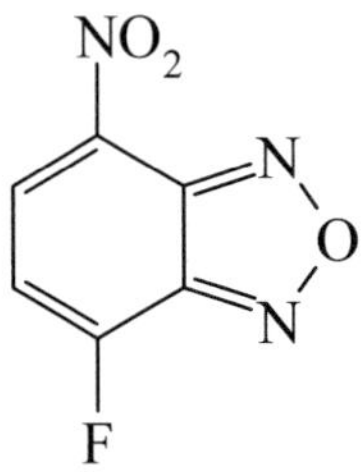

3

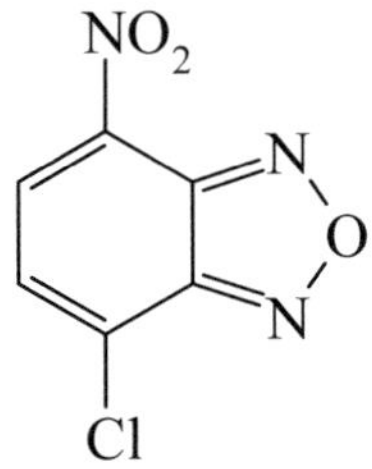

4

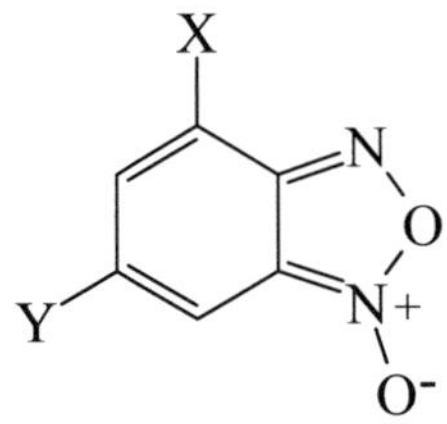

A $X = Y = NO_2$ (DNBF)
B $X = NO_2, Y = CF_3$
C $X = NO_2, Y = CN$
D $X = NO_2, Y = SO_2CF_3$
E $X = CF_3, Y = NO_2$
F $X = CN, Y = NO_2$
G $X = SO_2CF_3, Y = NO_2$

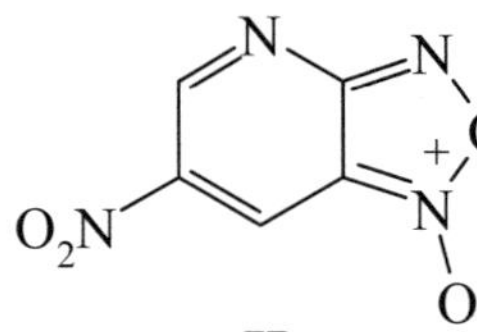

H

i.e. the 4-aza-6-nitro analogue of DNBF (ANBF, **H**). We demonstrated that highly electrophilic benzofuroxans, benzofurazans and related heteroaromatic substrates have also the potential to react in a variety of pericyclic patterns being able to contribute as dienophiles, heterodienes or carbodienes depending upon the experimental conditions and the reaction patterns at hand. Recently, it has been convincingly recognized that the exceptional electrophilic character of nitrobenzofuroxans is closely related to the low aromaticity of the carbocyclic ring. Crucial evidence for this relationship has been the discovery that the nitro-activated double bonds of this ring behave similarly to nitroalkene fragments in a variety of Diels-Alder processes, acting as dienophiles or heterodienes depending upon the reaction partner and the experimental conditions at hand.[10-16] A first illustrative sequence refers to the reaction of ANBF with cyclohexadiene. Reflecting the potential 1-oxide/3-oxide interconversion of benzofuroxans through the intermediacy of an *o*-dinitroso intermediate,[15] diadducts **5** resulting from normal electron-demand Diels-Alder (NEDDA) processes involving the N=O double bonds of such intermediates as the dienophile contributors have also been isolated. Treatment of ANBF with cyclohexadiene in $CHCl_3$ affords a 2:1 mixture of two products which were readily separated by column chromatography and isolated as pale yellow solids. The ORTEP view in Scheme 1 leaves no doubt that the major product is the diadduct **5** whose formation can only be accounted for in terms of two NEDDA processes in which the N=O double bonds of the *o*-dinitroso intermediate **6** play the role of the dienophiles contributors (Scheme 1). In view of the ^{1}H and ^{13}C NMR spectra, the minor product can be formulated as the cycloadducts **7**, which results from a regioselective and diastereoselective NEDDA process involving the C6-C7 double bond of **H**.

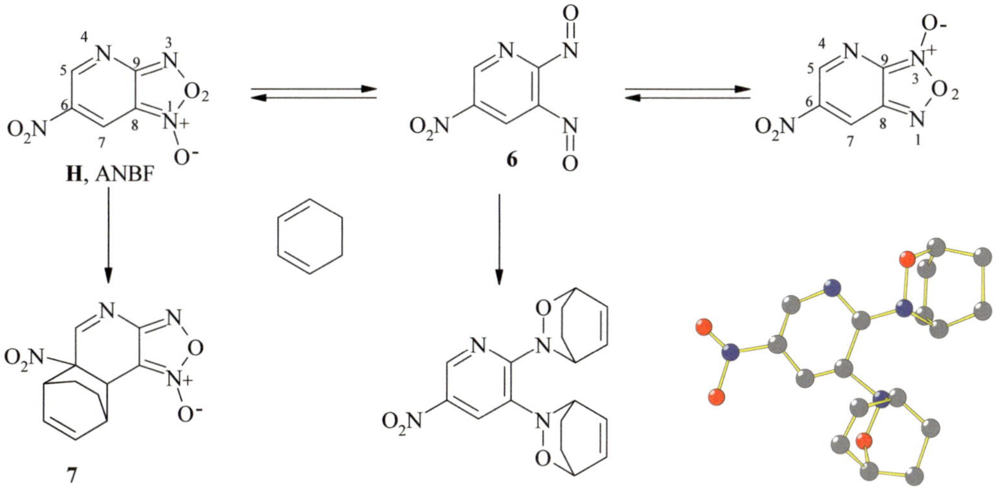

Scheme 1. Diels-Alder Trapping of the o-dinitroso intermediate **6**.

Some selected interactions will be presented in the first part of this review to illustrate that versatile and synthetically very promising Diels-Alder reactivity. It will be shown that NMR is a useful tool to determine the regioselectivity and the stereochemistry of the pericyclic processes. In many cases, the finding of characteristic couplings and/or signals with typical chemical shifts allows a fast determination of the regioselectivity of the Diels-Alder reactions. A short discussion of the NMR chemical shifts of the starting neutral materials (**A-H**) will show the influence of the substituent and of the position of this substituent on the chemical shifts. In some cases, ^{15}N labelling of nitro group has been used to determine unambiguously chemical assignments.

The considerable interest in the study of the high susceptibility of nitrobenzofuroxans to undergo covalent addition or substitution processes has led to a numerous synthetic, analytical and biological applications. A prototype example of this behaviour are the facile carbon-carbon coupling reactions of 4,6-dinitrobenzofuroxan (DNBF, **A**) - the reference compound in the series - with a number of benzenoid aromatics (phenols, anilines) or π-excessive heteroaromatics (pyrroles, indoles, thiophenes...) whose carbon basicities are associated with large negative pk_a values. In all of these reactions, covalent addition takes place at C-7 of the carbocyclic ring of DNBF to give stable σ-adducts of type **8** or **9**. Quantitative evaluation of thermodynamic reactivity is afforded from a comparison of pK_a values for H_2O addition to yield the respective σ-complexes, for example **C-A,OH**.

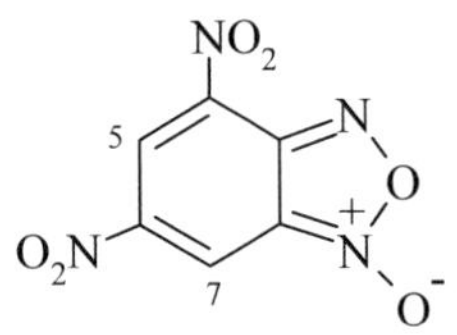

DNBF, **A**

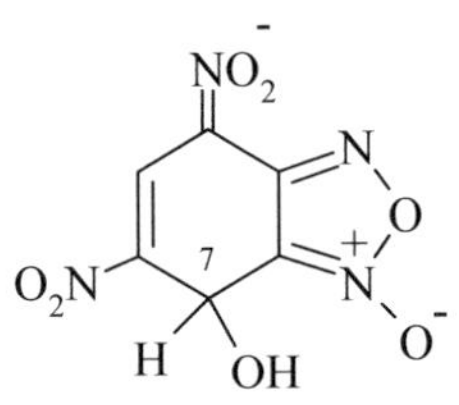

C-A,OH

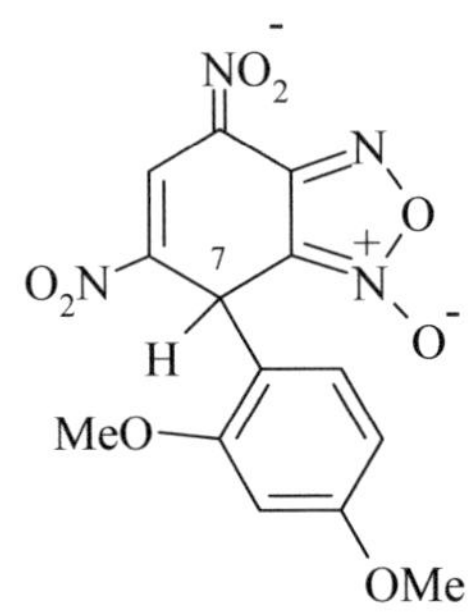

8

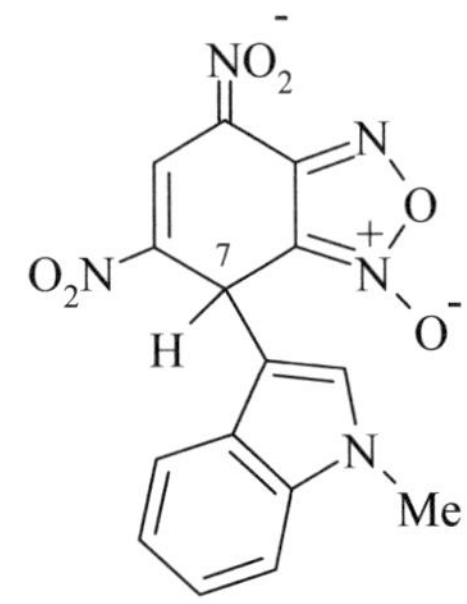

9

Thus the $pK_a^{H_2O}$ value for hydration of 4,6-dinitrobenzofuroxan (DNBF) according to (eq. 1) is equal to 3.75 in water, as compared with a $pK_a^{H_2O}$ value of 13.43 for hydration of TNB (eq. 2). It is this large difference in the thermodynamic ease of σ-complexation of DNBF and TNB, which has been the starting point for the discovery of a superelectrophilic dimension in the field of σ-complexation processes. On this basis, DNBF **A** and some related derivatives (**B-H**) have been termed superelectrophiles.[1,2]

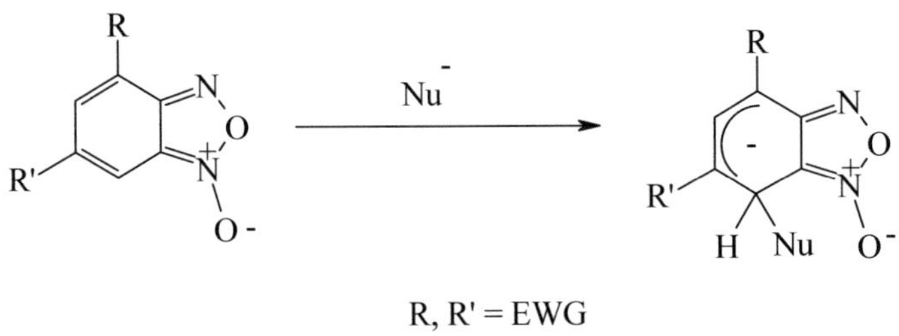

(1)

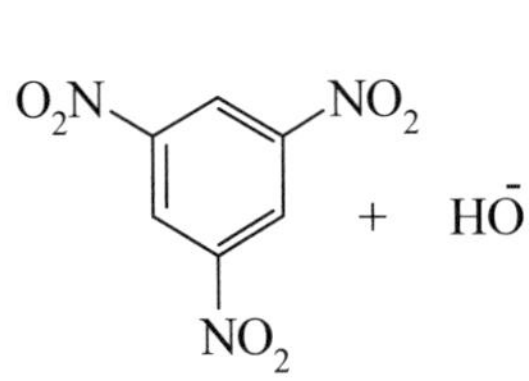

TNB

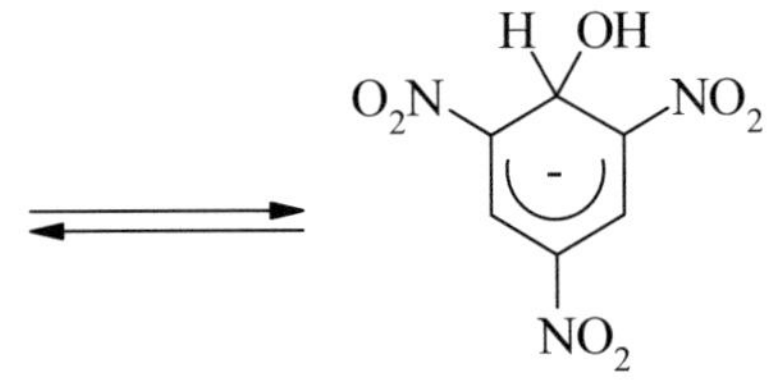

TNB,OH

(2)

The second part of this review will be closely related to the structure of σ-complexes and to the role of the various substituents in the stabilization of the negative charge. Interestingly, their inductive or mesomeric effect will be discussed in terms of NMR chemical shifts. Indeed, the variation of the chemical shift on going from the starting neutral materials (**A-H**) to the σ-complexes is a nice reflection of the electron-withdrawing effect of the substituent (eq. 3, EWG = electron-withdrawing group). The special case of the trifluoromethanesulfonyl (SO_2CF_3) group will be extensively discussed.

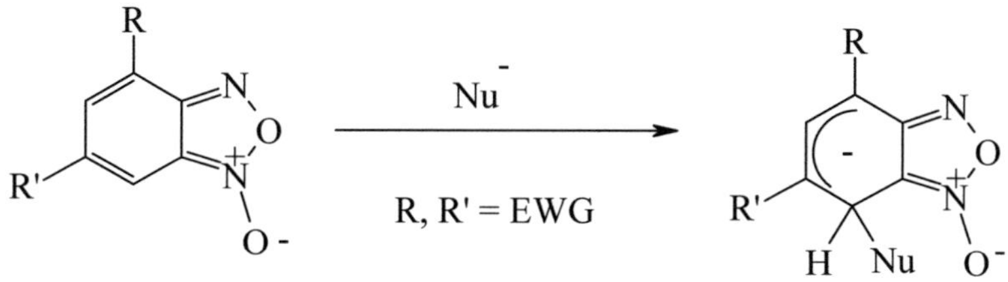

(3)

2. NMR investigation of substituted benzofuroxans and benzofurazans

The ^{1}H NMR spectra of these heterocycles are characterized by two deshielded protons at around 9 ppm. The signals of these two protons are, in the most cases, doublets with a coupling constant from 1Hz to 2 Hz, depending of the position and of the nature of the substituent (see Table 1). Interestingly, the signal of H_7 is at lower field than that of H_5. But it has to be noticed that the position of these signals are largely dependent of the solvent and unambiguous attributions can be performed using ^{15}N labelling of nitro groups as it was the case for DNBF (**A**).[17] The ^{1}H spectrum of DNBF (**A**) shows the H_A and H_X doublets of the AX system at 9.27 and 8.94 ppm, respectively, in dimethylsulfoxide (DMSO, J_{AX} = 1.9 Hz). On ^{15}N labelling of the 6-NO_2 group, the H_A and H_X resonances show coupling with the nitrogen atom and coupling constant may be readily determined from the spectra (J_{N6HA} = 2.4 Hz and J_{N6HX} = 1.6Hz). On further ^{15}N labelling at the 4-NO_2 group, the H_A resonance remains unaffected while that of H_X undergoes an additional splitting: J_{N4HX} = 2.9 Hz. These observations show unambiguously that H_A is H_7 and H_X is H_5 in DMSO. Similar experiments have been carried out in various solvents (Table 2). In THF and acetone, it is the high field resonance of the observed AX or AB patterns, respectively, that is split on the ^{15}N-labelling of the 4-NO_2 group. That indicates a sequence of the H_5 and H_7 resonances in these solvents that is the same as that found in DMSO. In contrast, it is the H_A resonances that is affected by labelling the 4-NO_2 group in nitromethane, methylene chloride, chloroform, benzene and acetonitrile. This shows that the low field doublet of the AX (or AB) system is ascribable to H_5 in these solvents. A particular situation is found in methanol where the two protons have quite identical chemical shifts.

Compounds	**H_5**	**H_7**	**CF_3***	**Coupling constants (Hz)**
A (DNBF)	8.94	9.27	-	$^4J_{5/7}$ = 1.9
B	8.74	8.87	-61.4	$^4J_{5/7}$ = $^4J_{5/F}$ 1.2
C	8.92	9.10	-	-
D	8.60	9.40	-76.2	-
E	8.70	9.07	-61.7	$^4J_{5/F}$ = 1.1
F	9.03	9.11	-	$^4J_{5/7}$ = 1.5
G	8.70	9.21	-76.9	$^4J_{5/7}$ = 1.8

*Internal reference: $CFCl_3$

Table 1. ^{1}H NMR data for the Benzofuroxans **A-G** (DMSO-d6)

solvent	H_5	H_7
DMSO	8.94	9.27
THF	9.04	9.16
Acetone	9.11	9.14
Methanol	9.07	9.07
Nitromethane	9.14	8.96
Acetonitrile	8.98	8.90
Methylene chloride	9.13	8.86
chloroform	9.12	8.82
benzene	8.08	7.29

Table 2. Solvent effect on ^{1}H NMR data for ^{15}N labelled DNBF

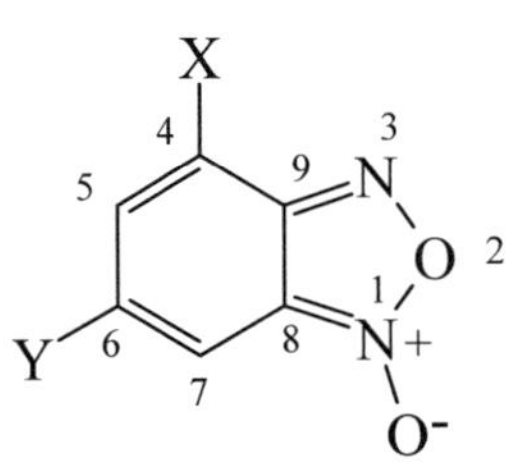

A X = Y = NO_2 (DNBF)
B X = NO_2, Y = CF_3
C X = NO_2, Y = CN
D X = NO_2, Y = SO_2CF_3
E X = CF_3, Y = NO_2
F X = CN, Y = NO_2
G X = SO_2CF_3, Y = NO_2

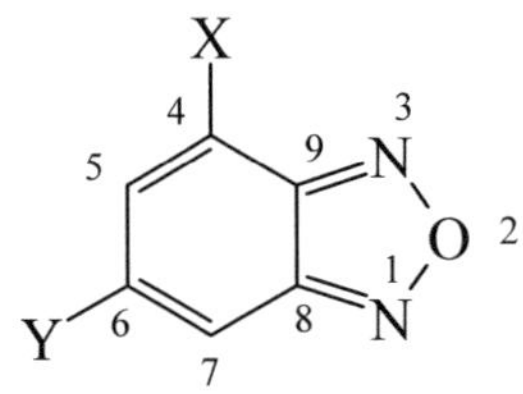

I X = Y = NO_2 (DNBZ)
J X = NO_2, Y = CF_3
K X = NO_2, Y = CN
L X = NO_2, Y = SO_2CF_3
M X = CF_3, Y = NO_2
N X = CN, Y = NO_2

The ^{13}C NMR spectra of benzofuroxans **A-F** show some characteristic features. The complete ^{13}C NMR assignment of these compounds has been obtained using one- and two-dimensional NMR techniques including HMQC and HMBC experiments. So, the two resonances pertaining to C_5 and C_7 are readily determined while the resonances of the C_9 and C_8 appear to be the key features of the ^{13}C NMR spectra of benzofuroxans. With chemical shift of 145 and 115 ppm, respectively, the signals of C_9 and C_8 are quite independent of the position and of the nature of the substituent (see Table 3). The position of the signal pertaining to C_8 with compare to that of C_9 could be explained by the mesomeric effect of the N-oxide functionality.[17-18]

This substituent effect has been attributed to the presence of a partial negative charge on C_8 resulting from a significant contribution of the second resonance form described in Scheme 2, while C_9, more distant from the N-oxide function, remains unaffected or only slightly affected.

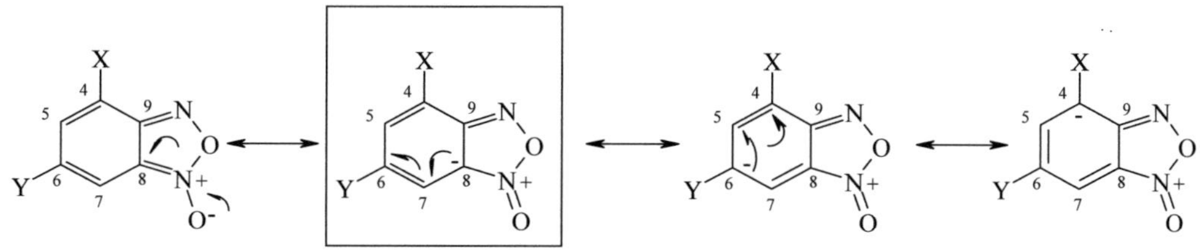

Scheme 2. Resonance forms of substituted benzofuroxans.

Compounds	C_4	C_5	C_6	C_7	C_8	C_9	CN	CF_3
A (DNBF)	136.7	126.5	144.8	120.8	116.6	145.02	-	-
B	137.9	128.1	127.1	122.5	116.8	145.2	-	121.9
C	137.0	133.1	110.0	130.8	117.1	147.7	115.6	-
D	138.1	128.4	127.6	132.1	118.0	145.2	-	119.0
E	118.8	127.2	145.6	118.5	114.9	147.68	-	121.3
F	102.5	135.9	146.0	119.0	114.6	150.2	112.5	-
G	124.3	135.3	144.7	121.5	114.4	146.2	-	119.4

Table 3. ^{13}C NMR data for the Benzofuroxans **A-G** (DMSO-d6)

HMBC spectra recorded for these compounds exhibited characteristic correlations. For example, two correlations between C_9 (δ = 145 ppm) and H_7 (J_{C9H7} = 5 Hz) and H_5 (J_{C9H5} = 7-9 Hz), respectively, can be observed while C_8 (δ = 115 ppm) is only correlated with H_7 (J_{C8H7} = 2-3 Hz). In the particular case of **B** and **E**, the couplings between the fluorine atoms of the CF_3 moiety and the various carbons are helpful to assign unambiguously the chemical shifts.

In most cases, the signals of the carbon atoms substituted by a NO_2 group at the 4 or 6 position are very broad due to long relaxation time.

To remove the N-oxide functionality of benzofuroxans, in order to obtain the benzofurazan analogues **I-N** may be easily achieved using triphenylphosphine in boiling toluene. Benzofurazans are obtained in fair to moderate yields and NMR spectra have been recorded (Table 4 and 5). The removal of the N-oxide functionality is going along with the disappearance of its electron-releasing effect and has two major effects:

- the resonances of H_5 and H_7 pertaining to **I-N** are at lower field than those of **A-F** (δ_{H5} = 8.94 and δ_{H7} = 9.27 for **A**, δ_{H5} = 9.04 and δ_{H7} = 9.80 for **I**, in DMSO).
- the C_8 resonance is now at lower field than that of C_9 (δ_{C9} = 145.0 and δ_{C8} = 116.6 for **A**, δ_{C9} = 143.3 and δ_{C8} = 150.0 for **I**, in DMSO).

Compounds	H_5	H_7	CF_3*	Coupling constants (Hz)
I (DNBZ)	9.04	9.80	-	$^4J_{5/7} = 1.9$
J	8.83	9.38	-62.1	$^4J_{5/7} = {}^4J_{5/F}$ 1.2
K	9.04	9.55	-	-
L	8.84	9.24	-76.7	$^4J_{5/7} = 1.3$
M	8.62	9.63	-61.8	$^4J_{5/7} = {}^4J_{5/F}$ 1.0
N	9.15	9.65	-	$^4J_{5/7} = 1.8$

*Internal reference: $CFCl_3$

Table 4. ^1H NMR data for the Benzofurazans **I-N** (DMSO-d6)

Compounds	C_4	C_5	C_6	C_7	C_8	C_9	CN	CF_3
I (DNBZ)	136.8	125.1	148.7	122.5	150.0	143.3	-	-
J	138.1	126.6	131.3	124.9	150.1	143.2	-	122.0
K	137.2	133.3	115.8	131.3	149.9	142.9	114.7	-
L	135.5	132.1	138.5	126.3	149.8	143.2	-	119.4
M	118.1	126.5	149.1	120.4	149.3	145.8	-	121.4
N	101.6	135.2	149.5	121.9	148.5	148.3	113.2	-

Table 5. ^{13}C NMR data for the Benzofurazans **I-N** (DMSO-d6)

3. NMR as a tool in the elucidation of Diels-Alder processes

In the introduction, we have mentioned that benzofuroxans are involved in a variety of Diels-Alder processes, acting as dienophiles or heterodienes depending upon the reaction partner, the position and the nature of the substituent of the carbocyclic ring and of the experimental conditions at hand (solvent and temperature). *In situ* NMR studies are very informative to understand the regioselectivity of the Diels-Alder process and to collect informations on the global reaction sequence. For example, does the Diels-Alder interaction involve the formation of any detectable short-live intermediates? Many studies have been carried out at low temperature (from -50°C to -20°C), using various amounts of dienes to investigate the formation of transient species which can only be characterized by NMR.

3.1 Elucidation of the reaction of DNBF, a with cyclopentadiene[13]

As it was mentioned below, the reaction of DNBF with cyclopentadiene leads to the stereoselective formation of the diadduct **12**. Informations on the reaction sequence leading to **12** was obtained by carrying out a series of experiments at -30°C, using lower concentrations of the reagents to overcome solubility problems.

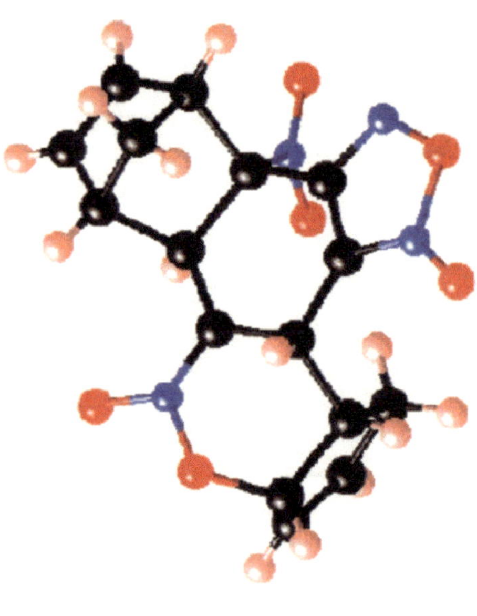

ORTEP view of **12**

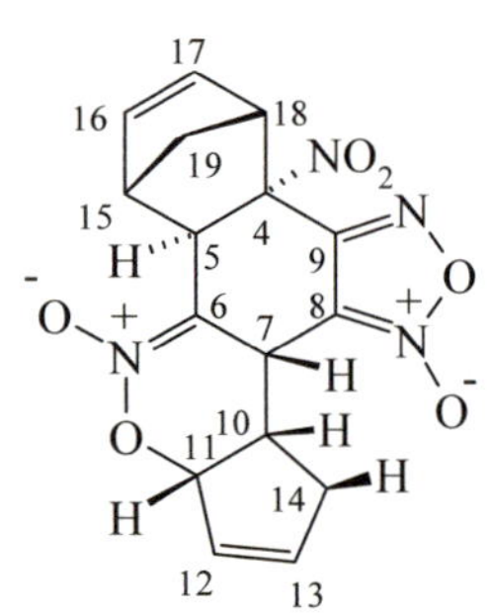

12

In this instance, the spectra recorded immediately after the mixing showed the formation of two new products, **X** and **Y**, in a 9:1 ratio. Raising the temperature to -10°C favors the formation of **Y** at the expense of **X**, both species being present in similar quantities after 30 minutes at this temperature, when the formation of **12** at the expense of **X** end **Y** begins to be detectable. Warming the solution to 0°C accelerated the appearance of **12**, which was the only product eventually present at the completion of the reaction process. On the basis of the collected ^{1}H NMR information, there is little doubt that **X** and **Y** are the monoadducts **10** and **11**, respectively.

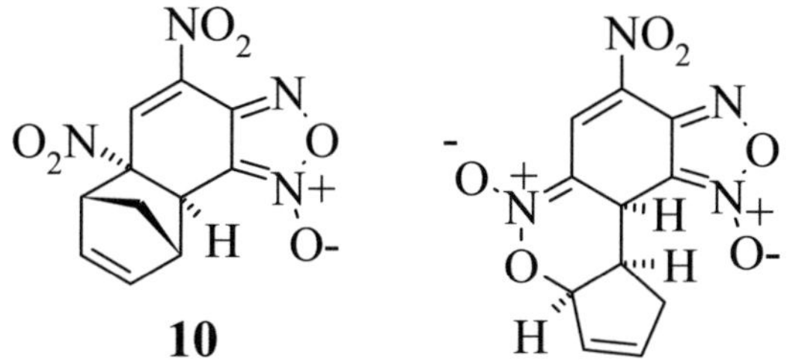

10 **11**

This implies that we are dealing with two highly regioselective and diastereoselective normal and inverse electron-demand Diels-Alder condensations. The regioselectivity at the C_6-C_7 double bond was readily demonstrated through ^{15}N labelling of the 4-NO_2 group of DNBF. In this instance, the only low filed proton observed in the ^{1}H NMR spectra of **11** and **10** is coupled with the ^{15}N atom indicating that this proton is H_5. In addition, the observed $^{3}J_{N4H5}$ coupling constants of 3.3 and 2.6 Hz, respectively, for **10** and **11** compare well with those previously reported for the parent DNBF molecule ($^{3}J_{N4H5}$ = 2.9 Hz).[17] Regarding the adduct **11**, the first strong, though indirect, evidence for the proposed stereochemistry is that this structure is the only one which can be viewed as a precursor of the diadduct **12**.

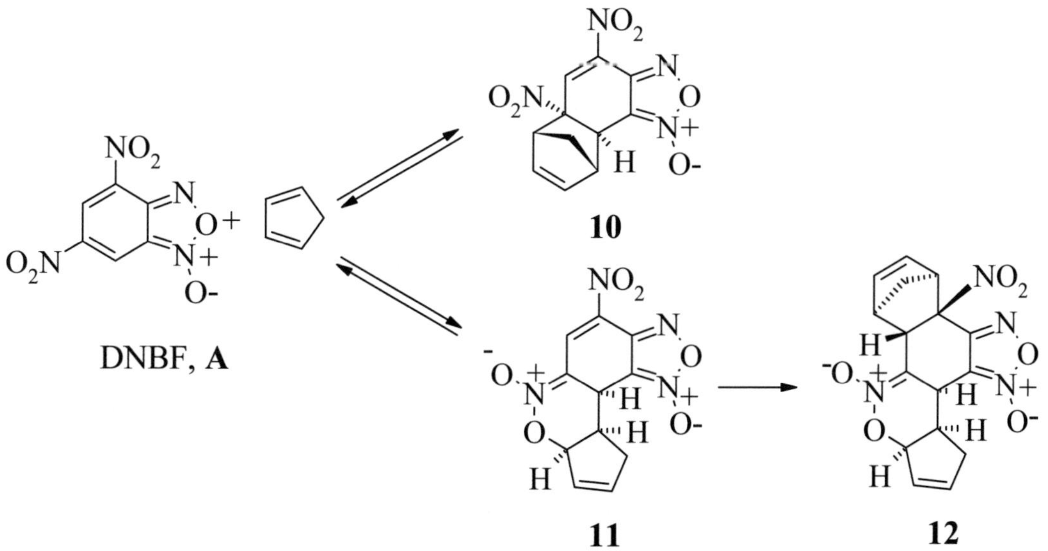

Scheme 3. Mechanism of the reaction of DNBF, A with cyclopentadiene.

NOE experiments have been carried out which have confirmed experimentally that the H_7 and H_{10} protons of **11** are in a cis arrangement, as found in **12**. The details of this mechanism are summarized in Scheme 3.

In as much as the C_6-C_7 double bond of DNBF is involved in the two initial normal and inverse electron-demand Diels-Alder processes, the formation of the NEDDA and IEDDA adducts **10** and **11** is a clear-cut example of the potentially ambident nitroalkene Diels-Alder reactivity of DNBF. On the other hand, the preferred formation of the unsymmetrical IEDDA-NEDDA adduct **12** implies a greater dienophilic reactivity of the remaining nitroolefinic moiety in the IEDDA adduct **11** than in the NEDDA adduct **10**.[10-16]

3.2 Elucidation of the reaction of DNBF with 2,3-dimethylbutadiene.[10,15]

Information on the reaction sequences leading to **14** was also obtained by recording a series of ^1H and ^{13}C spectra within a few minutes after mixing equimolar amounts of DNBF and 2,3-dimethylbutadiene. At this stage, the spectra showed the partial disappearance of the signals due to the starting materials and the concomitant appearance of a new set of resonances indicating the formation of a new product. The evidence is that this product can be formulated as the monoadduct **13** resulting from a regioselective NEDDA process involving the C_6C_7 double bond of the DNBF as the dienophile contributor.

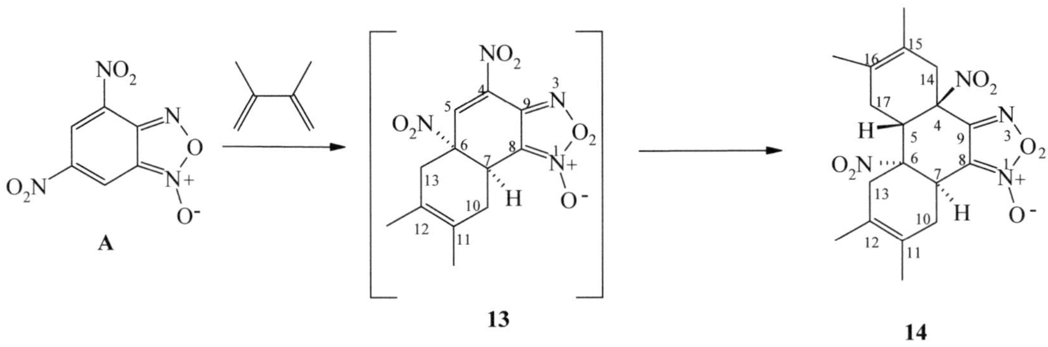

Scheme 4. Reaction of DNBF, A with 2,3-dimethylbutadiene.

The regioselectivity of the addition was demonstrated through ^{15}N labelling of the 4-NO_2 group of DNBF. In this instance, the only low-field proton δH_5 = 7.54 ppm observed in the ^1H spectra of **13** is coupled with the ^{15}N atom ($^3J_{N4H5}$ = 3 Hz), confirming that this proton is H_5. In contrast, the *cis* configuration of **13** could not be unambiguously confirmed from the collected NMR data. However it is clear that structure **13** with the 6-NO_2 group and H_7 being on the same side of the two rings is the only one which can be viewed as a precursor of the diadduct **14** (Scheme 4).

3.3 Time dependence of the ^1H NMR spectra of the adduct 15 obtained from the interaction of DNBF with isoprene[10,15-16]

Treatment of DNBF with a large excess of isoprene (10 equiv.) in dichloromethane at room temperature for 2 days afforded two compounds in a 1/1 ratio (overall yield 90%) which were readily separated by taking advantage of their different solubilities in pentane (Scheme 3). As shown by the ORTEP views of Figure 1, these two compounds correspond to diadducts which are only formed as the diastereomers **15** and **16**. The stereochemistry of **15** in the crystal agrees well with the structural information provided by a detailed analysis of the ^1H and ^{13}C NMR spectra recorded in $CDCl_3$ via COSY and HETCOR, as well as J-modulation experiments. Among other notable diagnostic features for **15**, there is the observation that the disappearance of the low field proton and carbon resonances associated with the $C_4C_5C_6C_7$ fragment of the DNBF structure goes along with a strong deshielding of the two sp^3 carbons C_6 and C_{15}. Both benefit from the strong electron-withdrawing inductive effect exerted by a NO_2 group and a $O\text{-}N^+\text{-}O^-$ fragment of a dihydrooxazine N-oxide ring. Also typical is the presence of the three vinylic protons H_{16}, H_{17a} and H_{17b} at 5.97, 5.45 and 5.35 ppm, respectively, in the ^1H spectra. NOE experiments have revealed the close space proximity of the protons H_5 and H_{14b} as well as of H_7 and H_{10b}.

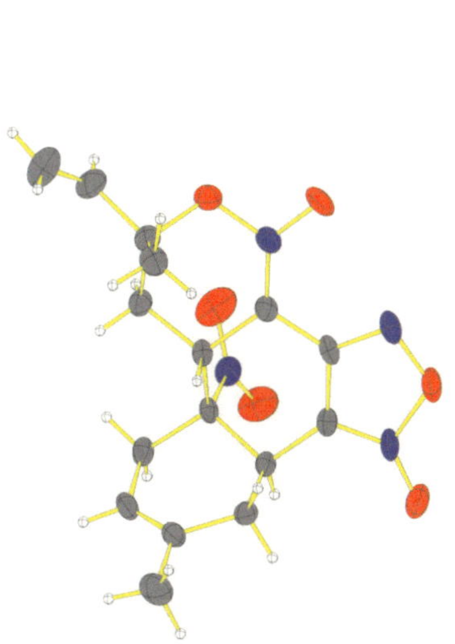

ORTEP view of **15**

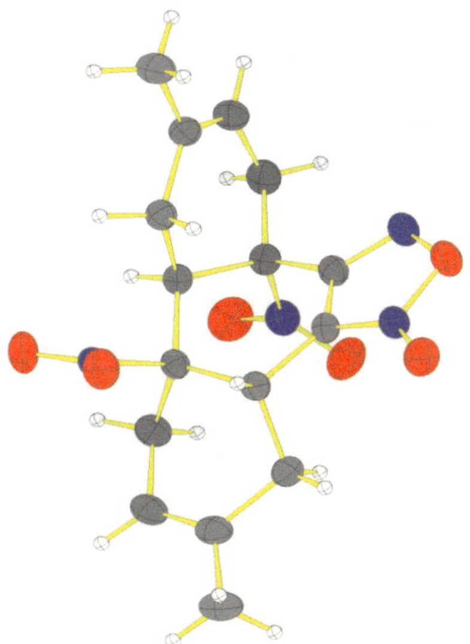

ORTEP view of **16**

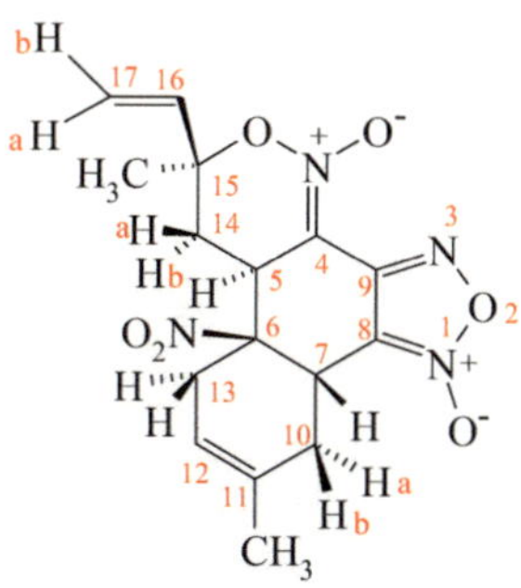

15

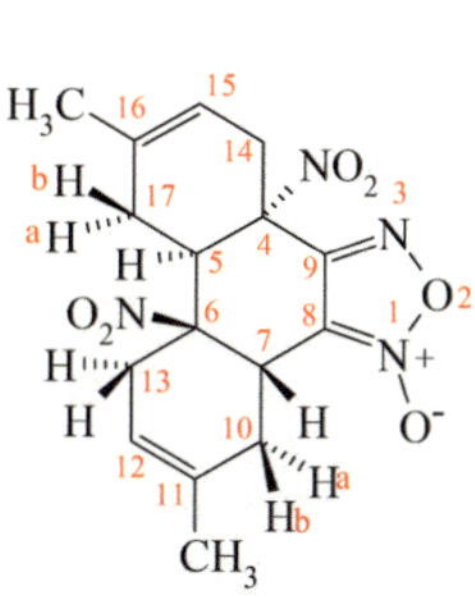

16

Fig. 1. Structures of Diels-Alder adducts **15** and **16**.

Despite its remarkable stability in the solid state, the diadduct **15** is not the thermodynamically stable product of the reaction of DNBF with isoprene. Major changes in the ^{1}H and ^{13}C spectra occurred with time when a $CDCl_3$ solution of **15** is kept at room temperature, with in about a month, an essentially complete disappearance of the resonances due to **15** and a concomitant development of new sets of proton or carbon signals ascribable to **16**. At completion of the interconversion, the recorded ^{1}H and ^{13}C spectra were in fact totally identical to those obtained after dissolution of a few crystals of **16** in the same solvent.[15-16]

In accordance with its greater olefinic character, the C_6-C_7 double bond of DNBF has been found to be more reactive than its C_4-C_5 counterpart in all Diels-Alder condensation pathways so far studied. Based on this, one could anticipate that the diadducts **15** and **16** are the result of competitive inverse and normal electron-demand reactions involving the remaining nitroalkene-like C_4-C_5 fragment of an initially formed NEDDA monoadduct of type **17** (Scheme 5 and Figure 2).

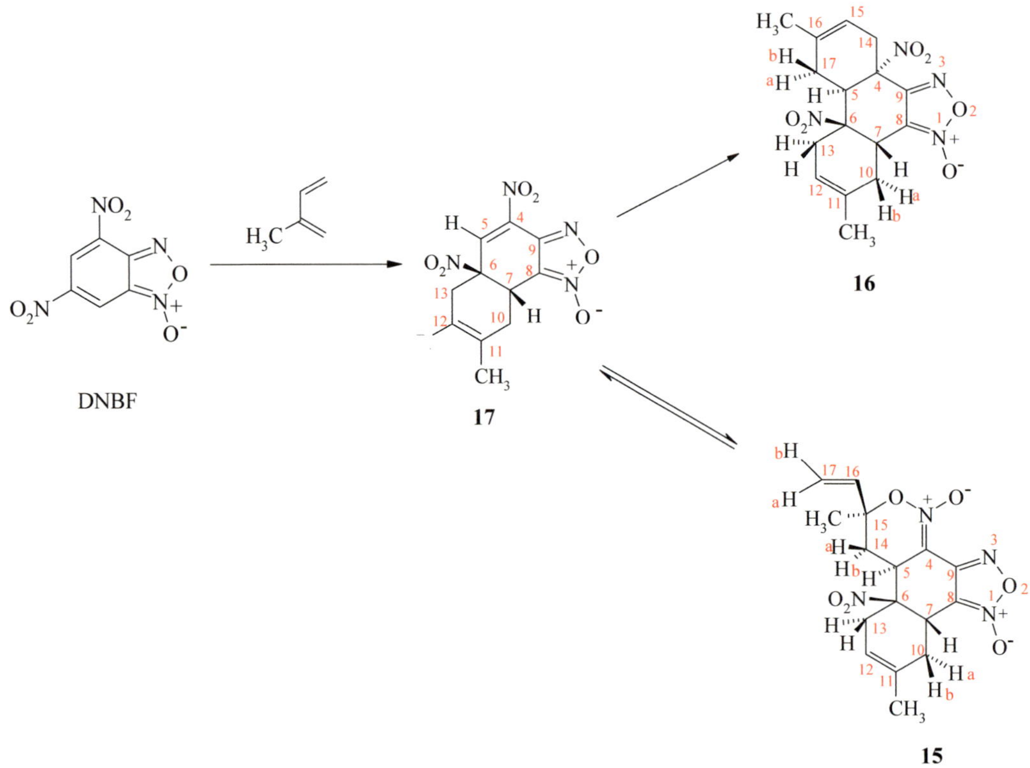

Scheme 5. Reaction of DNBF, A with isoprene.

Because of a more favorable thermodynamic driving force for formation of **16** than **15**, the complete equilibrium system of Scheme 5 is progressively shifted towards the obtention of the NEDDA-NEDDA diadducts **16**. There is little doubt that these species correspond to the products isolated in 1973 by Kresze and Bathelt.[10] At this time, however, no attempt was made to elucidate the stereochemistry and the mechanistic course of the reactions.

That the addition of the second molecule of isoprene and 2,3-dimethylbutadiene to the monoadducts **17** occurs through competitive normal and inverse electron-demand pathways to give a mixture of the NEDDA-NEDDA and NEDDA-IEDDA diadducts **16** and **15**, respectively, is an unprecedented finding in the chemistry of DNBF.

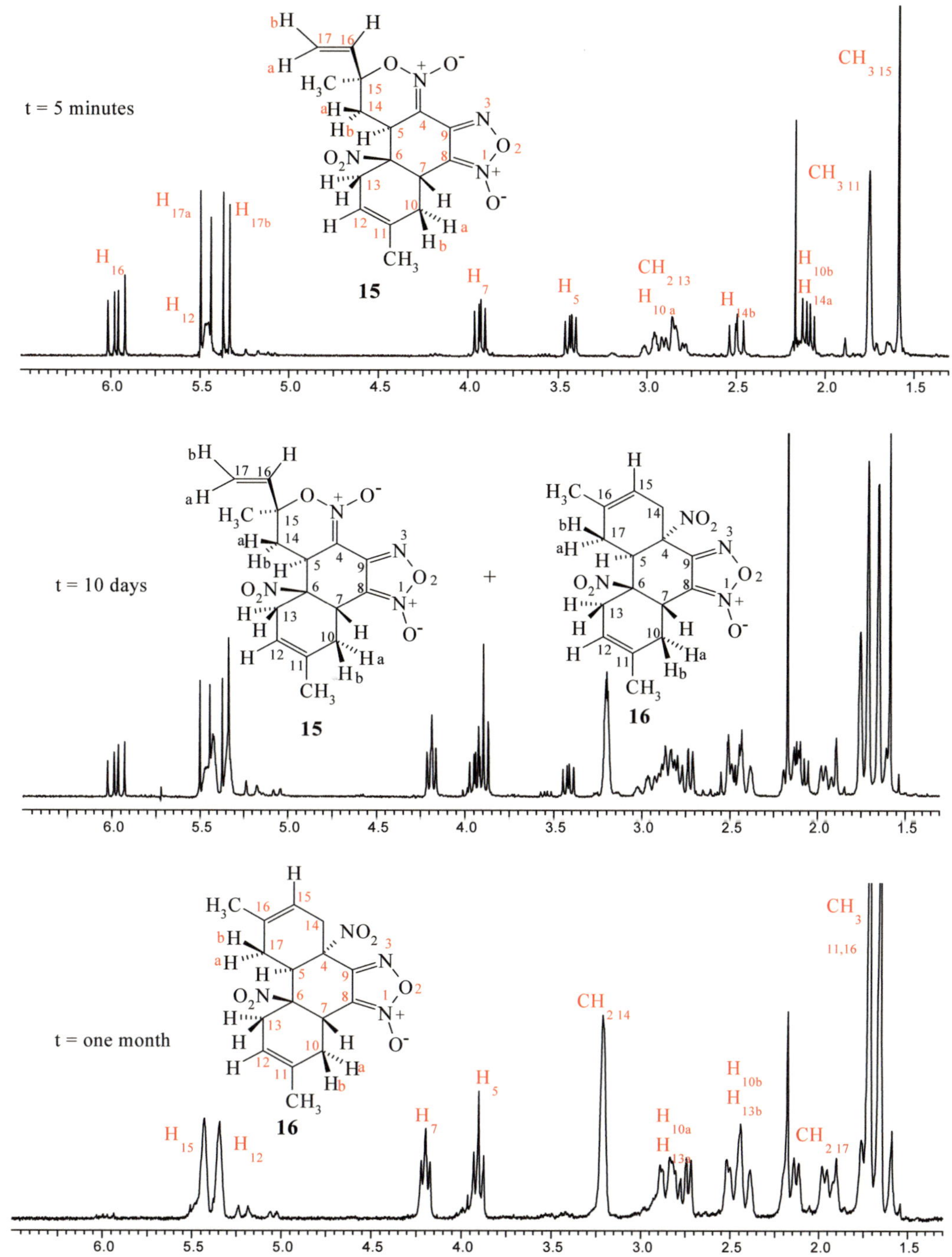

Fig. 2. Time dependence of the ¹H NMR spectra of a pure sample of **15** in $CDCl_3$.

The comprehensive and extensive study of the interactions between benzofuroxans and various dienes (cyclic or linear) highlights characteristic NMR data allowing to quickly determine if an adduct is the result of a Normal Electronic Demand Diels-Alder (NEDDA) reaction or of an Inverse Electronic Demand Diels-Alder (IEDDA) reaction. For example, for an IEDDA adducts, the ^{1}H NMR spectra show a deshielded signal at 6 ppm typical of H_{11} and a multicoupled signal at 4 ppm typical of H_{10} (see Figure 3) while ^{13}C NMR spectra show that the signals pertaining to carbon 7, 10, 14 are found to be at higher field in the case of IEDDA adducts than in the case of NEDDA adducts. For these latter adducts, the ^{1}H NMR spectra exhibited broad signals at 3.5 ppm pertaining to H_{10} and H_{13} (Figure 3).

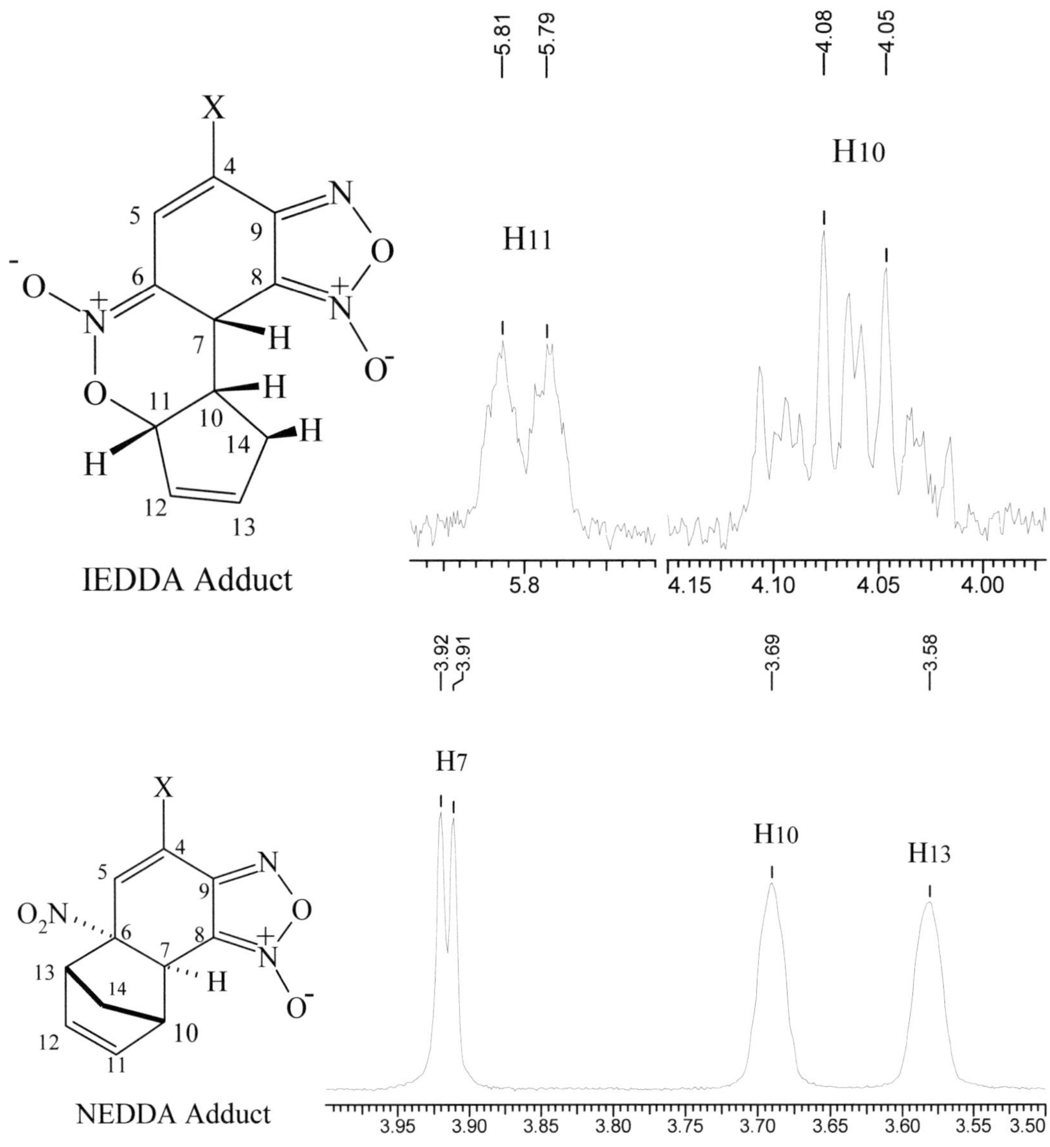

Fig. 3. Characteristic signals of Diels-Alder Adducts.

4. NMR in the study of the stability of σ-complexes

Besides the potentiality of the versatile behaviour of DNBF in terms of new synthetic approaches to heterocyclic chemistry, the results obtained are in themselves evidence that the carbocyclic ring of this superelectrophilic heterocycle has a poor aromatic character relative to TNB. This suggests the existence of a significant relationship between aromaticity on the one hand, electrophilicity in σ-complex formation and pericyclic reactivity on the other hand.

Benzofuroxans **A-H** represent a class of neutral 10-π-electron deficient heteroaromatic substrates which exhibit an extremely high electrophilic character in many covalent nucleophilic addition and substitution processes.[13-18] More importantly, **DNBF, A** reacts quantitatively at room temperature with such weak carbon π-nucleophiles, as benzenoid aromatics (phenols, anilines) or π-excessive heteroaromatics (indoles, pyrroles, thiophenes) to afford stable anionic C-bonded σ-adducts which are formally the products of S_EAr substitution on the benzene or hetarene ring. Coupling to weakly activated enolic double bonds is also a process that is readily achieved with **DNBF, A**. Based on these findings, **DNBF, A** can be used as a convenient probe to assess the C-basicity of a number of very weak carbon nucleophiles, e.g. anilines, 3-aminothiophenes….

4.1 Regioselectivity of the covalent nucleophilic addition to DNBF, A

The addition of sodium hydroxide solution to a solution of DNBF, **A** resulted in the immediate and quantitative formation of a σ-complex **18**, which can be seen as the two regio-isomeric Meisenheimer complexes **18a** or **18b**. Many NMR studies have been carried out to determine accurately the structure of this salt.[19-21]

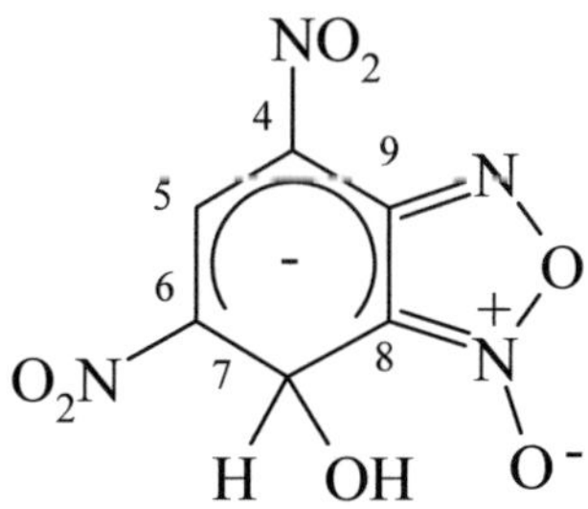

18a

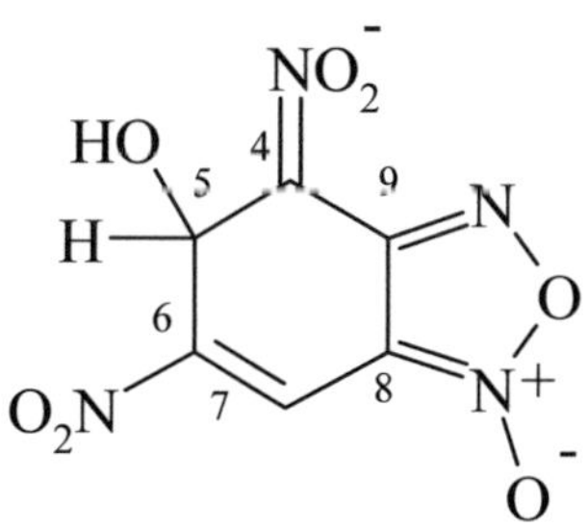

18b

^{1}H nmr spectra exhibit three signals at δ = 8.93, 6.20 (doublet, J = 7Hz) and 6.55 (doublet, J = 7 Hz) ppm. When the salt is prepared with deuterium oxide, only two signals at 8.93 and 6.20 ppm (doublets, J = 1 Hz) are obtained. The use of the deuterated salts permits assignments of the chemical shifts for all protons (structures **19** and **20**).

Unfortunately structures **18a** and **18b** are both consistent with the NMR data and it's not possible to discriminate between the two structures on this basis. Moreover, interconversion between **18a** and **18b** may exist in solution and is possible by two different pathways. One path is by a reversible hydroxylation at the 5- and 7-position (path a, scheme 6) and the other path involves a Boulton-Katritzky rearrangement (path b, Scheme 6).

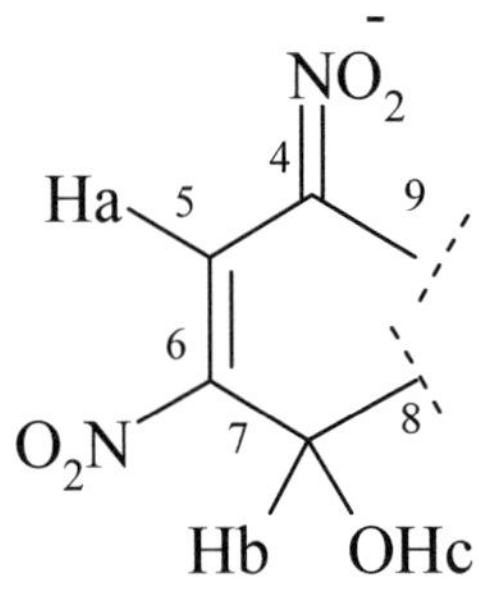

19

$H_a = 8.97$ ppm
$H_b = 6.20$ ppm (J = 7Hz)
$H_c = 6.55$ ppm (J = 7Hz)

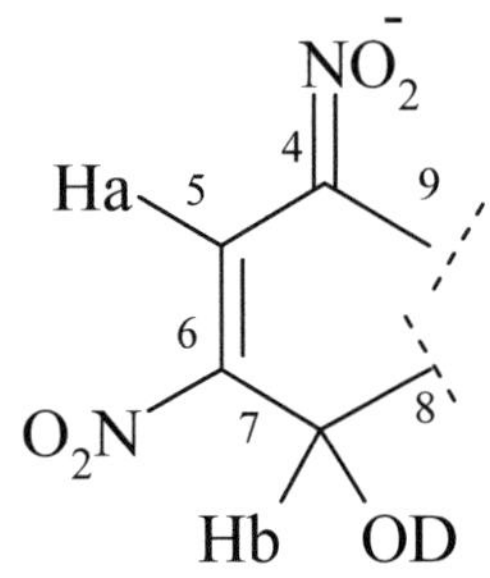

20

$H_a = 8.97$ ppm (J = 1 Hz)
$H_b = 6.20$ ppm (J = 1Hz)

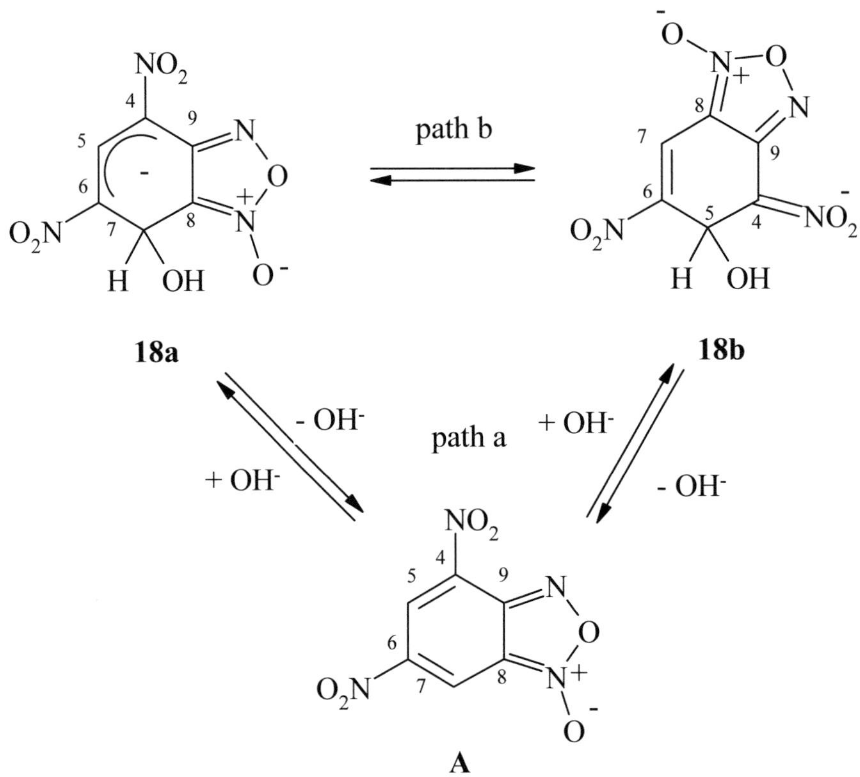

Scheme 6. Interconversion between **18a** and **18b**.

The NMR spectra indicate only one product. If a second substance is present, its NMR spectrum is identical with the other or is present in too small amount to be detectable or the two are exchanging at a rapid state. However, consideration of resonance forms indicates that **18a** (delocalization of the negative charge into the two nitro groups) should be more stable than **18b** (delocalization of the negative charge into only one nitro group). The correct structure for the Meisenheimer complex formed by the reaction of DNBF, **A** with aqueous base is considered to be **18a**. Confirmation of this result has been further confirmed by the study of the case of nitrobenzofuroxan **21**, which react very similarly with water and OH^- to afford hydroxy σ-adducts in aqueous solution. An analogous situation holds in methanol when there is a remarkable analogy between the rate and equilibrium parameters governing the ambident reactivity of 4-nitrobenzofuroxan **21** according to scheme 7 in this solvent.

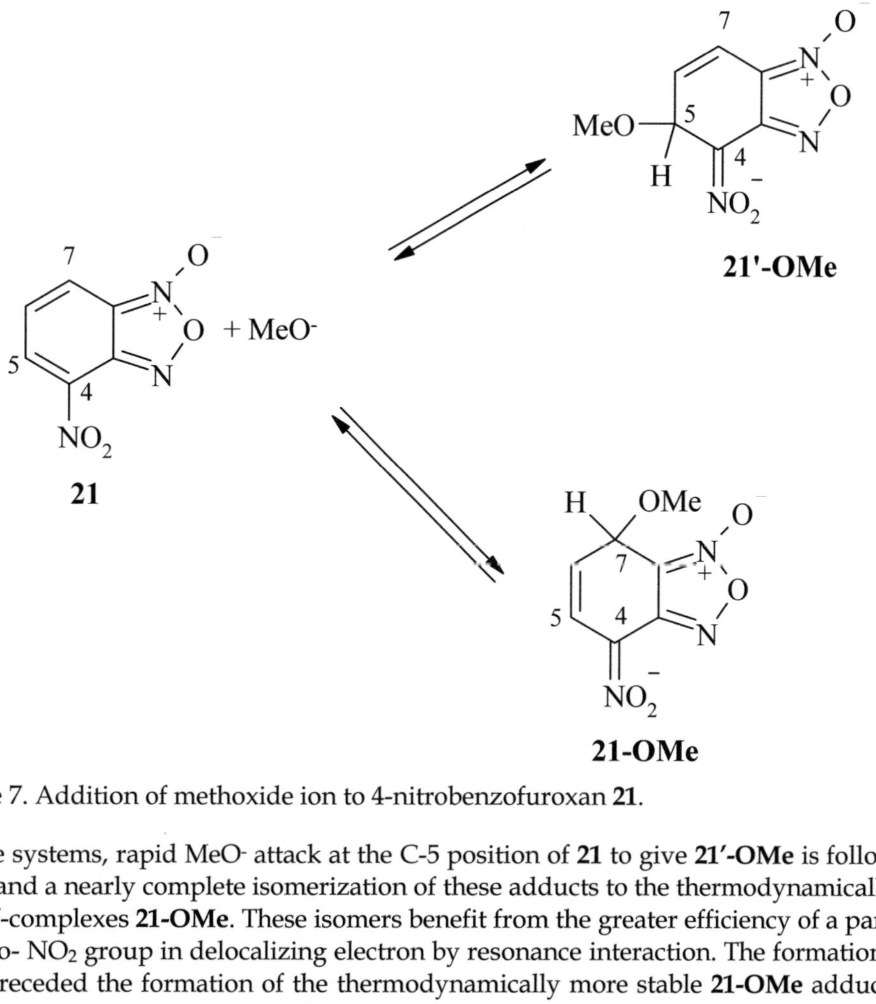

Scheme 7. Addition of methoxide ion to 4-nitrobenzofuroxan **21**.

In these systems, rapid MeO^- attack at the C-5 position of **21** to give **21′-OMe** is followed by a slow and a nearly complete isomerization of these adducts to the thermodynamically more stable 7-complexes **21-OMe**. These isomers benefit from the greater efficiency of a para- than an ortho- NO_2 group in delocalizing electron by resonance interaction. The formation of **21′-OMe** preceded the formation of the thermodynamically more stable **21-OMe** adduct. Only the C-7 adduct could be observed by room temperature NMR spectroscopy, it was necessary to cool the system at low temperature prior to start of the reaction in order to detect and characterize the C-5 adduct as the product of kinetic control. In as much as it occurs with other nucleophiles but is restricted to **21**, the ambident electrophilic behaviour depicted in scheme 7 is a typical feature of the chemistry of nitrobenzoxadiazoles. Because of a very fast interconversion between the C-5 and the C-7 adduct or because of a very high thermodynamic stability of the C-7 adduct, it has not been possible to detect and to characterize **18b,** the C-5 hydroxy-σ-adduct of DNBF, even at low temperature.[22-23]

4.2 NMR characterization of the C-7 adducts of DNBF, A and its derivatives B-H[24]

We have succeeded in obtaining new spectroscopic data on the Meisenheimer complexes of DNBF, **A** in looking at the interaction of this compound with 2-nitropropane anion. As a major diagnostic feature in the ^1H NMR spectra of **22** is the H_7 resonance which appears at 5.27 ppm, being in the range commonly found for many C-bonded DNBF adducts, e.g. δ = 5.40 ppm for **23**.[3,8] The shielding of the H_7 resonance (δH_7 = 9.27 ppm for DNBF, $\Delta\delta H_7$ = 4 ppm) is due to the $sp^2 \rightarrow sp^3$ rehybridization of the carbon 7 (Table 6). Also in accord with previous observations showing that the chemical shift of the H_5 proton located between the two NO_2 groups of the negatively charged DNBF moiety depends very little on the nature of the C-bonded structure, the H_5 resonance for **22** is δ = 8.69 ppm and close to those found for related adducts, e.g. δ = 8.62 ppm for **24**.[4] This slight shielding may be interpreted in terms of loss of the aromatic character and of appearance of a negative charge on the DNBF moiety.

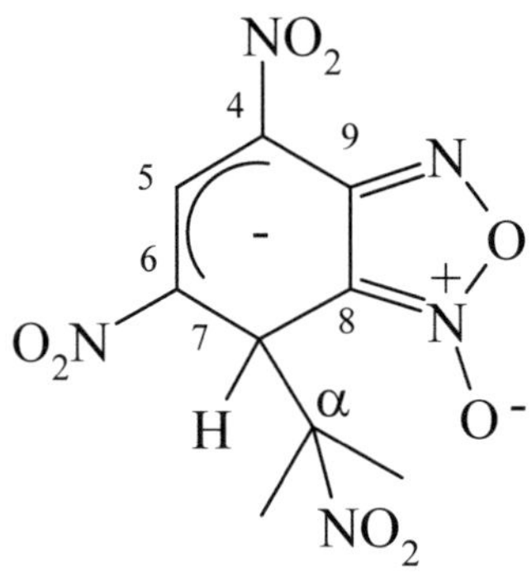

22

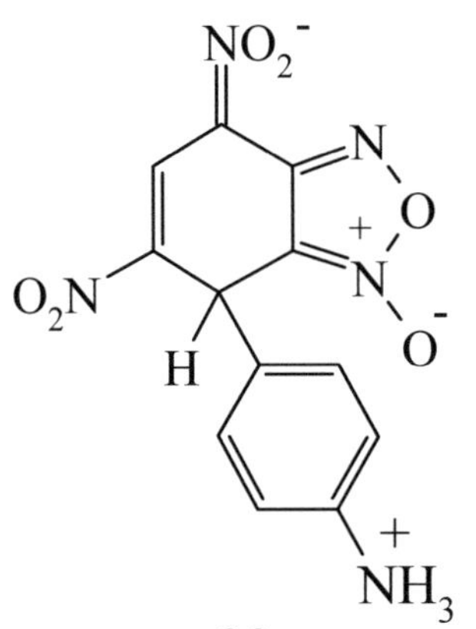

23

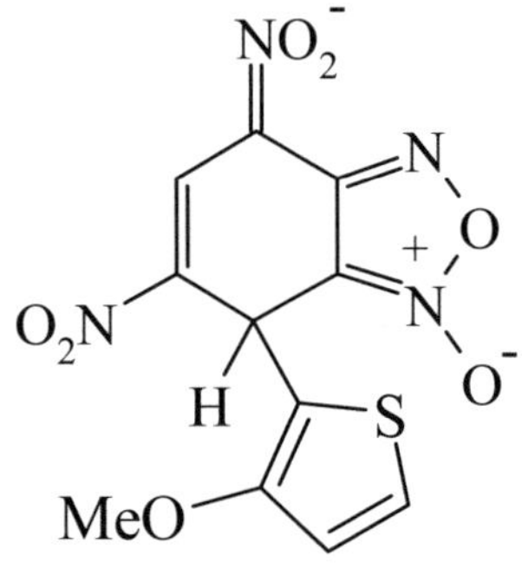

24

Regarding ^{13}C data, there are two noteworthy results: a) in accord with the $sp^2 \rightarrow sp^3$ rehybridization resulting from the complexation of the DNBF moiety, there is a strong upfield shift of the C_7 resonance (from 120.80 for DNBF to ~ 32 ppm for **22**); b) the substitution of 2-nitropropane (δC_α = 79.10 ppm) by DNBF induces a significant low-field shift of the resonance of the C_α carbon of the nitroalkane moiety (δC_α = 92.0 ppm for **22**, $\Delta\delta$ ~ 13 ppm). This latter result is mainly the reflection of the fact that a negatively charged DNBF structure exerts a notable – I effect. HMBC spectra recorded for these salts exhibited characteristic correlations. For example, one correlation between C_9 (δ = 150 ppm) and H_5 (J_{C9H5} = 6 Hz) while C_8 (δ = 110 ppm) is only correlated with H_7 (J_{C8H7} = 9 Hz). This latter correlation is a nice support that the covalent addition of the nucleophile takes place at C-7 of the carbocyclic ring of DNBF (Table 7).[24]

Compounds	H_5	H_7	CH_3	CF_3^*
22	8.69	5.27	1.51 1.49	-
25	7.68	4.73	1.54 1.44	-57.3
26	7.73	4.58	1.61 1.56	-
27	8.22	4.56	1.54 1.52	-78.7
28	7.97	5.30	1.51 1.46	-58.8
29	8.09	5.30	1.49 1.46	-

Table 6. ^1H NMR data for the adducts **22** and **25-29** (DMSO-d6)

Compounds	C_4	C_5	C_6	C_7	C_8	C_9	CN	CF_3	C_α	Me
22	110.6	133.3	121.0	41.3	110.1	149.8	-	-	92.1	23.3 23.2
25	106.4	132.7	99.7	40.2	110.0	150.8	-	124.5	92.6	24.9 21.3
26	108.7	140.4	80.5	42.5	109.3	150.0	121.1	-	92.6	23.5 22.9
27	113.3	144.2	90.4	41.3	109.1	149.8	-	120.2	92.5	23.0 22.8
28	91.0	134.2	110.9	41.5	109.6	151.4	-	123.9	92.7	23.8 23.2
29	73.8	141.1	115.1	41.3	109.2	153.6	117.8	-	92.5	23.5 22.9

Table 7. ^{13}C NMR data for the adducts **22** and **25-29** (DMSO-d6)

All the NMR data pertaining to **22** are summarized in Tables 6 and 7 together with the NMR data of the Meisenheimer complexes deriving from benzofuroxans **B-H**.

The delocalization of this negative charge over the DNBF moiety and over the two nitro groups is the main factor governing the outstanding stability of these Meisenheimer complexes. What will be the effect of the replacement of a nitro group by another electron-withdrawing group on the stability of the Meisenheimer complexes?

The first message emerging from the data, recorded for σ-adducts **25-29** and collected in Tables 6 and 7, is that the resonances of C_7 (from 40.2 to 42.5 ppm), C_8 (from 109.2 to 110.1 ppm), C_9 (from 149.8 to 153.6 ppm) and C_α (from 92.1 to 92.7 ppm) are independent of the position and of the nature of the substituent and are consistent with those reported for the adduct **22**. It could be through evaluation of the chemical shift variations brought about by the complex formation that reliable information on the structural reorganization which accompanies the formation of the σ-adduct may be obtained. Such variations (Δδ) are the result of a high field shift caused by the presence of the negative charge. On the basis of the above reasoning, a comparison in Table 8 of the $\Delta\delta H_5$, $\Delta\delta C_4$ and $\Delta\delta C_6$ associated with the complexes formation is very informative regarding the structure of the σ-adducts. As can be seen, large upfield shifts of H_5 ($\Delta\delta H_5$ ~ 0.2-1.2 ppm), of C_6 ($\Delta\delta C_6$ ~ 25-32 ppm) and of C_4 ($\Delta\delta C_4$ ~ 24-38 ppm) occur upon σ-complex formation (see Table 8). Such Δδ agree well with the presence of the negative charge, with the loss of the aromatic character and with a $sp^2 \rightarrow sp^3$ rehybridization. The large upfield shifts of C_6 for salts **25-27** and of C_4 for salts **28-29** is a large reflection that the resonance forms $C\text{-}Y^-$ and $C\text{-}X^-$, respectively, play a major role in the stabilization of the negative charge (Scheme 8). Because of a large inductive effect of the cyano and trifluoromethyl groups, the negative charge is retained on the C_4 or on the C_6 carbon. In the case of the trifluoromethanesulfonyl group, the inductive effect is larger than for the two latter groups and is going along with the smallest $\Delta\delta H_5$ (0.38ppm) and the largest $\Delta\delta C_6$ (37 ppm) leaving no doubt that the SO_2CF_3 group is capable to stabilize a negative charge by a strong polarization effect. The negative charge is largely retained on the C_6 carbon and is less delocalized through the carbocyclic ring.

Compounds	$\Delta\delta H_5$	$\Delta\delta C_4$	$\Delta\delta C_6$
22	0.25	26.1	23.8
25	1.06	31.5	27.4
26	1.19	28.3	29.5
27	0.38	24.8	37.2
28	0.73	27.8	34.7
29	0.94	29.7	31.6

Table 8. Changes in chemical Shifts ($\Delta\delta H_5$, $\Delta\delta C_6$ and $\Delta\delta C_4$) upon σ-complex formation in DMSO-d6

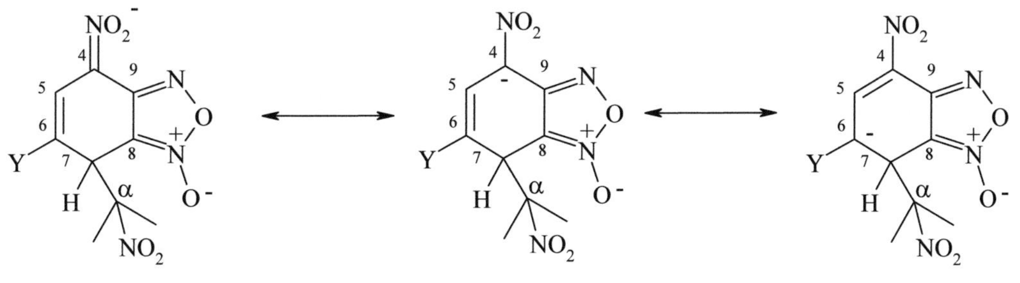

C-NO$_2^-$ **C-4$^-$** **C-Y$^-$**

Y= CF_3, **25**
Y = CN, **26**
Y= SO_2CF_3, **27**

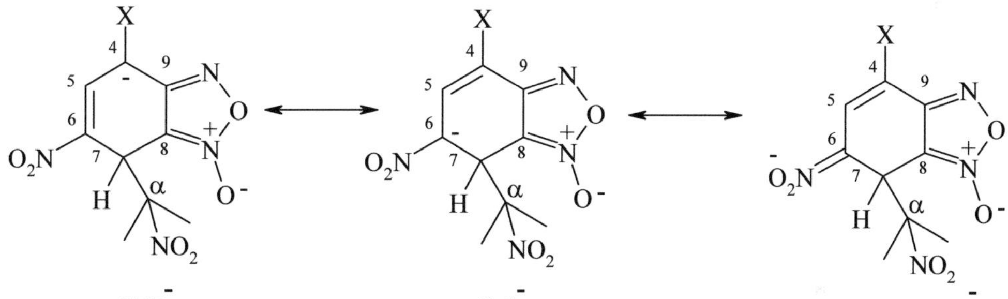

C-X$^-$ **C-6$^-$** **C-NO$_2^-$**

X = CF_3, **28**
X = CN, **29**

Scheme 8. Resonance forms of sigma-complexes **25-29**.

4.3 ^{15}N NMR characterization of the N-adduct of DNBF, A with 4,5-dimethylthiazole

Treatment of DNBF, **A** with a two-fold excess of **30** in acetonitrile solution, followed by addition of diethylether, resulted in the precipitation of an orange solid corresponding to the 4,5-dimethylthiazolium salt of the adduct **N-30** (Scheme 9). Because of the strong acidifying effect exerted by a negatively charged DNBF moiety,[24] the deprotonation of the NH_2^+ group of the initially formed zwitterion **N-30** by **30** acting as a base reagent is a facile process, accounting for the adduct salt **N-30;30,H$^+$** being the thermodynamically stable product of the interaction and therefore for the need of two moles of **30** to drive the overall equilibrium process to completion in acetonitrile solution.

The bonding of DNBF at a nitrogen center is supported by the presence of a relatively low-field $H_{7'}$ resonance ($\delta H_{7'}$ = 6.00 ppm) in the ^{1}H nmr spectra. The evidence, however, is that this resonance is very sensitive to the nature of the atom or group bonded to that position, the shielding increasing with decreasing the electronegativity of the attached atom, i.e. according to the sequence O < N < C.

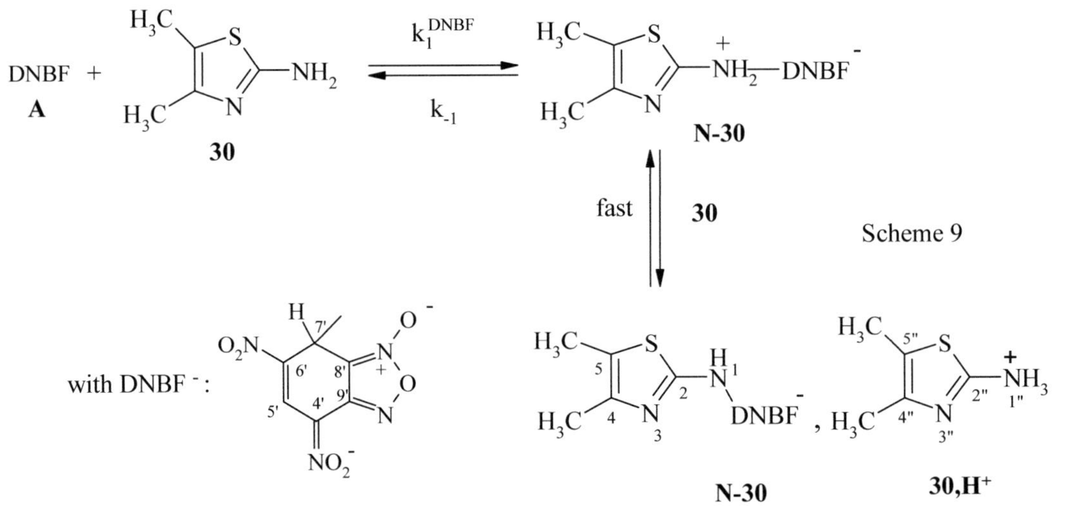

Scheme 9

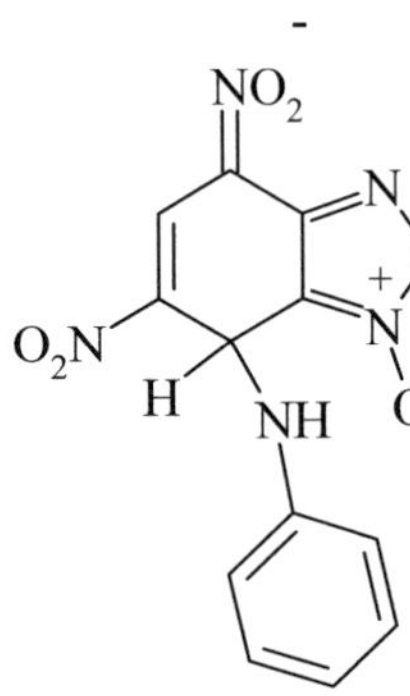

N-31

On this ground, the finding of a $H_{7'}$ resonance at 6.00 ppm and a $C_{7'}$ resonance at 46.1 ppm leaves little doubt regarding the N-bonded structure of the DNBF adduct of 4,5-dimethyl-2-aminothiazole **30**. As a matter of fact, the $H_{7'}$ resonance of **N-30** is very similar to that of the anionic aniline complex N-**31** ($\delta H_{7'}$ = 6.08 ppm).[3] ^1H-^{15}N correlations based on long-range coupling are clearly in favour of structure **N-30**. In the spectra, correlations can be observed between the exocyclic nitrogen N_1 (δ = 87.1 ppm) and $H_{7'}$ (δ = 6.00 ppm), between the endocyclic nitrogen N_3 (δ = 245.0 ppm) and the methyl group at C-4 (δ = 2.05 ppm); concomitantly, the correlation between the endocyclic nitrogen $N_{3''}$ (δ = 180.5 ppm) and the methyl group at C-4″ (δ = 2.08 ppm) of the thiazolium counterpart is observed (Figure 4a). This latter correlation is similar to that observed with the 4,5-dimethylaminothiazolium bromide (Figure 4b). To be noted is that all the ^{15}N nmr data collected from the various correlations are in full agreement with a recent review on the use of long-range ^1H-^{15}N correlations in the structural determination of organic compounds.[25-26]

The formation of the nitrogen adduct of DNBF is strongly supported by the ^{15}N NMR and especially through the ^1H -^{15}N correlations.

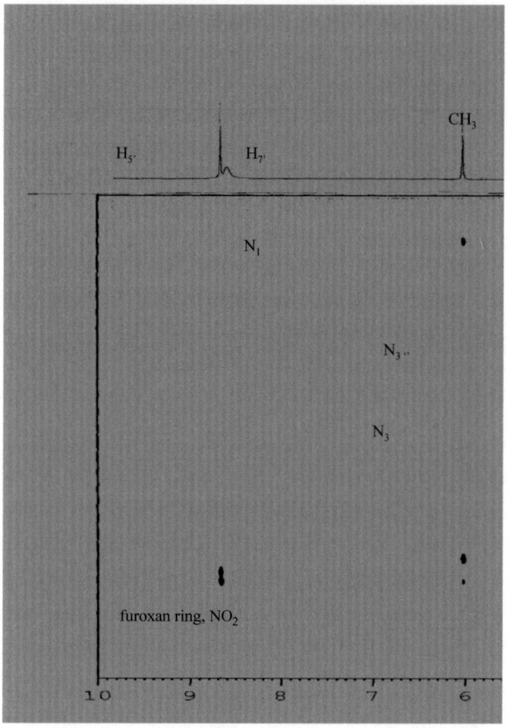

Fig. 4a. ^1H-^{15}N correlation for the adduct **N-30;30,H⁺**

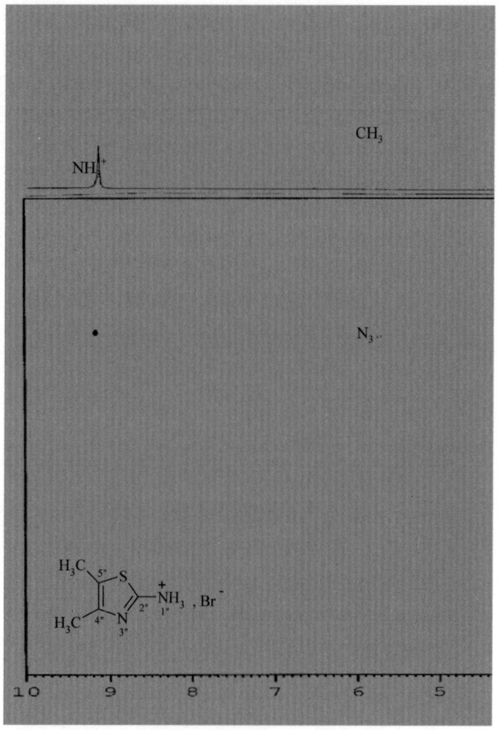

Fig. 4b. ^1H-^{15}N correlation for 4,5-dimethylaminothiazolium bromide

5. Conclusion

In this article we have highlighted some of the most significant examples where NMR spectroscopy brought important informations in the domain of the reactivity of benzofuroxans in synthetic applications (Diels-Alder, Meisenheimer Complexes formation). NMR strongly supports the structure of σ-complexes and informations on the capability of electron withdrawing groups to stabilize these complexes have been obtained. When σ-complexes are stabilized by electron-withdrawing inductive effect (CF_3, CN, SO_2CF_3), a large part of the negative charge is retained on the C_4 or C_6 carbon and is less delocalized through the carbocyclic ring. Moreover, the regioselectivity of the covalent nucleophilic addition can be unambiguously determined. The H_7 resonance is a key feature to see if DNBF is bonded at a nitrogen ($\delta H_7 \sim 6$ ppm) or carbon ($\delta H_7 \sim 4$ ppm) center. In the case of Diels-Alder reactions, NMR appears to be a useful tool, and especially using ^{15}N labelling, to highlight short-live species involved in complicated mechanisms.

6. References

[1] Terrier, F. In *Nucleophilic Aromatic Displacement*; Feuer, H, Ed.; VCH: New York, 1991. Terrier, F *Chem. Rev.* 1982, *82*, 77. Buncel, E.; Dust, J. M.; Terrier, F *Chem. Rev.* 1995, *95*, 2261.

[2] Terrier, F; Millot, F.; Norris, W. P. *J. Am. Chem. Soc.* 1976, *98*, 5883. Terrier, F.; Chatrousse, A. P.; Soudais, Y; Hlaibi, M. *J. Org. Chem.* 1984, *49*, 4176. Terrier, F.; Pouet, M. J.; Kizilian, E.; Hallé, J. C.; Outurquin, F.; Paulmier, C. *J. Org. Chem.* 1993, *58*, 4696.

[3] Strauss, M. J.; Renfrow, R. A.; Buncel, E. *J. Am. Chem. Soc.* 1983, *105*, 2473. Buncel, E.; Renfrow, R. A.; Strauss, M. J. *J. Org. Chem.* 1987, *52*, 488. Buncel, E.; Dust, J. M.; Manderville, R. A. *J. Am. Chem. Soc.* 1996, *118*, 6072. Buncel, E.; Manderville, R. A.; Dust, J. M. *J. Chem. Soc. Perkin Trans 2.* 1997, 1019 and references therein.

[4] Crampton, M. R.; Rabbitt, L. C. *J. Chem. Soc. Perkin Trans 2.* 1999, 1669. Crampton, M. R.; Rabbitt, L. C.; Terrier, F. *Can. J. Chem.* 1999, *77*, 639. Crampton, M. R.; Rabbitt, L. C. *J. Chem. Soc. Perkin Trans 2.* 2000, 2159. Atherton, J. H.; Crampton, M. R.; Duffield, G. L.; Stevens, J. A. *J. Chem. Soc. Perkin Trans 2.* 1995, 443.

[5] Kind, J.; Niclas, H. J. *Synth. Commun.* 1993, *23*, 1569. Niclas, H. J.; Göhrmann, B. *Synth. Commun.* 1989, *19*, 2141. Niclas, H. J.; Göhrmann, B.; Gründemann *Synth. Commun.* 1989, *19*, 2789.

[6] Ghosh, P. B.; Ternai, B.; Whitehouse, M. W. *Med. Res. Rev.* 1981, *1*, 159 and references therein.

[7] Lowe-Ma, C. K.; Nissan, R. A.; Wilson, W. S. *J. Org. Chem.* 1990, *55*, 3755.

[8] Terrier, F.; Kizilian, E.; Hallé, J. C.; Buncel, E. *J. Am. Chem. Soc.* 1992, *114*, 1740. Kizilian, E.; Terrier, F.; Chatrousse, A. P.; Gzouli, K.; Hallé, J. C. *J. Chem. Soc. Perkin Trans 2.* 1997, 2567. Terrier, F.; Pouet, M. J.; Hallé, J. C.; Kizilian, E.; Buncel, E. *J. Phys. Org. Chem.* 1998, *11*, 707. Terrier, F.; Pouet, M. J.; Gzouli, K.; Hallé, J. C.; Outurquin, F.; Paulmier, C. *Can. J. Chem.* 1998, *76*, 937.

[9] Spear, R. J.; Norris, W. P.; Read, R. W. *Tetrahedron Lett.* 1983, *23*, 1555. Norris, W. P.; Spear, R. J.; Read, R. W. *Aust. J. Chem.* 1989, *36*, 297.

[10] Kresze, G.; Bathelt, H.; *Tetrahedron* 1973, *29*, 1043.

[11] Hallé, J. C.; Vichard, D.; Pouet, M. J.; Terrier, F. *J. Org. Chem.* 1997, *62*, 7178. Pugnaud, S.; Masure, D.; Hallé, J. C.; Chaquin, P. *J. Org. Chem.* 1997, *62*, 8687.

[12] Vichard, D.; Hallé, J. C.; Huguet, B.; Pouet, M. J.; Riou, D.; Terrier, F. *Chem. Commun.* 1998, 791.

[13] Sepulcri, P.; Hallé, J. C.; Goumont, R.; Riou, D.; Terrier, F. *J. Org. Chem.* 1999, *64*, 9254. Sepulcri, P.; Goumont, R.; Hallé, J. C.; Riou, D.; Terrier, F. *J. Chem. Soc. Perkin Trans. 2.* 2000, 51.

[14] Sebban, M.; Goumont, R.; Hallé, J. C.; Marrot, J.; Terrier, F. *Chem. Commun.* 1999, 1009. Terrier, F.; Sebban, M.; Goumont, R.; Hallé, J. C.; Moutiers, G.; Cangelosi, I. Buncel, E., *J. Org. Chem.* 2000, *65*, 7391.

[15] Goumont, R; Sebban, M; Sepulcri, P; Marrot, J. and Terrier, F., *Tetrahedron* 2002, *58*, 3249; Goumont, R; Sebban, M. and Terrier, F., *Chem. Commun.* 2002, 2110.

[16] Goumont, M. Sebban, J. Marrot, F. Terrier, ARKIVOC, 2004, 85.

[17] Terrier, F.; Hallé, J. C.; MacCormack, P. and Pouet, M. J., *Can. J. Chem*, 1989, *67*, 50.

[18] Anet, F. A. L and Yavari, I., *Org. Magn. Reson.*, 1976, *8*, 158.

[19] Boulton, A. J. And Clifford D. P., *J Chem. Soc.*, 1965, 5414.

[20] Norris, W. P. and Osmunden, J., *J. Org. Chem.* 1965, *30*, 2407.

[21] Brown, W. E. and Keyes, R.T., *J. Org. Chem.* 1965, *30*, 2452.

[22] Terrier, F; Millot, F. and Chatrousse, A. P., *J. Org. Chem.* 1980, *45*, 2666.

[23] Terrier, F; Millot, F. ; Chatrousse, A. P. ; Pouet, M. J. and Simonnin, M., *Org. Magn. Reson.*, 1976, *8*, 56.

[24] Terrier, F.; Goumont, R.; Hallé, J. C. and Pouet, M. J., *J. Chem. Soc. Perkin Trans. 2.* 1995, 1629.

[25] Martin, G.E.; Hadden, C.E. *J. Nat. Prod.* 2000, 63, 543.

[26] Levy, G.C.; Lichter, R.L. *Nitrogen 15N NMR Spectroscopy*, Wiley : New York, 1978.

11

NMR Spectroscopy for Studying Integrin Antagonists

Nathan S. Astrof[1] and Motomu Shimaoka[2*]
[1]Mount Sinai School of Medicine
[2]Department of Molecular Pathobiology and Cell Adhesion Biology, Mie University Graduate School of Medicine
Japan

1. Introduction

The expansion of the modern pharmacopeia is driven by advances in structural genomics that enable the detailed understanding of drug - protein interactions necessary for the identification of novel compounds as well as improved variants of existing drugs. Our research has centered on understanding the mechanism by which a critical class of transmembrane receptor proteins, the integrins, become activated in healthy and disease states. An important component of this research has been in identifying novel inhibitors of integrin function and their mechanism of action. As we describe in the following sections, nuclear magnetic resonance spectroscopy (NMR) has been an essential tool in advances in this area, and is the major focus of this review.

Integrins are a family of cell surface receptor proteins that mediate cell-matrix and cell-cell adhesion (Hynes, 2002). Integrin mediated adhesion is critical in multiple phases of development and maintenance of tissue physiology. Conversely, aberrant integrin function that can arise due to inappropriate increase or decrease in expression levels as well as inappropriate levels of activation is implicated in many diseases including cancer, neurological and immunological disorders (Shimaoka and Springer, 2003). The critical role of integrins in maintenance of healthy physiology has stimulated intense efforts to understand the mechanism of integrin mediated adhesion and identify pharmacological agents that can alter integrin function and thus restore the appropriate levels of cellular adhesion. Although the focus of this review is on NMR spectroscopy, as opposed to the related technique of magnetic resonance imaging (MRI), many of the compounds identified as integrin antagonists are also of interest as probes for MRI, particularly in the area of cancer imaging (Dijkgraaf et al., 2009). Thus, although we confine ourselves to understanding the interactions between antagonists and integrins by NMR in vitro, many of these results are directly applicable to the study of integrin expression and function by MRI *in vivo*.

Nuclear magnetic resonance (NMR) spectroscopy has played a central role in understanding the mechanism of integrin activation and providing insight into the nature and dynamic

* Corresponding Author

consequences of known small molecule modulators of integrin function (Beglova et al., 2002; Kallen et al., 1999). However, integrins are large (~2 megadalton), poly-glycosylated, membrane-associated receptor proteins and NMR studies of systems of such complexity are exceptionally challenging. Fortunately, (at least some of) the ecto- domains of the integrin heterodimer can be expressed in the absence of the transmembrane segments and retain ligand binding function and specificity (Xiong et al., 2007). In particular, the ligand binding I-domain, is found in half of all vertebrate integrins and can be expressed (and isotope labeled) using conventional bacterial over-expression systems (Kriwacki et al., 2000; Lambert et al., 2008; Legge et al., 2000). Many potent integrin antagonists that target the I domain have been developed drawing on the structural insights of NMR investigations into I-domain : antagonist structure, and this remains an active and promising area of research (Constantine et al., 2006; Crump et al., 2004; Liu et al., 2001; Winn et al., 2001; Weitz-Schmidt et al., 2001).

Although there has been great progress in understanding integrin biology using recombinantly expressed fragments, there is also considerable interest in studying the regulation of integrin function *in situ*. Integrins are regulated by signals originating both outside and within the cell on which they are expressed and a pure *in vitro* system can-not fully recapitulate the complex dynamics of cellular signaling. The large size and transmembrane linkage limits the use of routine solution experiments for NMR observation of the integrin in the native environment. However, techniques described in this review, including saturation transfer difference NMR (STD-NMR), allow for a detailed investigation into the binding mechanism from the perspective of the ligand (Mayer and Meyer, 1999). Although the integrin is not directly observed in these techniques, these investigations bridge the gap between structural studies of integrin ligands in solution by NMR and high-resolution structures of integrins obtained both by crystallography and advanced modeling techniques (Wagstaff et al., 2010b; Claasen et al., 2005; Meinecke and Meyer, 2001). These methods are useful both in large scale screening programs and also to understand conformational changes in ligands associated with integrin binding.

2. Integrin function in physiology and disease

Integrins are a family of metazoan specific transmembrane proteins that mediate cell adhesion (intercellular and cell-matrix) and transmit signals associated with attachment into the cell (Hynes, 2002). Integrins are expressed on all cell types and have a panoply of physiological roles in development, as evidenced by the dramatic phenotype(s) observed in transgenic knock-out models of many integrins or their protein ligands e.g. (George et al., 1993; Yang et al., 1993). Some integrins, though less critical during development, are absolutely required for survival of the mature organism. For example, knockout of the leukocyte restricted integrin LFA-1 results in pronounced but selective immune deficits, underscoring the importance of LFA-1 in multiple phases of the immune response (Ding et al., 1999).

Integrins can rapidly up and down regulate their affinity for ligands from the basal to fully activated state (Shamri et al., 2005). This differs from other adhesion molecules that require changes in cell surface expression and in-membrane diffusion to modulate the adhesive properties of the cells on which they are expressed. Cells utilize the dynamic nature of integrin adhesion to dynamically modulate their interaction with the surrounding environment on a timescale much shorter than possible with other cell adhesion molecules. Conversely, the dynamic nature of integrin-mediated adhesion requires a precision regulatory apparatus since even small perturbations in integrin activity regulation can have pronounced effects. This is strikingly evident in murine transgenics in which constitutively active variants are 'knocked-in' to replace the normal wild-type variants. These knock-in mice display phenotypes often as severe as the transgenic knock-out of the same gene (Imai et al., 2008; Park et al., 2007; Semmrich et al., 2005).

Each integrin is formed from the non-covalent association of 1 of 18 alpha subunits and 1 of 8 beta subunits with 24 known combinations expressed on mammalian cells excluding splice variants (Hynes, 2002). For example, the integrin LFA-1 is formed from the alphaL subunit and the beta2 subunit, designated αLβ2. A third commonly encountered nomenclature is the cluster of differentiation where LFA-1 is designated CD11a/CD18. The integrin Mac-1, found predominantly on neutrophils, is formed from the common beta2 (CD18) subunit but uses the CD11b alpha chain and is designated as αMβ2 or CD11b/CD18. The complete array of mammalian integrins is shown in **FIGURE 1**.

Each integrin has a unique, but overlapping, ligand binding profile (Campbell and Humphries, 2011). Most integrin ligands are extracellular matrix molecules including fibronectin, vitronectin and collagen. Other ligands are cell surface proteins, such as the Intercellular Adhesion Molecules (ICAMs). A canonical recognition motif for many integrins is Arg-Gly-Asp (RGD), with residues flanking either end of the triplet responsible for specifying the correct conformation to bind to distinct integrins (Ruoslahti, 1996). Other integrins recognize unique motifs found in a select group of protein(s). While many integrins do not recognize the RGD motif, an acidic moiety is a common feature of all integrin ligands (Plow et al., 2000).

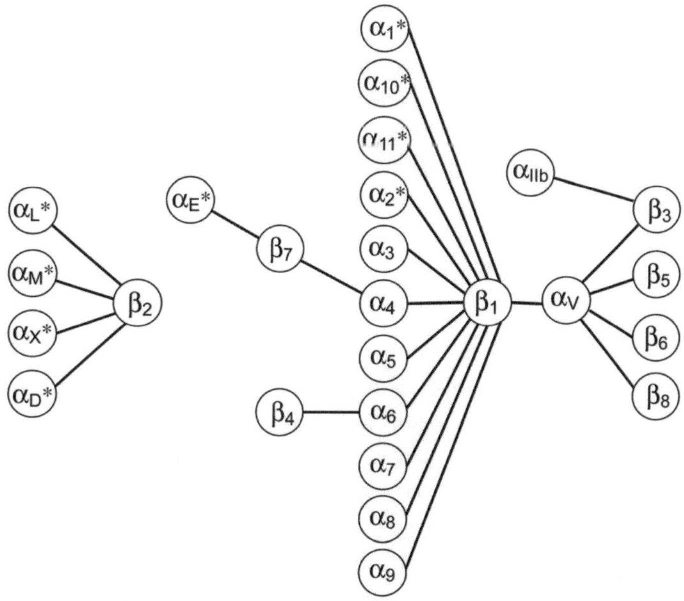

Fig. 1. Integrin subunit combinations. 18 alpha and 8 beta subunits form 24 integrin heterodimers. Asterisks denote alpha subunits containing an inserted (I) domain.

2.1 Disease

Integrins are involved in all aspects of mammalian physiology. It is not surprising that integrins are also involved in the pathogenesis of numerous diseases. Integrins involvement in disease initiation and progression may result either via direct perturbation of integrin expression or function. Alternatively, integrin function may be exploited to circumvent ordinary protection against disease physiology. One of the central challenges of pharmacology is to selectively alter integrin function that promotes the disease state in the much greater background of normal integrin activity (Shimaoka and Springer, 2003).

Cancer: Several Integrins play a crucial role in cancer development and the specific integrins varies depending upon the primary origin of the cancer (Jin and Varner, 2004). Down regulation of integrin expression is required to migrate to secondary tissues as well as establish a secondary site of growth. The high metabolic needs of cancer cells also requires extensive angiogenesis, the growth of blood vessels. Two αV integrins (αVβ3 and αVβ8) have received considerable interest due to their role in cell survival and promoting angiogenesis(Nemeth et al., 2007). Appreciation of the critical role of these integrins in cancer has led to the development of inhibitors targeting αV integrins as chemotherapeutics. One example, the cyclic RGD-f(NMet) peptide, is currently in clinical trials for glioblastoma (Reardon et al., 2008).

Thrombosis: Integrin αIIbβ3 binding to ligand fibrinogen is required for the process of blood clot formation. Aberrant clot formation is occurring within blood vessels is called thrombosis, a life-threatening condition (Coller and Shattil, 2008). Thrombosis may be treated with drugs such as eptifibtide, a cyclic peptide derived from a snake venom protein barbourin with a KGD sequence that acts as an αIIbβ3 competitive antagonist (Scarborough, 1999).

Autoimmunity: Integrins play multiple roles within the immune system including mediating migration to and from the source of infections, stabilizing contacts between immune cells, delivering key co-stimulatory signals required for immune cell development and function, as well as mediating opsonization of foreign organisms (Evans et al., 2009). Autoimmune disorders, including multiple sclerosis, psoriasis and colitis, involve physiological integrin function being co-opted by dysfunctional immune cells, facilitating the propagation of disease. Developing selective inhibitors of leukocyte expressed integrins, particularly the β2 family and the α4 integrins is a major focus of anti-inflammatory effector research (Shimaoka and Springer, 2003).

Infection: Although integrin function is obligate for normal immune homeostasis, several integrins are also exploited for the establishment and maintenance of several diseases. Integrins act as receptors or co-receptors for several viruses, including paploma virus (α6β4) (Yoon et al., 2001), rotavirus (α2β1 and α4β1) (Fleming et al., 2007), Ebola virus (α5β1) (Schornberg et al., 2009) and adenoviruses (Cuzange et al., 1994). These interactions may be with the canonical ligand binding regions or with other regions of the integrins, a critical consideration in the design of selective inhibitors of pathogen - intergrin interactions. Some integrins may also facilitate the formation of a virological synapse and promote the spread of lentiviruses such as HIV (Cicala et al., 2011).

3. Integrin structure

Both α and β integrin subunits are complex, multidomain single-span type-I transmembrane glycoproteins with short (but critical) cytoplasmic sequences excluding β4 which has a large intracellular domain (**FIGURE 2A-C**). High-resolution structural techniques including x-ray crystallography, cryo-electron microscopy (cryo-EM) and NMR spectroscopy have converged on a model of the individual integrin domains and their role in the transition from inactive to active state. Of particular importance is the high level of sequence conservation within the integrin family, such as the location and number of critical disulphide bonds (Luo et al., 2007). Thus, although high-resolution structures have only been obtained for two intact members of the β3 family and a single β2 integrin, the structural insights gained are applicable to other integrins (Xie et al., 2004; Xiong et al., 2001).

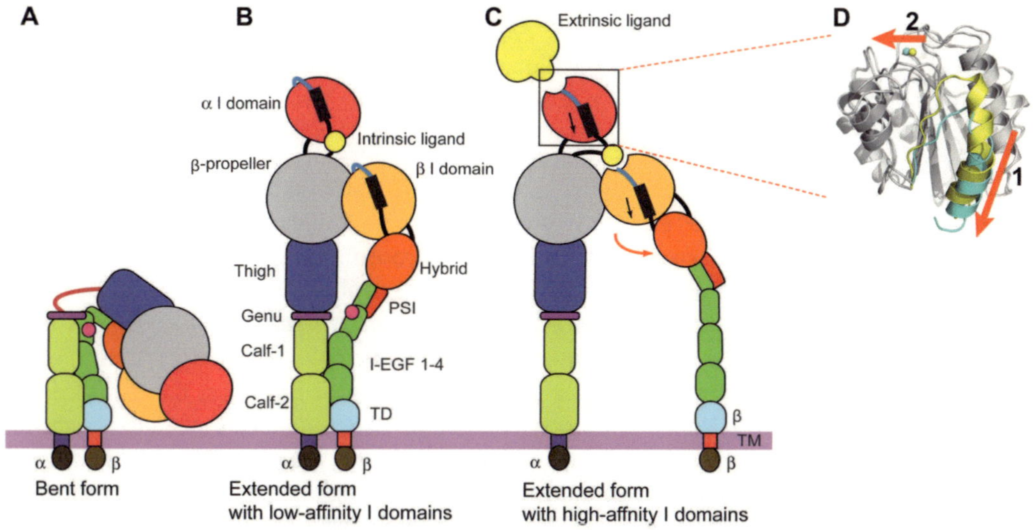

Fig. 2. Integrin structures and domains and conformational changes. (**A-C**) Global conformational changes between the bent (**A**), intermediate (**B**), and extended (**C**) conformations. Blow-ups showing the structures of the high- and low-affinity conformations of the alpha I domains (**D**). A piston-like downward shift of the C-terminal helix (arrow 1) is allosterically linked to the conversion of the MIDAS to the high-affinity configuration (arrow 2). Superposition of the high- (blue) and closed low- (yellow) affinity I domains is shown. Regions undergoing significant conformational changes are colored, whereas regions not undergoing significant conformational changes are in gray.

3.1 Extracellular domain

3.1.1 α-subunit

Integrin alpha subunits are organized in 4 or 5 domains and are approximately 1000 amino acids in length. The N-terminus forms a β-propeller with each strand of the propeller formed from a 4-stranded antiparallel β-sheet. C-terminal to the β-propeller is the thigh, calf-1 and calf-2 domains, all β-sandwich domains that bear topological similarity with immunoglobin domains. A short disulphide bonded loop, the genu, is positioned between the thigh and calf-1 domains; the genu can form a calcium coordinating site although this is not observed in all integrins (Xie et al., 2004). A furin protease cleavage site, located in calf-2 that separates the alpha subunit into light and heavy chains is found in a subset of integrins (α3, α5, α6, α8, αV, and αIIb) (Campbell and Humphries, 2011).

In half of all mammalian integrin subunits (α1, α2, α10, α11, αL, αX, αM, αD, αE) an additional domain is inserted between blades 2 and 3 of the β-propeller. When present the Inserted (I-) domain forms all or part of the ligand-binding site (Shimaoka et al., 2002). Multiple crystal, and one NMR structure, have been determined of isolated I domains from several integrins. The I-domain is built from seven α-helices wrapping five parallel and one anti-parallel strands that generally alternate in the protein sequence. On the 'top' face of the I domain, five amino acids side chains form a divalent cation binding site (the metal ion dependent adhesion site, MIDAS) (Lee et al., 1995b; Qu and Leahy, 1995). A ring of hydrophobic residues (the hydrophobic cup) surrounds the MIDAS site (Shimaoka et al., 2002). The N- and C- termini of the I domain are in close proximity and form flexible linkers to the β-propeller, as revealed in a recent crystal structure of the integrin αXβ2 (Xie et al., 2004).

The I domain from integrin αM crystallizes in two conformations, termed open and closed (Lee et al., 1995a; Lee et al., 1995b). The two conformations, which are thought to represent endpoints of a conformational continuum, differ in the coordination sphere surrounding the MIDAS (**FIGURE 2D**). In the open conformation, one of the acidic residues coordinating the metal is replaced by a water molecule, the effect of which is to increase the electrophilicity of the metal. Since physiological integrin ligands contain acidic residues, reorganization of the MIDAS promotes ligand binding, as does the repositioning of loops on the top face that occurs in the open state. Also, in the open conformation the C-terminal helix is shifted downward by approximately two turns with respect to the position in the closed conformation. It is thought that conformational changes C-terminal helix acts as an allosteric switch regulating the conformation of the ligand binding face, a hypothesis that is supported by additional biochemical evidence and computer simulations (Jin et al., 2004; Xiong et al., 2000).

Unlike αM, the I domain from αL does not crystallize naturally in the open conformation; this is consistent with the observation that the isolated wild-type αM I domain retains affinity for ligand while the I domain from αL does not (Lu et al., 2001b; Qu and Leahy, 1995). However, using the open structure of αM as a template, is has been possible to engineer disulphide bonds in the αL sequence that stabilize the conformation of the open state (Lu et al., 2001a). Locking the αL I domain in the open conformation results in a 10^4 increase in affinity for ligand. In a co-crystal of the high affinity αL I domain with a two domain fragment of the ligand Intracellular Adhesion Molecule-1 (ICAM-1-D1D2), the C-terminal helix is found in the (expected) downward conformation and the ligand binding face, including the MIDAS, has undergone the appropriate conformational changes to facilitate binding to ligand. A number of polar and electrostatic interactions adjacent to the hydrophobic cup (and absent in αM) confer specificity of the I-domain : ICAM-1 interaction (Shimaoka et al., 2003).

3.1.2 β-subunit

The β subunits are ~640 amino acids in length, organized into 8 discrete extracellular domains. The N-terminus is a 54 residue, 2 stranded antiparallel β-sheet linked by disulphide bonds to pair of short α helices. The structure is homologous to the plexins and semaphorins and is thus called the Plexin-semaphorin-integrin (PSI) domain. Notably, the fourth disulphide bond is actually to a stretch of amino acids C-terminal to the adjacent hybrid domain, an immunoglobulin - like structure, such that the hybrid domain is inserted within the PSI domain (Luo et al., 2007).

Inserted within the hybrid domain is the βA or I - like domain, which is structurally homologous to the I-domain found in half of mammalian integrin α subunits. The peculiar topology of the I-like domain, a domain inserted into a domain inserted into a domain, is critical for the mechanism of integrin activation. In addition to the MIDAS, there are two additional coordination sites whose occupancy regulates the affinity of the MIDAS metal for ligand through shared coordination residues. These two metal binding sites (the Adjacent to MIDAS, ADMIDAS, and Ligand Induced Biniding Site, LIMBS) may also selectively directly coordinate some ligands (Xiao et al., 2004; Xiong et al., 2002).

The residues C-terminal to the I-like domain are organized into four- cysteine rich Epidermal Growth factor like (EGF) domains. The integrin-EGF (I-EGF) domains are highly homologous to the canonical domain but have additional numbers and/or placements of the disulphide bonds (Beglova et al., 2002; Takagi et al., 2001; Wouters et al., 2005). The most C-terminal ecto domain is the β-terminal domain (βTD), a novel fold with an N-terminal helix facing a mixed parallel/antiparallel β-strand.

Transmembrane: The transmembrane (TM) domains of integrins form a critical nexus between the extracellular and intracellular domains. Despite the great importance of the domains to the mechanism of integrin mediated adhesion and signaling, they are the least well-understood domains of integrin heterodimers. NMR of isolated transmembrane domains (in detergent solutions), disulphide cross-linking studies and molecular modeling studies have been used to identify the interface between the two chains. These studies converge on a right-handed coil-coil structure, which persists into the cytoplasm, similar to the previously determined structure of the TM protein glycophorin (Gottschalk, 2005; Li et al., 2002; Luo et al., 2004).

Cytoplasmic: Integrin cytoplasmic domains play a role in integrin function that is disproportionate to their generally small size. Interactions between the α and β cytoplasmic domains help constrain integrins in the inactive conformation (Vinogradova et al., 2002). Phosophorylation of the cytoplasmic domains regulates indirect interactions with the cytoskeleton and protein signaling complexes (Fagerholm et al., 2004). The cytoplasmic tail complexes of two integrins, αIIbβ3 and αLβ2 have been extensively studied by NMR (Vinogradova et al., 2002). The αIIb tail forms a short N-terminal a helix followed by a turn and a C-terminal loop that collapse back onto the N-terminal helix. The β3 tail also forms an N-terminal helix while the majority of the tail lacks persistent structure. A salt bridge between residue arginine 995 in the αIIb chain (αR-995) forms with the aspartic acid 723 in the β3 tail (βD-723). Prior biochemical studies of integrins using heterologous expression suggested the existence of a stabilizing salt bridge interaction as a critical element in regulating the affinity state of integrins (Lu et al., 2001c). Notably, the cytoplasmic tail structure of the integrin αLβ2, also determined by NMR, is significantly different (Bhunia et al., 2009). The αL is folds into three defined α-helical segments with compact tertiary structure and the β2 tail into a single helix followed by unstructured segments. Like the αIIbβ3 tail complex, the αLβ2 association incorporates a prominent electrostatic interaction. Both similarities and differences in the two structures highlight the strengths, but also limitations, of extrapolating limited structural studies of one integrin to another, particularly in regions of lower sequence homology such as the tail domains.

4. Architecture and activation mechanism

Overall, in both α and β chains the integrin architecture can be divided into distinct structural elements. The integrin "head", which includes the canonical ligand-binding site, is formed from the β-propeller in the α-subunit and the I-like domain in the β- subunit. In a subset of integrins, the Inserted (I-) domain is also present in the integrin head. The headpiece includes both the head domains as well as the thigh domain in the α chain and the plexin-semaphorin- integrin (PSI), and hybrid domains in the β subunit. The tailpiece is formed in the alpha subunit by the calf -1 and calf-2 domains and 4 integrin-type epidermal growth factor like (I-EGF) domains in the β subunit. The tailpiece is connected to the transmembrane domains which each span the membrane a single time and the (generally) short cytoplasmic sequences.

In the crystal structure of αVβ3, the integrin is folded into a 'V 'shape; a 135 degree angle is found between the head and tailpiece domains with a bend between the thigh and calf-1 domains in the alpha subunit and the I-EGF-1 and I-EGF-2 in the beta subunit. Although neither the transmembrane, nor the cytoplasmic domains are present in the crystallized proteins, they are generally regarded as being fully associated in the conformation visualized in the crystal structure. In this conformation, which establishes substantial inter and intradomain buried interfaces, the ligand-binding headpiece is inaccessible to ligands on opposing surfaces (Xiong et al., 2001).

Integrins that lack I-domains use an interface between the β-propeller and the I -like domain to form the ligand-binding site. The architecture of a canonical ligand binding motif was first identified in a crystal structure of the integrin αVβ3 with P5, a RGD containing cyclic peptide [Arg-Gly-Asp-{D-Phe}-N-methyl-Val} (Xiong et al., 2002). P5 binds within a crevice formed from the β-propeller and the βA domain; 335 Å, or 45% of the peptide surface area, is buried within the crevice. In the bound structure, the arginine and aspartic acid are pointed in opposite directions, the (partially solvent exposed) Arg pointing towards the β-propeller, inserted into a narrow sub-groove where it is stabilized by a pair of aspartic acids that form a bidentate salt bridge. The Asp is fully buried with one of the carboxylates coordinating the MIDAS metal; the second oxygen establishes a network of polar interactions with backbone amides and the aliphatic side chain makes additional hydrophobic contacts with protein side chain. The medial glycine sits at the α/β interface, making hydrophobic contacts with the α chain. Both of the non-RGD residues are purely structural, establishing the correct disposition of the RGD and point away from the α/β interface.

The crystal structure of ligand bound integrins reveal a number of structural changes in the β chain I -like domain that are analogous to those that occur during activation of the I domain. The β6-α7 loop is repositioned and the C-terminal helix is shifted downward in a piston like motion. Subsequent structures reveal how ligand binding is coupled to activation of the holoreceptor (Xiao et al., 2004). Ligand binding to the αIIβ3 headpiece crystal structure shows a profound swing out motion of the hybrid domain/PSI, away from the α/β interface where the hybrid domain is tucked in the resting conformation. This motion propagates changes in the ligand-binding headpiece to the remainder of the integrin, and is a critical element of the *switchblade model* of integrin activation.

The switchblade model of integrin activation states that the integrin is in a conformational equilibrium between the bent state, observed in the crystal structure of αVβ3 and an extended conformation (or conformations) in which legs become separated and the headpiece becomes extended over the tailpiece (Luo et al., 2007). In this extended conformation, the headpiece is well disposed to bind ligands in the extracellular matrix or on the surface of opposing cells. Extension also favors dissociation of the transmembrane and cytoplasmic, facilitating the formation of signaling complexes on the tails. Integrin activation is bidirectional and can be driven either by ligand binding to the headpiece, favoring a swung out hybrid domain which in turn disrupts the stabilizing interfaces and favors receptor extension. Alternatively, activation may occur within the cell via binding of transiently exposed cytoplasmic tails which, stabilized in the dissociated conformation, can initiate conformational changes that propagate across the membrane, resulting in extension, swing out of the hybrid domain and an integrin primed for ligand binding.

In integrins that have an I domain in the a subunit (i.e. αLβ2), there is a conserved acidic residue in the linker connecting the C-terminal tail back into the β-propeller (Alonso et al., 2002). When the C-terminal helix is shifted downward, the acidic residue can coordinate the β subunit MIDAS metal. The downward motion of the C-terminal helix thus transmits the effect of ligand binding to the I domain across the α/β subunit interface with the acidic residue acting as an internal ligand. The subsequent steps of integrin activation are identical for both classes of integrins (Nishida et al., 2006).

5. NMR overview

NMR spectroscopy is an extensively used tool for the structural and dynamic characterization of proteins, small molecule ligands and their complexes. An exhaustive review of NMR theory and methodology is available in many organic and biological chemistry texts (e.g. (Cavanagh et al., 2006; Ege, 2003)); here, we selectively present information salient for understanding (and interpreting) published and future work on integrin and integrin - antagonist complexes.

NMR spectroscopy draws on quantum mechanical property of spin, the polarization of a subset of nuclear isotopes when placed in a magnetic field. This includes all three isotopes of hydrogen, the most abundant element in biomolecules. However, only the spin ½ nuclei – such as the ^{1}H (proton) nucleus is commonly studied by NMR. ^{2}H (deuterium) is a spin 1 nucleus; nuclei with spin >1/2 are generally low sensitivity and difficult to observe in solution. The radioactive ^{3}H (tritium) nucleus is not commonly observed, despite being spin ½ and the most sensitive NMR active nucleus. Fortunately, both carbon (^{13}C) and nitrogen (^{15}N) have a spin ½ isotope, albeit at low natural abundance (~1 % and ~0.4 % respectively). To utilize these nuclei for biomolecular investigations it is necessary, in general, to increase the enrichment levels. This can be accomplished by expressing proteins in organisms, typically *Escherichia coli,* that can grow in defined media containing appropriate isotopic precursors (i.e. ^{15}N labeled ammonium chloride, ^{13}C labeled glucose). Unfortunately, there is no spin ½ nucleus of oxygen, precluding direct observation in proteins and studies of hydrogen bonding in protein - ligand studies.

NMR experiments involve the perturbation of the equilibrium spin state by one or more appropriately tuned radio-frequency pulses and interspersed delay periods. This collection of pulses and delays is called a pulse sequence. A pulse sequence may be as simple as a single pulse applied to a single nucleus or involve hundreds of pulses and delays applied to as many as four nuclei. In both extremes, the resulting spectra (derived as the Fourier transform of the time dependent signal obtained by the NMR detector) are determined by the same set of three interactions: (1) chemical shift, (2) scalar (J-coupling) and (3) dipolar coupling that modulate the energy levels of the nuclear spins during the NMR experiment.

Local variations in electronic structure within the molecule result in the nucleus becoming more or less shielded from the spectrometer magnetic field, giving rise to small differences in nuclear magnetic energy levels. This phenomenon is known as the chemical shift and is the most readily observed effect in the NMR spectrum. Each peak in the NMR spectrum corresponds to the single type of nucleus in the molecule. Because each nucleus has a distinctive chemical shift, it is possible to obtain site-specific information throughout the molecule with the chemical shift of a particular nucleus acting as its molecular signature.

The J- coupling is an interaction between (directly or indirectly) covalently bonded NMR active nuclei. In the simple, one dimensional (1D) NMR experiment, the J-coupling between NMR active nuclei results in the NMR signals (peaks) to be split into multiple peaks. The number of peaks in the observed NMR spectrum is governed by the total number of coupled nuclei - each spin ½ nucleus coupled to n nuclei is split into n+1 peaks. The magnitude of the J coupling is determined by: (a) the chemical nature of the coupled nuclei (heteronuclear vs. homonuclear), the number of covalent bonds between coupled nuclei and the relative orientation between the two coupled nuclei.

Finally, the dipolar coupling between nuclei is a through space interaction that depends on the distance between the two NMR active nuclei, as opposed to covalent connectivity. In simple NMR experiments, the dipolar coupling largely contributes to the line width of the peaks in the spectrum, since each NMR active nucleus acts as its own magnet and thus perturbs the magnetic field of those nuclei around it. The dipolar coupling gives rise to the Nuclear Overhauser effect (NOE), the perturbation of the energy state of one spin by another through space.

With simple organic molecules, it is possible to determine the molecular structure using one-pulse (i.e. ^{1}H and ^{13}C) NMR experiments. Most organic groups have defined chemical shift ranges and, in conjunction with other spectroscopic techniques, the chemical shift and J-coupling provide suitable information to determine the molecular structure. For more complicated molecules - and especially large biopolymers, the enormous number of nuclei results in a complex, highly degenerate and uninterpretable NMR spectrum. The general approach to obtain resonance assignments for complex molecules is based upon a technique known alternatively as correlation or multidimensional NMR spectroscopy (nD NMR). In nD NMR, the NMR interactions, obtained by a suitably designed pulse sequence are displayed along two (n = 2) or more orthogonal axis. For example, the chemical shifts of two J-coupled nuclei can be obtained by an NMR experiment that first detects the chemical shift of the first nucleus, then allows for transfer between the two nuclei by the J coupling and then finally detects the chemical shift of the second nucleus. Alternatively, the same experiment can be performed by with transfer arranged via the NOE effect. Then, the chemical shifts of all nuclei close in physical space, but not necessarily covalently connected, can be obtained. Together, these techniques permit both the assignment of complex organic molecules as well as a determination of three- dimensional structure.

For moderately sized proteins (<= 100 amino acids), homonuclear (2D) ^{1}H-NMR spectroscopy provides sufficient information to obtain resonance assignments, secondary and tertiary structural constraints suitable for the determination of high-resolution structure (Wuthrich, 1986). The resonance assignments phase proceeds in two steps. First, individual amino acids are assigned using J-coupling experiments to identify coupled sets of spins (spin systems), taking advantage of the characteristic proton fingerprint spin topologies of the natural amino acids. As there are no strong proton J-couplings between adjacent amino acid, this results in exclusively intra-residue assignments. Inter-residue connectivities are obtained via through space NOE experiments that allow correlations between protons that are close in space (i.e. on adjacent amino acids) but which are not necessarily detectably J-coupled.

2D-^{1}H spectra of protein encode both distance and angle restraints that can be extracted from the spectra. The magnitudes of multi-bond scalar couplings (i.e. the three bond J coupling along the peptide backbone between the alpha and amide protons, $^3JC\alpha_H$-N_H) are a function of the intervening angles. The intensity of the cross peaks in ^{1}H-NOE type experiments are proportional to the inverse sixth power of the distance between the two nuclei. Additional structural information is available from the pattern of chemical shifts that deviate in a regular pattern from that of an unstructured peptide depending upon the type of secondary structural element they are found in. Furthermore, during the NMR experiment, amide protons from the protein backbone can exchange with solvent if not protected by stable hydrogen bond formation. If deuterated water is used during the NMR experiment, hydrogens that have undergone exchange disappear from the spectrum. Thus, by dissolving the protein in ^2H_2O, it is possible to identify amino acids that are located in regions of stable secondary structure, since they are protected from exchange with ^{2}H. The data obtained can then be used to compute a family of NMR structures that satisfy the measured constraints.

The greater number of resonances, and higher molecular weight of larger proteins (which results in broader and less well resolved NMR signals) necessitates the use of heteronuclear (^{13}C and ^{15}N) multidimensional (nD > 2) spectroscopy for resonance assignments and structure to be obtained. Numerous pulse sequences have been developed to obtain chemical shifts, scalar couplings and distances using the ^{15}N and ^{13}C chemical shifts to provide additional resolution for the spectra. Despite the additional complexity associated with performing these experiments (including the need to prepare isotopically labeled protein samples), the basic building blocks of structure determination are essentially the same as described for homonuclear ^{1}H protein spectroscopy: obtain resonance assignments from intra- and inter-residue correlations, determine distance and spatial (angular) constraints, incorporate additional parameters such as amide protection and patterns of chemical shifts and convert experimental constraints into energy terms for computational refinement.

NMR experiments involve the perturbation of the collection of spins from their equilibrium, a process that is opposed by relaxation effects that restore the collection of spins back to their equilibrium state. Although spontaneous relaxation is an inefficient process, the motion of the protein in solution (both overall tumbling and low barrier transitions) gives rise to local magnetic fields that can result in the loss of the NMR signal. In general, there are two relaxation processes that are of interest. T_1 (transverse) relaxation is the true relaxation of the spins to equilibrium state. T_2 (longitudinal) relaxation is the loss of NMR coherence between two otherwise identical spins in different molecules. Both are a result of global and internal protein motions and place limits on the length (and complexity) of a given NMR experiment. While great care can be taken to minimize the effects on the NMR spectra (such as designing the shortest possible pulse sequences necessary to obtain required information) the relaxation processes also provide valuable information both on the overall shape of the protein (from tumbling effects) or internal conformational transitions (dynamics). The latter information is of increasing importance as it is recognized that proteins, rather than being static entities, exist in multiple inter-converting sub-states and that agonists and antagonist may function by favoring (or disfavoring) one or more of these states. Site specific information on protein dynamics is thus of both basic interest to understanding protein function but also of practical interest to the design of improved pharmaceuticals.

NMR experiments specifically designed to measure protein dynamics have been developed (Mittermaier and Kay, 2006). These include the aforementioned amide proton protection experiments, since transient opening of the protein structure permits the exchange of ^1H with ^2H which can be directly measured in a 2D ^1H,^{15}N J-coupling correlation experiment (the heteronuclear single quantum coherence, HSQC experiment) for each amide nucleus in the protein backbone and some side chains as well. More quantitative information on backbone protein dynamics can be obtained by measuring the T_1 and T_2, as well as the ^1H-^{15}N NOE. Methods have been developed to interpret these parameters in terms of the angular fluctuations and timescales of motion of the protein backbone. Similar experiments have been developed to monitor the dynamics of protein side chains using heteronuclear relaxation of isotopically labeled side chains.

Motions slower than that contributing to nuclear relaxation are also apparent in the NMR spectrum of proteins. For example, if the protein inter-converts between two or more conformations slower than the NMR data is recorded; two sets of resonances will appear in the spectrum. When this chemical exchange is faster, a single set of resonances may appear but the exchange parameters may be extracted from appropriately designed NMR experiments. Because these experiments measure biologically relevant timescale motions (μs-ms) they are of special interest in understanding protein function, and its perturbation by ligand binding (Palmer and Massi, 2006).

NMR dynamics and exchange experiments are excellent of examples of NMR investigations where high-resolution structure determination is not necessarily the key endpoint. Other examples include measuring one or more NMR parameters, such as protein ^1H and ^{15}N chemical shifts in an HSQC experiment as a function of ligand concentration to identify binding sites (and in some cases binding constants). These experiments are particularly valuable when structure of the biomacromolecule of interest has already been obtained and the goal is restricted to identifying novel ligands, ligand variants or the mode of ligand binding. This approach, namely measuring a subset of crucial NMR parameters and utilizing previously available information on the structure of the target molecule, is employed by many of the studies summarized in this review.

6. NMR of integrin I domain antagonists

The I domain from integrin LFA-1 has been the primary objective of numerous investigations to identify novel integrin antagonists. This is due both to the critical role of LFA-1 in mediating multiple phases of the immune response, as well as the capacity to produce large quantities of pure, soluble isotopically labeled protein to exploit the full range of tools of structural biology. An NMR structure of the αL I domain was obtained using assignment and structural determination methods described in the prior section (Legge et al., 2000). In general, the topology is identical to that determined by x-ray crystallography. Most significantly, the C-terminal helix (α7), which shows the greatest variation in crystallographic structures, is highly flexible, as determined both by absence of long-range ^{1}H-^{1}H NOEs, weak ^{1}H-^{15}N NOEs as well as limited protection against amide proton exchange, compared to the core of the protein. These observations validate the biophysical model and computer simulations of a flexible C-terminus acting as a ratchet or switch regulating the conformation and ligand binding activity of the protein (Jin et al., 2004).

The ligand for αLβ2 is the five-domain cell surface molecule Intracellular Adhesion Molecule (ICAM)-1. Titration of a soluble two domain ICAM-1 fragment (sICAM-1-D1-D2) into the protein labeled with ^{15}N and / or ^{15}N, ^{13}C revealed unique, concentration dependent behavior of the pattern of heteronuclear and proton chemical shifts (Huth et al., 2000). At high concentrations of ligand, extensive broadening in the NMR spectrum was observed, consistent with formation of a high molecular weight complex. At sub-saturating concentrations, however, the broadened residues were largely confined to two regions of the protein. Line broadening at residues around the MIDAS could be expected due direct chemical exchange with ligands. A second region of greater than average broadening was observed in the C-terminal helix and the opposing β-strand. The cleft between the two secondary structural elements was termed the I domain activation site (IDAS) as the basal and inducible ligand binding activity of several holoreceptors bearing mutations in the cleft was enhanced when compared to wild-type LFA-1 receptors.

6.1 Lovastatin

The allosteric regulation of I domain function by residues in the MIDAS suggests that some anti-LFA-1 antagonists may work via an allosteric mode of pharmacological intervention distinct from competitive inhibition. A high-throughput screen for small molecule antagonists of LFA-1 identified one such compound, lovastatin, which is the prototypical member of a class of small molecule allosteric integrin antagonists (Kallen et al., 1999).

Lovastatin, a fungal metabolite was earlier identified as competitive inhibitor of a 3-hydroxy-3'-methyl glutaryl coenzyme A (HMG CoA) reductase, an enzyme in the cholesterol biosynthetic pathway and is used clinically for the reduction of high serum cholesterol. However, lovastatin also has (potentially) beneficial immunosuppressive properties that may be independent of the role in lowering serum cholesterol. Together, the observation of immune-modulation properties of lovastatin and its identification in a screen for LFA-1 antagonists suggests that the novel effects may be obtained directly via inhibition of LFA-1 (Weitz-Schmidt et al., 2001).

Using a cell based assay, lovastatin inhibits the adhesion of LFA-1 expressing cells to ICAM-1 substrate with an IC50 ~25 μM. Using a cell free assay with purified receptor and ligand proteins, the IC50 obtained was ~ 2.5 μM, demonstrating that the inhibition is a property of the proteins and does not involve the HMG-CoA reductase activity. Because lovastatin contains a lactone moiety that may be prone to hydrolysis, it was hypothesized that direct coordination of lovastatin acid to the MIDAS as the mechanism of inhibiting LFA-1 / ICAM-1 adhesion. Contrary to this suggestion, the hydroxyacid has weaker inhibition potential (>100 μM and ~14 μM for the cell based and cell free assays, respectively).

The mechanism of lovastatin inhibition of LFA-1 was directly addressing using soluble I domain labeled with ^{15}N using an E. coli expression system (Kallen et al., 1999). ^{1}H,^{15}N HSQC spectra were obtained for the free protein and in the presence of increasing concentrations of lovastatin-lactone or lovastatin-hydroxyacid. When the chemical shift differences between the free and drug added forms are mapped onto the structure of the I domain, a clear pattern became evident. The most significant perturbation in chemical shifts both in intensity and position are in the crevice between the C-terminal helix and the opposing beta sheet. Computer simulations further support the conjecture that lovastatin, and its derivatives, act as allosteric antagonists of LFA-1 function, preventing the obligate downward motion of the C-terminal helix (Gaillard et al., 2007).

A family of related statin derivatives was subsequently screened for binding to the I domain using a ^{1}H,^{15}N - HSQC . By obtaining spectra as a function of ligand concentration (with fixed protein) it is possible to estimate the binding dissociation constant (K_D) between statin derivative and I domain. The K_Ds range from ~2.0 μM for lovastatin and simvistatin to ~ 8 μM for mevastatin. Previstatin, with a hydroxylated terpenoid ring has an K_D > 100 μM, presumably due to the energetic costs of burying a polar residue in the largely hydrophobic crevice. The tightest binding inhibitor identified by NMR in this study was the synthetic derivative LFA703, which bound with ~0.2 μM affinity. Most significantly, these changes in K_D directly parallel the IC50 measured in using the intact holoreceptor in cell based assays, demonstrating that the I domain is the principle, and likely exclusive, source of the inhibitory effect and that screening allosteric antagonists by binding to isolated I domains is a valid approach to determining the affinity, and indirectly the efficacy, of I domain allosteric antagonists. Also, although the dynamics of the I -domain / lovastatin complex was not quantitatively measured, the spectra all showed signs of conformational exchange, consistent with fast binding and release kinetics of lovastatin or its derivatives from the I domain.

The demonstration of potent allosteric inhibition of the I domain has driven additional screens for LFA-1 antagonists derived from alternative chemotypes. One successful cell based screen identified a diaryl sulphide with an IC50 of ~2.3 μM, comparable to lovastatin (Crump et al., 2004). The addition of drug to ^{1}H,^{15}N labeled protein results in chemical shift and intensity changes in the spectra (due to chemical exchange) that were analogous to those for lovastatin, demonstrating that the two dissimilar chemotypes utilized a common mechanism for inhibition of function. Additional synthetic diaryl sulfides were prepared and also shown to bind to the same position of the I domain, albeit with dramatically greater efficacy (IC50 ~44 nM). Unlike lovatatin and the parent compound, however, no chemical exchange broadening was observed in the spectrum, consistent with tighter binding of the derivative; this indicates that the improved efficacy is a function of better binding to the I domain, as opposed to acting on a second site on the intact receptor.

Although the HSQC spectra are a rapid means of identifying and characterizing compounds that bind to the I domain, the process of drug design is greatly enhanced by having a high-resolution structural model of the drug - protein complex. Towards this aim, a comprehensive study of an I -domain allosteric inhibitor complex to the I domain was undertaken, initially with the determination of the ^{1}H, ^{15}N and ^{13}C chemical shifts assignments of the full complex. The authors subsequently obtained multiple NOE distance based constraints between drug and protein, facilitating a high-resolution structure of the complex that could be used to rationalize the enhanced efficacy of the drug. As expected, the parent compound binds within the IDAS with a pocket formed by strands one, three and four of the central beta sheet and helices one and seven. Excellent superposition of the model with a crystal structure of the I domain - lovastatin complex validates the principle of using distinct molecular scaffolds to identify optimal allosteric inhibitors of I domain function.

6.2 SAR by NMR

Structure activity relationships by NMR (SAR by NMR) is an NMR based screening technology for discovering *de novo* or enhanced variants of existing protein inhibitors (Shuker et al., 1996). A library of small molecules is screened for binding to a protein target, typically by monitoring chemical shifts in a ^{1}H,^{15}N HSQC experiment. Although most small fragments in the library bind to protein weakly, when joined synthetically the binding affinity and hopefully, efficacy of the composite molecule is improved dramatically. SAR by NMR may be used to identify completely novel combination of appropriate molecular fragments. Alternatively, the approach can be used to selectively enhance the affinity of one segment of a small molecule while leaving another fixed. In this context, the invariant moiety is added first to the NMR tube; subsequently, a library is screened to find appropriate binders with enhanced binding potential at the variable portion of the molecule. Finally, the novel molecular fragment is tethered synthetically to the fixed portion and the molecule is tested for the desired biological activity.

SAR by NMR was used to successfully improve the binding and efficacy of inhibitors based on an aryl cinnamide moiety (Liu et al., 2001; Winn et al., 2001). After identifying fragments that could potentially improve the inhibitor, the authors next obtained ^{1}H-^{1}H NOEs of the ternary complex. The introduction of this additional step was a significant advance over simpler NMR screening protocols since it was possible to conclusively demonstrate that both fragments could bind to proximate but distinct regions on the protein. This extra step validated the potential of the separate fragments to mutually enhance protein binding when synthetically fused. These efforts led to the identification of a number of LFA-1 inhibitors with EC50s between 20 and 800 nM. In several cases the enhanced affinity was much less than anticipated based on the estimated binding affinity of the two fragments. However, this is not an unexpected phenomena since the linkers can both directly, through interactions with the protein, and indirectly, by forcing unfavorable orientation/steric effects on the protein, lower the combined binding potential of the linked fragment with respect to that of the individual chemical moieties.

6.3 Peptides

Peptides, with sequences derived from the canonical binding protein ligand are an alternative source of integrin binding reagents. Generally, short peptides are unstructured in aqueous solution. Cyclization of the peptide through the backbone or appropriate side chain chemistries enhances the population of one or more structured states. Artificial non-genetically encoded amino acids are also introduced into the sequence as structural promoting agents or to add additional side chain chemistries.

Peptides, however, are particularly difficult to crystallize, particularly from aqueous solution. Also, crystal structures of small molecules and peptides are modulated by strong packing forces and the observed structure may be different from that in free solution or bound to a target protein. NMR spectroscopy can capture the full range of conformations sampled by the peptide and in appropriate systems, such as the I domain, also permits direct observation of both receptor free and receptor bound forms.

Two cyclic peptides, cIBR, derived from ICAM-1 $_{12\text{-}21}$, (Cyclo1,12-Pen-PRGGSVLVTGC-OH) and cIBC, derived from ICAM-1$_{6\text{-}15}$, (Cyclo1,12-Pen-PSKVILPRGGC) have been shown to inhibit homotypic and heterotypic cell adhesion mediated by LFA-1 in a concentration dependent manner (Anderson et al., 2004). The peptides were cyclized through disulphide formation between the penicillamine moiety in position one and the cysteine at position twelve. Both peptides work, at least in part, via interactions with the I domain since their binding can be inhibited by the anti-αL-I domain antibody R3.1. Direct binding to intact soluble, TM free LFA-1 was demonstrated using a colorimetric ELISA binding assay. It is critical to note that although both peptides are derived from the authentic ligand, neither contains the canonical acidic group (in this case Glu34 of ICAM-1), suggesting an alternative mode of inhibition.

The structure of cIBR was determined by NMR spectroscopy in aqueous solution (Gursoy et al., 1999). The resonances were assigned using conventional through- bond (J-mediated) 2D-1H NMR spectra and inter-residue correlations from NOESY type experiments which were also used to obtain distance based constraints. Technically, the authors used a related pulse sequence called ROESY, a pulse sequence more suitable for obtaining distance constraints in low molecular weight systems. One experiment was performed to obtain the $^3J_{NH\text{-}HC\alpha}$ constants, another to determine the temperature dependence of the amide proton chemical shifts that are related to hydrogen bonding strength and thus indicative of presence of stable secondary structure. Molecular dynamics was used to obtain a set of structures for structural analysis. During the simulation, all the peptide bonds except the first (between Pen-1 and Pro-2) were held in the trans conformation. Final analysis of the structural ensemble revealed that a cis-conformer was present, albeit at low population and this form was not further studied.

Interactions between proximate amide protons observed in the ROESY spectrum suggest as many as 3 β-turns about Pro2-Gly5, Gly5-Leu8, and Val9-Cys12 in the peptide structure, although it is unclear of all three turns are present in the structure simultaneously or are inter-converting on a timescale slower than the NMR experiment. Additional data, namely the temperature dependence of amide protein chemical shift, suggests that the hydrogen bonds are weak and the structures are transiently populated.

In total, six structural families were obtained consistent with the NMR data, with each family containing 20 structures. Remarkably, some of the structures in the ensemble are in good agreement with the sequences in the context of the full-length domain 1 of ICAM-1. For example, the Pro-Arg-Gly-Gly sequence is derived from the β-hairpin turn connecting strands A and B of domain 1 of ICAM-1. Other regions of structural homology were also identified between peptide and full length protein, demonstrating that the small, cyclized peptide has captured at least some of the authentic architecture of the full-length ligand.

The binding site of both ICAM-1 derived peptides was measuring using the perturbation in 2D-NMR heteronuclear chemical shifts approach previously described. As anticipated by the absence of an acidic group in the ligand, the NMR data suggest an alternative, allosteric mode of inhibition for the two peptides. Specifically, the binding site was identified as the IDAS, the binding pocket for small molecule antagonists (Zimmerman et al., 2007).

Although high resolution structural data was not obtained, the authors utilized the existing peptide structures, as well as the known structure of the I domain, to dock the peptides individually into the IDAS performing energy minimization to obtain a structural model which could reveal key interactions between peptide and protein. Intriguingly, despite being of entirely distinct classes of chemical moieties, it was possible to superimpose segments of the peptide on the known position of the lovastatin. The superposition revealed that common amino acids in the I domain contact the two distinct types of inhibitor. The model of the peptide - I domain revealed that, much like lovastatin, the hydrophobic residues of the peptide Gly 5- Gly 11 of cIBR are buried into the crevice with numerous hydrophobic contacts between the apolar core and the peptide. In general, the polar peptide regions of the peptide are exposed to solvent; however there is a putative salt bridge interaction between the arginine residue and Glu301 of the protein. Future high resolution studies will be required to provide important insight into the mechanism of recognition between peptide and I domain, the role of the flexible, hydrophilic peptide sequence in inhibiting integrin function, and to rationalize the superior performance of cIBR over cIBC as an LFA-1 antagonist. However, the cyclic ICAM-1 peptides were first designed using the rational that competitive antagonists could be obtained using appropriately constrained elements of the native ligand sequence. These studies then demonstrate the power of basic, readily accessible NMR technology to test and refute mechanistic hypothesis of integrin antagonism.

6.4 Volatile anesthetics

General anesthesia is administered to ~40 million patients undergoing surgery in the United States every year (Suttner et al., 2002). Volatile anesthetics (VAs), a group of lipophilic small molecules that induce general anesthesia, are a major component of the anesthetics drugs currently used in operating rooms worldwide. Nevertheless, our understanding of the mechanisms by which these small-molecules alter the activity of the CNS, thereby leading to the loss of consciousness, remains limited. The established molecular targets of VAs in the CNS include membrane-embedded ion channels; e.g., γ-aminobutyric acid (GABA) type A receptors, two-pore-domain potassium channels, and N-methyl-D-aspartate (NMDA) receptors. The aggregate of biochemical evidence suggests that VAs modulate ion channel functions in an allosteric, as opposed to a competitive, manner (Hemmings et al., 2005). The lack of high-resolution structural information regarding ion channels has made it impossible to determine the exact VA binding site(s) or mechanisms at work.

A unique feature of volatile anesthetic drugs is that the blood concentration at which these drugs exert pharmacological activities (i.e., induction of general anesthetic states) is high (0.1 to 1 mM). At these concentrations, anesthetics have been reported to affect not only neuronal cells but also diverse types of cells including leukocytes, platelets, endothelial cells, myocardial cells, bronchial epithelial cells, and cancer cells (McBride et al., 1996). Therefore, these secondary effects of VAs are of enormous clinical relevance and concern.

We investigated integrin interactions with volatile anesthetics for three reasons (Yuki et al., 2010; Yuki et al., 2008). First, we rationalized that the promiscuous nature of VA - protein interactions, in conjunction with the important role of LFA-1 function in the immune system made the protein a potential candidate for modulation by VA. Second, the I domain is a well-characterized, soluble protein amenable to biophysical and structural analysis. Beyond the direct physiological relevance of LFA-1 : VA interactions, we viewed the I domain as an ideal model system to understand how weakly binding VA could modulate protein function. Finally, the availability of NMR techniques would allow us to obtain a molecular mechanism for our observation that two volatile anesthetics, isoflurane and sevoflurane act as antagonists of LFA-1 binding to ICAM-1, both in cell and cell- free assays. NMR spectroscopy has been utilized in earlier studies of VA : protein interactions and demonstrated that it is possible to identify VA binding sites on proteins using NMR (Yonkunas et al., 2005). A critical difference between our studies and earlier investigations, is in the ability to perform activity assays on the I domain and directly compare anesthetic interactions with effect on biological functions. Previous studies have utilized model proteins that lack catalytic or adhesive activity and such comparisons were unavailable.

To map potential isoflurane binding site(s) in the LFA-1 I domain, we utilized heteronuclear $^{1}H,^{15}N$-HSQC-NMR spectroscopy, an established technique for the identification of small-molecule interaction sites on isotopically labeled biomolecules, including anesthetic interactions with soluble protein domains (Yuki et al., 2008). An overlay of two HSQCs taken at the endpoints of an isoflurane titration (0 and 12 mM isoflurane, because high concentrations are preferred in order to fully occupy the binding site) not only revealed that a number of resonances undergo shifts in resonance frequency, but also identified the LFA-1 I domain as a potential binding site for isoflurane. The chemical shift of most residues was unchanged whether at the lowest (0 mM) or the highest (~12 mM) concentration of drug However, several resonances, such as threonine 291 at top the loop that connects to the C-terminal helix, underwent a dose-dependent shift in resonance frequency, indicating an interaction and/or change in the electronic environment or local structure of the protein.

The magnitude of the isoflurane-induced shift was mapped onto the sequence and secondary structure (FIGURE 3). Significant chemical-shift perturbation occurred in six regions of the protein sequence: 1) the N-terminal segment; 2) the C-terminal portion of β1; 3) the loop between β2 and β3; 4) β3; 5) β5; and 6) the C-terminal segment incorporating β5-α7. Residues perturbed by the addition of the LFA-1 I allosteric antagonist lovastatin (visible as a uniform yellow background, **FIGURE 3***)* showed a good correlation with those by isoflurane. The largest deviation in chemical shifts occurred with the aromatic resonances

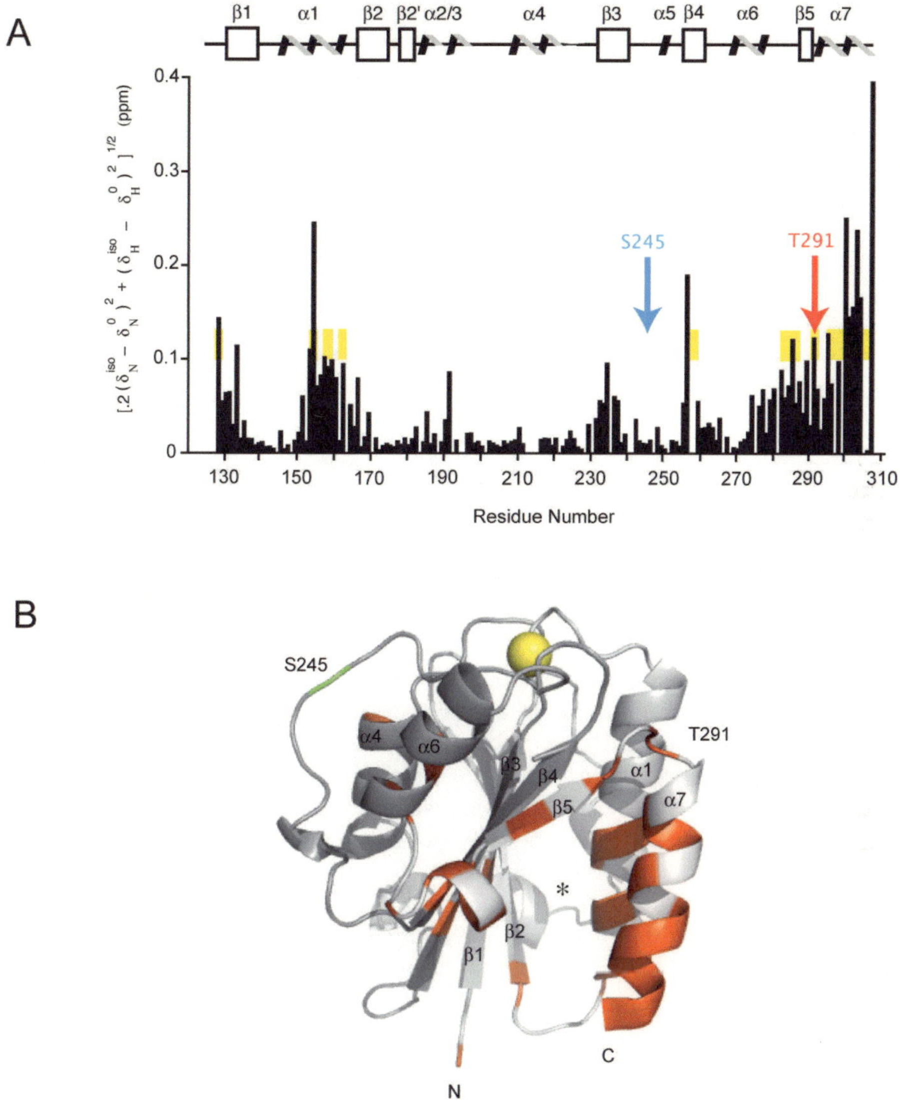

Fig. 3. NMR spectroscopy to study isoflurane-binding site(s) in the LFA-1 I (**A**) Scaled chemical-shift perturbation of 12 mM isoflurane mapped onto the LFA-1 I domain protein sequence and secondary structure. (**B**) Structure of the LFA-1 I domain showing amide nitrogen residues affected (Δppm = 0.05 ppm) by the addition of 12 mM isoflurane. Gray represents residues unperturbed by isoflurane while red represents residues that met or exceeded the threshold for perturbation. Helices and strands are labeled. Residues T291 (red) and S245 (green) are labeled. The yellow spheres represent the Mg^{2+} ion at the ICAM-1 binding site, termed the metal ion-dependent adhesion site (MIDAS). Note that the residues near the MIDAS were not affected and that the affected residues clustered near the cavity formed between the α1 and α7 helices and the central β strands. This figure was adopted from Yuki et al. 2008.

phenylalanine 153 (F153) and tyrosine 307 (Y307), which could indicate a direct interaction between the halogenated hydrocarbons and the aromatic moieties, as previously suggested. We note that Y307 is also an interacting residue in the derived model of cILB peptide with theI domain, suggesting a common mechanism of inhibition by the two remarkably different chemotypes. To generalize these results to other VA, we performed the same experiment using the VA sevoflurane (Yuki et al., 2010). Sevoflurane induced chemical shift perturbation in a subset of residues located at the C-terminal portion. This is consistent with the NMR data that we previously obtained from isoflurane's interaction with the LFA-1 I domain thereby suggesting that sevoflurane also binds to the C-terminal portion of the LFA-1 I domain, in which it blocks LFA-1 in the same allosteric manner that isoflurane does. By contrast, propofol, a distinct class of VA, induced perturbations to many residues spread over the I domain. The data is consistent with the idea that a high concentration of propofol inhibits LFA-1 in a mixed competitive and allosteric manner (NSA and MS, unpublished).

7. Saturation-Transfer Difference NMR (STD) and transferred NOE NMR studies

One of the central challenges faced in the study of integrin- antagonist interactions, particularly in the study of agonists which may interact with integrin domains that can-not be expressed in isolation such as the β- I like domain, is to determine the structure of the ligand bound complex. While docking and modeling studies, such as those described above, are valuable, changes in the conformation of the ligand and receptor can contribute to uncertainty in the molecular nature of complex formation. Saturation transfer difference NMR spectroscopy (STD-NMR), a technique originally developed to identify the carbohydrate epitope of protein lectins, has emerged as a powerful approach to overcome this difficulty (Mayer and Meyer, 1999). Because STD-NMR can be performed on proteins expressed in the native environment and does not require substantial quantities of protein, it is ideally suited to studying the interaction of cell surface transmembrane receptor interactions with potential antagonists. In fact, the high molecular weight of integrin in cell membranes - and even within cells - is advantageous since the saturation transfer effect improves with the molecular weight of the complex.

STD-NMR is based on the NMR effect of saturation. Prolonged irradiation of one or more spins by a long pulse or pulse train results in loss of signal intensity from the spectra of the irradiated spin. This saturation can propagate to neighboring spins through the dipolar interaction; the kinetics of the spread is favored in systems with high molecular weight. Because the transfer effect is through the dipolar coupling, the nuclei do not need to be covalently joined on the same molecule for saturation to spread between the spins. Thus saturation will result in the loss of signal intensity both for irradiated peaks and those spatially proximate. The saturation time can be manipulated to allow for propagation to proximate as opposed to distal spins, allowing for the mapping of direct binding epitopes between high-molecular weight protein systems and their ligands.

The STD-NMR experiment requires two sequential NMR spectra be obtained - one with and one without saturation. Because the experiment is performed with a large excess of ligand over protein, the saturation free spectrum is effectively identical to the spectrum of the free ligand. The high molecular weight of the membrane preparations or cells renders them undetectable by solution NMR. The second spectrum is acquired with saturation pulse(s) applied selectively to a protein resonance. The saturation is then transferred to the ligand from the protein by the dipolar coupling. If the two spectra are subtracted, the difference spectrum only contains peaks from ligand resonances that were in contact with the protein during the saturation period. The STD effect is useful for characterizing protein-ligand complexes with weak-moderate binding constants ($K_D \sim 1X10^{-3}$ - $K_D \sim 1X10^{-8}$). This technique can be used to both validate the specificity of a binding interaction and map the epitope of nuclei that are directly bound to the protein since they undergo the greatest saturation effect.

STD-NMR was first applied to the study of cyclic-RGD peptides binding to purified αIIbβ3 integrin reconstituted into liposomes (Meinecke and Meyer, 2001). Using STD-NMR the authors determine an affinity K_D of 30-60 μM for the peptide cyclo(RGDfv) complex with reconstituted integrin. No saturation effect was observed for liposomes free of integrin or non-ligand peptides with integrin containing liposomes, validating the specificity of the approach. Furthermore, a mixture of linear and cyclic RGD peptides gave rise only to spectra of the cyclic peptides, consistent with a previously established greater affinity for the cyclic versus linear peptide analogs. Analysis of the spectra and concentrations allowed for an estimate of ~1mM for the K_D of the linear peptide. By comparison, the linear RGDS peptide, with a known K_D of 55 μM was shown by STD-NMR to be an effective competitor of the cyclic-RGD peptide.

The authors further mapped the binding epitope of the peptide using the intensity of the resonances as a measure of proximity to the proteins surface. The largest signals were from the aromatic proteins of the D-Phe followed by the Arg Hα, ArgHβ/Hγ, Asp Hβ and the β-proteins of the unnatural amino acid D-Hph residue as well as the γ-protons of Val, the Hα protein of Gly, demonstrating that these were the atoms directly contact with integrin. Prior studies on the conformation of the RGDfV cyclic peptide in DMSO by 2D-NMR structural methods was used to interpret the epitope mapping investigation (Aumailley et al., 1991). In the NMR structure, the side chains of Arg, Asp and Val are disposed perpendicular to the plane of the peptide and point to one side. The D-Phe side chain is located in an equatorial conformation. These suggest that the ligand interactions on one side of the peptide ring with the Phe in the equatorial position making further stabilizing interactions. The pattern of the Arg alkyl side chain suggests that strongly hydrophobic interactions are predominant while the Arg δ-protons, which would be indicative of the tight interaction of the guanidine group, are only weakly saturated. Although this is at first surprising, given the conservation of the Arg in the canonical binding motif, the L-amino acids norleucine, cyclohexylglycine, norvaline, tert-leucine and 4-hydroxyproline all have tighter affinity in the position occupied by Arg that the Arg itself, suggesting that the ionic interaction makes little or no contribution to the stability of the complex. Also, the high intensity of the D-Phe resonance is consistent with the fact that hydrophobic and aromatic residues that are adjacent to the Asp have greater inhibitory potential, both in natural disintegrin proteins and designed inhibitor peptides. This effect is exploited in αIIbβ3 specific platelet inhibitors including the cyclic hepta-peptide eptifibatdide, which has a L-homoarginine in the first position (Scarborough et al., 1993). Thus the extended alkyl chain in the first position and the aromatic in the fourth position of this optimized αIIbβ3 inhibitor are both consistent with the results of the STD-NMR studies of the binding epitope.

A comparison between STD-experiments obtained on liposomal preparations with αIIbβ3 on the surface of platelets was obtained with interesting results (Claasen et al., 2005). Although the binding epiotpe in the two experimental contexts is almost identical (with minor variations) the STD effect was much higher in the intact platelet preparation, despite the fact that the concentration of receptor in the liposomal sample is ~ 5 μM and only ~0.6 μM for the platelet sample, demonstrating the affinity, of αIIbβ3 for the ligand is significantly higher in the native context. This demonstrates the great utility of STD -NMR that can determine both epitopes and approximate measure of antagonist affinity on intact cells. Assuming 150,000 receptors/cell, 10^8 or fewer cells are required to obtain an STD-NMR spectrum with good signal to noise, a number that can readily be accommodated in a standard NMR tube.

A powerful feature of the STD-NMR experiment is consequently the ability to obtain binding information directly on the cells targeted by a therapeutic agent of interest (Potenza et al., 2011). One such study examined the binding of two closely related cyclic-RGD peptides with dramatically different IC50s to the integrin αVβ3 on EVC304, a bladder cancer cell line. The two cyclic peptides, with competitive IC50s of 6.4 nM versus 154 nM against echistastin binding differ in the configuration about two stereo-centers and are known, from earlier NMR studies of the free inhibitor, to have distinct conformations in the unbound state. The STD-NMR derived epitope of the stronger binding cyclic-peptide that has a μM IC50 for inhibiting cell adhesion to ECM ligands agrees with a previously derived docking model. The ligand interacts through a pair of ionic interactions (Arg-guandinium with αV-Asp218 and Asp-carboxyl with the β3-MIDAS), a π-π interaction (between a benzylic group on the ligand and an aromatic ring of β3-Tyr122) and an extended network of hydrogen bonds including the Asp-NH and C=O of β3-Arg216. The overall structure of the cyclic peptide closely resembles the high-resolution crystal structure of the peptide cingletide bound to αVβ3.

The authors used a second technique, transferred NOE (TR-NOE) spectroscopy, to obtain the conformation of the bound ligand. TR-NOE is an NMR experiment that permits the selective observation of ligand NOEs through space correlations present in the low population bound form of a complex to be observed in the high population free state. Using this technique, it was possible to identify conformational changes in the ligand that are required for ligand binding.

STD-NMR of the weaker binding cyclic peptide was also obtained using STD-NMR and revealed a distinct binding epitope. The most significant change, due to the altered conformation around the two stereocenters, was the loss of the hydrogen bonding network between ligand Asp and the β-subunit. The authors also using TR-NOE observed conformational changes between the ligand in the free and bound state. The bound conformation of the second inhibitor forms less favorable contacts with the integrin, accounting for the loss of inhibition efficacy.

One important extension of the STD-NMR experiments is the incorporation of heteronuclear 2D detection, which is required to determine the epitope of more complex peptides and proteins that would otherwise be difficult to study due to resonance overlap (Assadi-Porter et al., 2010; Wagstaff et al., 2010b). A recent investigation both demonstrated both the overall utility of STD-NMR for study of integrin-antagonist interactions and also the advantages of using 2D NMR to as opposed to 1D detection despite the added time and expense of preparing the requisite isotopic labeled sample(s). The authors studied a complex of αVβ6 with a peptide inhibitor derived from the surface loop of the foot and mouth virus capsid protein, which utilizes this integrin as a receptor. The peptide, A20FMDV2, has the sequence NAVPNLRGDLQVLAQKVART. Previous work showed that peptide inhibitors of αVβ6 utilize the extended sequence DLXXLRGD as an extended recognition motif. To obtain the isotopic labeled peptide, the authors utilized a commercial *E. coli* fusion peptide system whereby the peptide is fused to the insoluble ketosteroid isomerase protein with a methionine residue introduced between KSI and the peptide sequence. The insoluble fusion pair is readily separated from the soluble cell material and then can be cleaved using cyanogen bromide treatment (Wagstaff et al., 2010a).

The 2D-^{13}C STD-NMR experiments demonstrate a pronounced contribution from the DLXXL motif to the binding epitope and, surprising, a less substantial component from the RGD regions. Significantly, an earlier 1D-STD-NMR misidentified part of the binding epitope, due to uncertainty in the resonance assignments that occur due to overlap in the NMR spectrum. The primary interaction between peptide and protein is through ^{6}Leu, ^{12}Val and ^{13}Leu. Despite not obtaining any high resolution (i.e. NOE or J-coupling) constraints, the authors were able to utilize intensity and phase information (both sensitive to the saturation transfer efficiency) of resonances from the ^{1}H-^{13}C and ^{1}H-^{15}N detected STD-NMR experiments to construct a refined model of the peptide-integrin interaction which is of great utility in the design of novel peptide and peptide-mimetic inhibitors.

8. Conclusions

To build upon the advances described in this review, we have identified five critical areas which we feel will contribute to a greater understanding of the mechanism of integrin activation and the development of improved antagonists targeting integrin function.

Automation: Conventional NMR spectroscopy requires the determination of resonance assignments to extract meaningful spectroscopic data. The process of resonance assignment is, however, manually intensive and cumbersome, especially given the need to screen large number of potential binding reagents to a molecular target. There has, however, been recent progress in automating the assignment and structure determination and analysis process (Guerry and Herrmann, 2011). In particular, methods which permit partial assignments of putative ligand binding interfaces without resorting to total assignment or structure determination would greatly facilitate the utility of NMR as a high-throughput screening tool. One recent advance in this area applied to the development of integrin antagonists is the technique of Methyl Scanning. Because many I domain inhibitors contain aromatic rings that can induce large chemical shifts in proximal aliphatic side chain resonances, partial assignments of methyl carbons and protons can serve as a useful source of constraints probing ligand binding to suitable protein pockets. This technique was recently employed to study the mechanism of a tight binding (18.3 nM) arylthio allosteric inhibitor of the LFA-1 I domain (Constantine et al., 2006).

Expression and Labeling: Although the I domain can be produced in isolation of other integrin domains using standard *E. coli* expression systems, other critical integrin domains require domain- domain interactions for correct folding. This precludes the use of basic *E. coli* expression systems that are optimal for preparing the isotope labeled samples used in high resolution NMR studies. Recent advances in two areas promise to break though this bottleneck. First, the use of eukaryotic expression either in yeast or mammalian cells has been demonstrated to produce quantities of protein suitable for NMR studies. *In vitro* translation systems have also been optimized to produce suitable quantities of isotopic labeled proteins and represent a viable alternative approach to producing complex multidomain proteins of eukaryotic origin (Yokoyama, 2003).

Transmembrane and cytoplasmic domains: Separation of the transmembrane and cytoplasmic domains is a critical step in integrin activation. While existing integrin modulators work by stabilizing the inactive conformation of the ecto- domains, there has been recent interest in pharmacological targeting of transmembrane structure (Shandler et al., 2011). However, transmembrane domains pose a particular challenge for conventional solution NMR due to the large molecular weight of the bilayer required to maintain the protein in the correct conformation. Recent advances in solution NMR, particularly the development of membrane nanodiscs that preserve the authentic structure of the native bilayer, have begun to overcome this limitation and provide detailed, high-resolution structural details on association of transmembrane peptides (Warschawski et al., 2011).

Dynamics: While the role of protein dynamics in protein function, and inhibition have been widely appreciated, there has been renewed development in methods that can obtained with site-specific resolution. A major existing challenge is the incorporation of dynamics information into docking and screening protocols. In this area, improved computational protocols will be needed to parallel the increased ability to observe and quantify chemical exchange processes in proteins. New methods for incorporation of dynamics data into drug discover protocols will likely be of comparable importance to the introduction of structural constraints (Lin, 2011; Salsbury, 2010).

Crystal Structures: Paradoxically, the most urgent need in the area of NMR based integrin drug design is for additional crystal structures both of new integrins as well as drug - integrin complexes. While NMR is a powerful structural tool in its own right, the true power of NMR lies in the capacity to rapidly determine structural and dynamic information of ligands and their binding sites that can be integrated with existing structures using computational modeling tools. The most successful future structure based design approaches are likely to integrate multiple sources of information to identify the most optimal drug candidates for biological screening.

9. References

Alonso, J.L., Essafi, M., Xiong, J.P., Stehle, T., and Arnaout, M.A. (2002). Does the integrin alphaA domain act as a ligand for its betaA domain? Curr Biol 12, R340-342.

Anderson, M.E., Yakovleva, T., Hu, Y., and Siahaan, T.J. (2004). Inhibition of ICAM-1/LFA-1-mediated heterotypic T-cell adhesion to epithelial cells: design of ICAM-1 cyclic peptides. Bioorg Med Chem Lett 14, 1399-1402.

Assadi-Porter, F.M., Tonelli, M., Maillet, E.L., Markley, J.L., and Max, M. (2010). Interactions between the human sweet-sensing T1R2-T1R3 receptor and sweeteners detected by saturation transfer difference NMR spectroscopy. Biochim Biophys Acta 1798, 82-86.

Aumailley, M., Gurrath, M., Muller, G., Calvete, J., Timpl, R., and Kessler, H. (1991). Arg-Gly-Asp constrained within cyclic pentapeptides. Strong and selective inhibitors of cell adhesion to vitronectin and laminin fragment P1. FEBS Lett 291, 50-54.

Beglova, N., Blacklow, S.C., Takagi, J., and Springer, T.A. (2002). Cysteine-rich module structure reveals a fulcrum for integrin rearrangement upon activation. Nat Struct Biol 9, 282-287.

Bhunia, A., Tang, X.Y., Mohanram, H., Tan, S.M., and Bhattacharjya, S. (2009). NMR solution conformations and interactions of integrin alphaLbeta2 cytoplasmic tails. J Biol Chem 284, 3873-3884.

Campbell, I.D., and Humphries, M.J. (2011). Integrin structure, activation, and interactions. Cold Spring Harb Perspect Biol 3.

Cavanagh, J., Fairbrother, W., AG Palmer III, and Skelton, N. (2006). Protein NMR Spectroscopy, Second Edition: Principles and Practice (San Diego, CA, Academic Press).

Cicala, C., Arthos, J., and Fauci, A.S. (2011). HIV-1 envelope, integrins and co-receptor use in mucosal transmission of HIV. J Transl Med 9 Suppl 1, S2.

Claasen, B., Axmann, M., Meinecke, R., and Meyer, B. (2005). Direct observation of ligand binding to membrane proteins in living cells by a saturation transfer double difference (STDD) NMR spectroscopy method shows a significantly higher affinity of integrin alpha(IIb)beta3 in native platelets than in liposomes. J Am Chem Soc 127, 916-919.

Coller, B.S., and Shattil, S.J. (2008). The GPIIb/IIIa (integrin alphaIIbbeta3) odyssey: a technology-driven saga of a receptor with twists, turns, and even a bend. Blood 112, 3011-3025.

Constantine, K.L., Davis, M.E., Metzler, W.J., Mueller, L., and Claus, B.L. (2006). Protein-ligand NOE matching: a high-throughput method for binding pose evaluation that does not require protein NMR resonance assignments. J Am Chem Soc 128, 7252-7263.

Crump, M.P., Ceska, T.A., Spyracopoulos, L., Henry, A., Archibald, S.C., Alexander, R., Taylor, R.J., Findlow, S.C., O'Connell, J., Robinson, M.K., et al. (2004). Structure of an allosteric inhibitor of LFA-1 bound to the I-domain studied by crystallography, NMR, and calorimetry. Biochemistry 43, 2394-2404.

Cuzange, A., Chroboczek, J., and Jacrot, B. (1994). The penton base of human adenovirus type 3 has the RGD motif. Gene 146, 257-259.

Dijkgraaf, I., Beer, A.J., and Wester, H.J. (2009). Application of RGD-containing peptides as imaging probes for alphavbeta3 expression. Front Biosci 14, 887-899.

Ding, Z.M., Babensee, J.E., Simon, S.I., Lu, H., Perrard, J.L., Bullard, D.C., Dai, X.Y., Bromley, S.K., Dustin, M.L., Entman, M.L., et al. (1999). Relative contribution of LFA-1 and Mac-1 to neutrophil adhesion and migration. J Immunol 163, 5029-5038.

Ege, S. (2003). Organic Chemistry: Structure and Reactivity (Chicago, IL, Houghton Mifflin Harcourt).

Evans, R., Patzak, I., Svensson, L., De Filippo, K., Jones, K., McDowall, A., and Hogg, N. (2009). Integrins in immunity. J Cell Sci 122, 215-225.

Fagerholm, S.C., Hilden, T.J., and Gahmberg, C.G. (2004). P marks the spot: site-specific integrin phosphorylation regulates molecular interactions. Trends Biochem Sci 29, 504-512.

Fleming, F.E., Graham, K.L., Taniguchi, K., Takada, Y., and Coulson, B.S. (2007). Rotavirus-neutralizing antibodies inhibit virus binding to integrins alpha 2 beta 1 and alpha 4 beta 1. Arch Virol 152, 1087-1101.

Gaillard, T., Martin, E., San Sebastian, E., Cossio, F.P., Lopez, X., Dejaegere, A., and Stote, R.H. (2007). Comparative normal mode analysis of LFA-1 integrin I-domains. J Mol Biol 374, 231-249.

George, E.L., Georges-Labouesse, E.N., Patel-King, R.S., Rayburn, H., and Hynes, R.O. (1993). Defects in mesoderm, neural tube and vascular development in mouse embryos lacking fibronectin. Development 119, 1079-1091.

Gottschalk, K.E. (2005). A coiled-coil structure of the alphaIIbbeta3 integrin transmembrane and cytoplasmic domains in its resting state. Structure 13, 703-712.

Guerry, P., and Herrmann, T. (2011). Advances in automated NMR protein structure determination. Q Rev Biophys 44, 257-309.

Gursoy, R.N., Jois, D.S., and Siahaan, T.J. (1999). Structural recognition of an ICAM-1 peptide by its receptor on the surface of T cells: conformational studies of cyclo (1, 12)-Pen-Pro-Arg-Gly-Gly-Ser-Val-Leu-Val-Thr-Gly-Cys-OH. J Pept Res 53, 422-431.

Hemmings, H.C., Jr., Akabas, M.H., Goldstein, P.A., Trudell, J.R., Orser, B.A., and Harrison, N.L. (2005). Emerging molecular mechanisms of general anesthetic action. Trends Pharmacol Sci 26, 503-510.

Huth, J.R., Olejniczak, E.T., Mendoza, R., Liang, H., Harris, E.A., Lupher, M.L., Jr., Wilson, A.E., Fesik, S.W., and Staunton, D.E. (2000). NMR and mutagenesis evidence for an I domain allosteric site that regulates lymphocyte function-associated antigen 1 ligand binding. Proc Natl Acad Sci U S A 97, 5231-5236.

Hynes, R.O. (2002). Integrins: bidirectional, allosteric signaling machines. Cell 110, 673-687.

Imai, Y., Park, E.J., Peer, D., Peixoto, A., Cheng, G., von Andrian, U.H., Carman, C.V., and Shimaoka, M. (2008). Genetic perturbation of the putative cytoplasmic membrane-proximal salt bridge aberrantly activates alpha(4) integrins. Blood 112, 5007-5015.

Jin, H., and Varner, J. (2004). Integrins: roles in cancer development and as treatment targets. Br J Cancer 90, 561-565.

Jin, M., Andricioaei, I., and Springer, T.A. (2004). Conversion between three conformational states of integrin I domains with a C-terminal pull spring studied with molecular dynamics. Structure 12, 2137-2147.

Kallen, J., Welzenbach, K., Ramage, P., Geyl, D., Kriwacki, R., Legge, G., Cottens, S., Weitz-Schmidt, G., and Hommel, U. (1999). Structural basis for LFA-1 inhibition upon lovastatin binding to the CD11a I-domain. J Mol Biol 292, 1-9.

Kriwacki, R.W., Legge, G.B., Hommel, U., Ramage, P., Chung, J., Tennant, L.L., Wright, P.E., and Dyson, H.J. (2000). Assignment of 1H, 13C and 15N resonances of the I-domain of human leukocyte function associated antigen-1. J Biomol NMR 16, 271-272.

Lambert, L.J., Bobkov, A.A., Smith, J.W., and Marassi, F.M. (2008). Competitive interactions of collagen and a jararhagin-derived disintegrin peptide with the integrin alpha2-I domain. J Biol Chem 283, 16665-16672.

Lee, J.O., Bankston, L.A., Arnaout, M.A., and Liddington, R.C. (1995a). Two conformations of the integrin A-domain (I-domain): a pathway for activation? Structure 3, 1333-1340.

Lee, J.O., Rieu, P., Arnaout, M.A., and Liddington, R. (1995b). Crystal structure of the A domain from the alpha subunit of integrin CR3 (CD11b/CD18). Cell 80, 631-638.

Legge, G.B., Kriwacki, R.W., Chung, J., Hommel, U., Ramage, P., Case, D.A., Dyson, H.J., and Wright, P.E. (2000). NMR solution structure of the inserted domain of human leukocyte function associated antigen-1. J Mol Biol 295, 1251-1264.

Li, R., Babu, C.R., Valentine, K., Lear, J.D., Wand, A.J., Bennett, J.S., and DeGrado, W.F. (2002). Characterization of the monomeric form of the transmembrane and cytoplasmic domains of the integrin beta 3 subunit by NMR spectroscopy. Biochemistry 41, 15618-15624.

Lin, J.H. (2011). Accommodating protein flexibility for structure-based drug design. Curr Top Med Chem 11, 171-178.

Liu, G., Huth, J.R., Olejniczak, E.T., Mendoza, R., DeVries, P., Leitza, S., Reilly, E.B., Okasinski, G.F., Fesik, S.W., and von Geldern, T.W. (2001). Novel p-arylthio cinnamides as antagonists of leukocyte function-associated antigen-1/intracellular adhesion molecule-1 interaction. 2. Mechanism of inhibition and structure-based improvement of pharmaceutical properties. J Med Chem 44, 1202-1210.

Lu, C., Shimaoka, M., Ferzly, M., Oxvig, C., Takagi, J., and Springer, T.A. (2001a). An isolated, surface-expressed I domain of the integrin alphaLbeta2 is sufficient for strong adhesive function when locked in the open conformation with a disulfide bond. Proc Natl Acad Sci U S A 98, 2387-2392.

Lu, C., Shimaoka, M., Zang, Q., Takagi, J., and Springer, T.A. (2001b). Locking in alternate conformations of the integrin alphaLbeta2 I domain with disulfide bonds reveals functional relationships among integrin domains. Proc Natl Acad Sci U S A 98, 2393-2398.

Lu, C., Takagi, J., and Springer, T.A. (2001c). Association of the membrane proximal regions of the alpha and beta subunit cytoplasmic domains constrains an integrin in the inactive state. J Biol Chem 276, 14642-14648.

Luo, B.H., Carman, C.V., and Springer, T.A. (2007). Structural basis of integrin regulation and signaling. Annu Rev Immunol 25, 619-647.

Luo, B.H., Springer, T.A., and Takagi, J. (2004). A specific interface between integrin transmembrane helices and affinity for ligand. PLoS Biol 2, e153.

Mayer, M., and Meyer, B. (1999). Characterization of ligand binding by saturation transfer difference NMR spectroscopy. . Angewandte Chemie 38, 1784-1788.

McBride, W.T., Armstrong, M.A., and McBride, S.J. (1996). Immunomodulation: an important concept in modern anaesthesia. Anaesthesia 51, 465-473.

Meinecke, R., and Meyer, B. (2001). Determination of the binding specificity of an integral membrane protein by saturation transfer difference NMR: RGD peptide ligands binding to integrin alphaIIbbeta3. J Med Chem 44, 3059-3065.

Mittermaier, A., and Kay, L.E. (2006). New tools provide new insights in NMR studies of protein dynamics. Science 312, 224-228.

Nemeth, J.A., Nakada, M.T., Trikha, M., Lang, Z., Gordon, M.S., Jayson, G.C., Corringham, R., Prabhakar, U., Davis, H.M., and Beckman, R.A. (2007). Alpha-v integrins as therapeutic targets in oncology. Cancer Invest 25, 632-646.

Nishida, N., Xie, C., Shimaoka, M., Cheng, Y., Walz, T., and Springer, T.A. (2006). Activation of leukocyte beta2 integrins by conversion from bent to extended conformations. Immunity 25, 583-594.

Palmer, A.G., 3rd, and Massi, F. (2006). Characterization of the dynamics of biomacromolecules using rotating-frame spin relaxation NMR spectroscopy. Chem Rev 106, 1700-1719.

Park, E.J., Mora, J.R., Carman, C.V., Chen, J., Sasaki, Y., Cheng, G., von Andrian, U.H., and Shimaoka, M. (2007). Aberrant activation of integrin alpha4beta7 suppresses lymphocyte migration to the gut. J Clin Invest 117, 2526-2538.

Plow, E.F., Haas, T.A., Zhang, L., Loftus, J., and Smith, J.W. (2000). Ligand binding to integrins. J Biol Chem 275, 21785-21788.

Potenza, D., Vasile, F., Belvisi, L., Civera, M., and Araldi, E.M. (2011). STD and trNOESY NMR study of receptor-ligand interactions in living cancer cells. Chembiochem 12, 695-699.

Qu, A., and Leahy, D.J. (1995). Crystal structure of the I-domain from the CD11a/CD18 (LFA-1, alpha L beta 2) integrin. Proc Natl Acad Sci U S A 92, 10277-10281.

Reardon, D.A., Fink, K.L., Mikkelsen, T., Cloughesy, T.F., O'Neill, A., Plotkin, S., Glantz, M., Ravin, P., Raizer, J.J., Rich, K.M., et al. (2008). Randomized phase II study of cilengitide, an integrin-targeting arginine-glycine-aspartic acid peptide, in recurrent glioblastoma multiforme. J Clin Oncol 26, 5610-5617.

Ruoslahti, E. (1996). RGD and other recognition sequences for integrins. Annu Rev Cell Dev Biol 12, 697-715.

Salsbury, F.R., Jr. (2010). Molecular dynamics simulations of protein dynamics and their relevance to drug discovery. Curr Opin Pharmacol 10, 738-744.

Scarborough, R.M. (1999). Development of eptifibatide. Am Heart J 138, 1093-1104.

Scarborough, R.M., Naughton, M.A., Teng, W., Rose, J.W., Phillips, D.R., Nannizzi, L., Arfsten, A., Campbell, A.M., and Charo, I.F. (1993). Design of potent and specific integrin antagonists. Peptide antagonists with high specificity for glycoprotein IIb-IIIa. J Biol Chem 268, 1066-1073.

Schornberg, K.L., Shoemaker, C.J., Dube, D., Abshire, M.Y., Delos, S.E., Bouton, A.H., and White, J.M. (2009). Alpha5beta1-integrin controls ebolavirus entry by regulating endosomal cathepsins. Proc Natl Acad Sci U S A 106, 8003-8008.

Semmrich, M., Smith, A., Feterowski, C., Beer, S., Engelhardt, B., Busch, D.H., Bartsch, B., Laschinger, M., Hogg, N., Pfeffer, K., et al. (2005). Importance of integrin LFA-1 deactivation for the generation of immune responses. J Exp Med 201, 1987-1998.

Shamri, R., Grabovsky, V., Gauguet, J.M., Feigelson, S., Manevich, E., Kolanus, W., Robinson, M.K., Staunton, D.E., von Andrian, U.H., and Alon, R. (2005). Lymphocyte arrest requires instantaneous induction of an extended LFA-1 conformation mediated by endothelium-bound chemokines. Nat Immunol 6, 497-506.

Shandler, S.J., Korendovych, I.V., Moore, D.T., Smith-Dupont, K.B., Streu, C.N., Litvinov, R.I., Billings, P.C., Gai, F., Bennett, J.S., and Degrado, W.F. (2011). Computational Design of a beta-Peptide That Targets Transmembrane Helices. J Am Chem Soc 133, 12378-12381.

Shimaoka, M., and Springer, T.A. (2003). Therapeutic antagonists and conformational regulation of integrin function. Nat Rev Drug Discov 2, 703-716.

Shimaoka, M., Takagi, J., and Springer, T.A. (2002). Conformational regulation of integrin structure and function. Annu Rev Biophys Biomol Struct 31, 485-516.

Shimaoka, M., Xiao, T., Liu, J.H., Yang, Y., Dong, Y., Jun, C.D., McCormack, A., Zhang, R., Joachimiak, A., Takagi, J., et al. (2003). Structures of the alpha L I domain and its complex with ICAM-1 reveal a shape-shifting pathway for integrin regulation. Cell 112, 99-111.

Shuker, S.B., Hajduk, P.J., Meadows, R.P., and Fesik, S.W. (1996). Discovering high-affinity ligands for proteins: SAR by NMR. Science 274, 1531-1534.

Suttner, S., Kumle, B., and Boldt, J. (2002). Pharmacoeconomic considerations in anaesthetic use. Expert Opin Pharmacother 3, 1267-1272.

Takagi, J., Beglova, N., Yalamanchili, P., Blacklow, S.C., and Springer, T.A. (2001). Definition of EGF-like, closely interacting modules that bear activation epitopes in integrin beta subunits. Proc Natl Acad Sci U S A 98, 11175-11180.

Vinogradova, O., Velyvis, A., Velyviene, A., Hu, B., Haas, T., Plow, E., and Qin, J. (2002). A structural mechanism of integrin alpha(IIb)beta(3) "inside-out" activation as regulated by its cytoplasmic face. Cell 110, 587-597.

Wagstaff, J.L., Howard, M.J., and Williamson, R.A. (2010a). Production of recombinant isotopically labelled peptide by fusion to an insoluble partner protein: generation of integrin alphavbeta6 binding peptides for NMR. Mol Biosyst 6, 2380-2385.

Wagstaff, J.L., Vallath, S., Marshall, J.F., Williamson, R.A., and Howard, M.J. (2010b). Two-dimensional heteronuclear saturation transfer difference NMR reveals detailed integrin alphavbeta6 protein-peptide interactions. Chem Commun (Camb) 46, 7533-7535.

Warschawski, D.E., Arnold, A.A., Beaugrand, M., Gravel, A., Chartrand, E., and Marcotte, I. (2011). Choosing membrane mimetics for NMR structural studies of transmembrane proteins. Biochim Biophys Acta 1808, 1957-1974.

Weitz-Schmidt, G., Welzenbach, K., Brinkmann, V., Kamata, T., Kallen, J., Bruns, C., Cottens, S., Takada, Y., and Hommel, U. (2001). Statins selectively inhibit leukocyte function antigen-1 by binding to a novel regulatory integrin site. Nat Med 7, 687-692.

Winn, M., Reilly, E.B., Liu, G., Huth, J.R., Jae, H.S., Freeman, J., Pei, Z., Xin, Z., Lynch, J., Kester, J., et al. (2001). Discovery of novel p-arylthio cinnamides as antagonists of leukocyte function-associated antigen-1/intercellular adhesion molecule-1 interaction. 4. Structure-activity relationship of substituents on the benzene ring of the cinnamide. J Med Chem 44, 4393-4403.

Wouters, M.A., Rigoutsos, I., Chu, C.K., Feng, L.L., Sparrow, D.B., and Dunwoodie, S.L. (2005). Evolution of distinct EGF domains with specific functions. Protein Sci 14, 1091-1103.

Wuthrich, K. (1986). NMR of Proteins and Nucleic Acids (New York, John Wiley and Sons).

Xiao, T., Takagi, J., Coller, B.S., Wang, J.H., and Springer, T.A. (2004). Structural basis for allostery in integrins and binding to fibrinogen-mimetic therapeutics. Nature 432, 59-67.

Xie, C., Shimaoka, M., Xiao, T., Schwab, P., Klickstein, L.B., and Springer, T.A. (2004). The integrin alpha-subunit leg extends at a Ca2+-dependent epitope in the thigh/genu interface upon activation. Proc Natl Acad Sci U S A 101, 15422-15427.

Xiong, J.P., Goodman, S.L., and Arnaout, M.A. (2007). Purification, analysis, and crystal structure of integrins. Methods in enzymology 426, 307-336.

Xiong, J.P., Li, R., Essafi, M., Stehle, T., and Arnaout, M.A. (2000). An isoleucine-based allosteric switch controls affinity and shape shifting in integrin CD11b A-domain. J Biol Chem 275, 38762-38767.

Xiong, J.P., Stehle, T., Diefenbach, B., Zhang, R., Dunker, R., Scott, D.L., Joachimiak, A., Goodman, S.L., and Arnaout, M.A. (2001). Crystal structure of the extracellular segment of integrin alpha Vbeta3. Science 294, 339-345.

Xiong, J.P., Stehle, T., Zhang, R., Joachimiak, A., Frech, M., Goodman, S.L., and Arnaout, M.A. (2002). Crystal structure of the extracellular segment of integrin alpha Vbeta3 in complex with an Arg-Gly-Asp ligand. Science 296, 151-155.

Yang, J.T., Rayburn, H., and Hynes, R.O. (1993). Embryonic mesodermal defects in alpha 5 integrin-deficient mice. Development 119, 1093-1105.

Yokoyama, S. (2003). Protein expression systems for structural genomics and proteomics. Curr Opin Chem Biol 7, 39-43.

Yonkunas, M.J., Xu, Y., and Tang, P. (2005). Anesthetic interaction with ketosteroid isomerase: insights from molecular dynamics simulations. Biophys J 89, 2350-2356.

Yoon, C.S., Kim, K.D., Park, S.N., and Cheong, S.W. (2001). alpha(6) Integrin is the main receptor of human papillomavirus type 16 VLP. Biochem Biophys Res Commun 283, 668-673.

Yuki, K., Astrof, N.S., Bracken, C., Soriano, S.G., and Shimaoka, M. (2010). Sevoflurane binds and allosterically blocks integrin lymphocyte function-associated antigen-1. Anesthesiology 113, 600-609.

Yuki, K., Astrof, N.S., Bracken, C., Yoo, R., Silkworth, W., Soriano, S.G., and Shimaoka, M. (2008). The volatile anesthetic isoflurane perturbs conformational activation of integrin LFA-1 by binding to the allosteric regulatory cavity. FASEB J 22, 4109-4116.

Zimmerman, T., Oyarzabal, J., Sebastian, E.S., Majumdar, S., Tejo, B.A., Siahaan, T.J., and Blanco, F.J. (2007). ICAM-1 peptide inhibitors of T-cell adhesion bind to the allosteric site of LFA-1. An NMR characterization. Chem Biol Drug Des 70, 347-353.

12

Review: Cyclodextrin Inclusion Complexes Probed by NMR Techniques

Francisco B. T. Pessine, Adriana Calderini and Guilherme L. Alexandrino
Department of Physical Chemistry, Chemistry Institute, State University of Campinas
Brazil

1. Introduction

Cyclodextrins (CDs) are cyclic oligomers of glucopyranose units that play an important role as a host in inclusion complexes, where non-covalent interactions are involved. They have been extensively studied in supramolecular chemistry. Because of its biocompatibility, relatively non-toxicity and relatively low price, CDs have been widely employed for encapsulation of several substances, being used in food, cosmetic and pharmaceutical industries. Nuclear Magnetic Resonance spectroscopy (NMR) is one of the most useful techniques to study interactions of cyclodextrins with guest compounds. It is relatively easy to apply, the experiments are fast and it is the only technique that provides information on the right orientation of the guest molecule inside the cavity and also on other important parameters related to the physico-chemical characteristics of the inclusion complexes. In this review, it will be discussed the study of inclusion complexes between drugs and cyclodextrins by different NMR techniques. Initially, a brief introduction of the properties of cyclodextrins, its importance as innovative drug carrier systems and its applicability is reviewed. Then different NMR techniques used for characterization of inclusion complexes are detailed, with examples studied in our group, which involves since simple measures of ^{1}H-NMR spectrum to more sophisticated experiments, e.g. Diffusion Ordered SpectroscopY (DOSY), NOE methods (ROESY), T1 measure and solid NMR by ^{13}C Cross-Polarization Magic Angle Spinning (CPMAS).

2. Properties of cyclodextrins

Cyclodextrins (CDs) as complexation agents and its study in supramolecular chemistry have been used in many areas (Steed & Atwood, 2002; Chen & Jiang, 2011). Cyclodextrins are cyclic oligosaccharides classified according to their number of glucopyranose units. The natural and most employed cyclodextrins are crystalline, homogeneous, non-hygroscopic substances and includes α-cyclodextrin (αCD, cyclohexaamylose, 6 units of glucopyranose), β-cyclodextrin (βCD, cycloheptaamilose, 7 units of glucopyranose) and γ-cyclodextrin (γCD, cyclooctaamylose, 8 units of glucopyranose), whose chemical structures are shown in Figure 1 (Szejtli, 1998). They are biocompatible, non-toxic in a wide range of concentration, relatively inexpensive and produced naturally by enzyme degradation of starch (Yorozu et al., 1982).

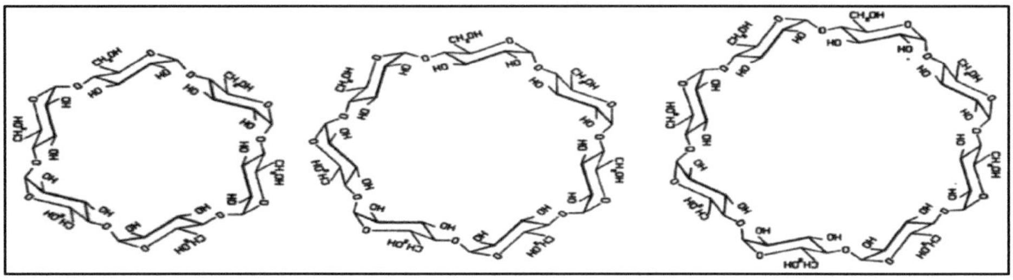

Fig. 1. Chemical structures of (a) αCD; (b) βCD; (c) γCD

These cyclodextrins have torus-like macro ring shape, are relatively low soluble in water and have a hydrophobic cavity. The main factors acting as driving force to form complexes and also responsible for the stability of these complexes are hydrophobic forces, the sizes of molecules/cavity and the guest properties (Griffiths & Bender, 1973).

The glucopyranosides units are in C1 conformation, where the OH groups are linked to the carbon atoms C2 and C3 around the bigger edge and the more reactive OH group (linked to C6) is in the smaller edge. The cavity is delined by the hydrogens atoms and by the glucosidal bridge. The non-ligant electron pairs of the oxygen atoms are inner of cavity, leading to a high electron density and resulting in an environment similar to that of Lewis bases (Szejtli, 1988).

Casu et al. (Casu et al., 1966, 1968), had applying Nuclear Magnetic Resonance and Rotatory Optical Dispersion techniques, to DMSO solution containing CDs, where there is a strong competition with the solvent molecules by the intramolecular hydrogen bridge, showing that the glucose residues kept their conformation and the hydrogen bridge bonds in both solid state and in solution, where this competition is much lower, although, in solution, there is much more conformational mobility than in the solid state.

Bergeron (1977) and Saenger (1980) studied the formation of hydrogen bridges between the OH groups of the C2 and C3 atoms and observed that the conformational mobility of the macro cyclic ring is restricted, contributing to its toughness, both in solid and solution. This array keeps the linkages directed to the core of the cavity, leading to a hydrophobic environment, although the outer surface is hydrophilic, as shown in Figure 2. Some CDs structural and physical-chemical parameters are in Table 1.

Properties	αCD	βCD	γCD
Number of glucopyranose units	6	7	8
Molar mass / (g/mol)	972	1135	1297
Solubility / (g/100 mL)	14.5	1.85	23.2
Inner cavity diameter / (Å)	4.7-5.2	6.0-6.4	7.5-8.3
Outer cavity diameter / (Å)	14.6	15.4	17.5
Cavity height / (Å)	6.7	7.0	7.0
Specific rotation $(\alpha)_D^{25*}$	150.5 ± 0.5	162.5 ± 0.5	177.4 ± 0.5
Volume of the cavity / (Å^3)	174	262	427
ΔH^0 (aq) / (kcal/mol)	7.67	8.31	7.73
ΔS^0 (aq) / (cal/(mol K))	13.8	11.7	14.7

Table 1. α, β and γCD water solubility (25°C) and structural parameters (Szejtli, 1988, 1998; Connors, 1997)

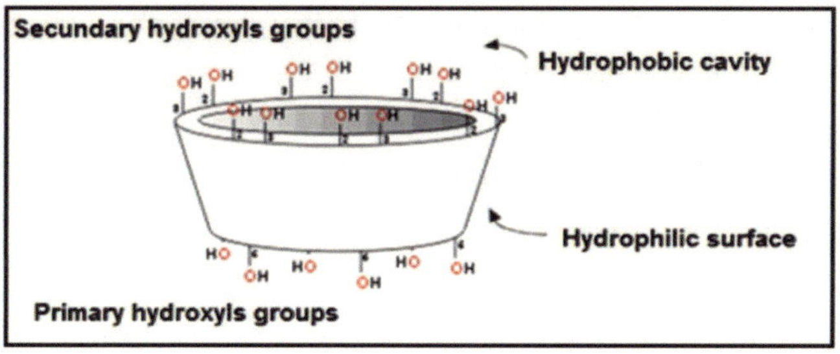

Fig. 2. CDs structure in torus-like macro ring shape, with the hydroxyls groups (Uekama et al., 1998)

The cavity size increases with the number of glucose units, although the height is constant (6.7-7.0 Å). The solubility do not follow this rule: βCD is considerably less soluble in water than αCD and γCD and this low solubility is due to the hydrogen bridges between OH groups of C2 and C3, leading to a rigid structure. In the αCD molecule, one glucose unit in distorted and only 4 of 6 possible hydrogen bridges are formed. In γCD, its glucose units are not in the same plane and its structure is more flexible; therefore, this CD have higher solubility in aqueous solutions (Uekama et al., 1998).

Although the solubility of βCD is smaller, the size of its cavity is more appropriate to encapsulate a great variety of molecules with biological and pharmacological properties. Chemical substitution of the OH groups in C2, C3 and C3 have been done to increase its solubility, as for example, the hydroxipropyl-βCD.

Some factors should be considered to choose the type of the CD for a given study: physical-chemical properties of the guest, size of the CD cavity, solubility, the preparation method and possibility of co-encapsulation. Basically, the inclusion complexes involves interactions of the molecules of both the host and the guest, and it is a combination of different non-covalent interactions as ionic, dipolar, electronic, van der Waals and the hydrophobic effect, besides the size and the shape of the molecules (Chen & Jiang, 2011).

The stability of the inclusion complex is due to, primarily, hydrophobic forces. The association constant is, usually, in the order of 10^{-3} M, typical of weak interactions (Griffiths & Bender, 1973). Hydrophobic molecules, or only the hydrophobic part of a polar molecule, are incorporated in the CD cavity promoting the shift of the water molecules from inside the cavity, which is favored by repulsions between the apolar guest and the water polar molecule. This process leads to the partial or total encapsulation of the guest molecule, increasing aqueous solubility of the sample. However, when the inclusion complex is diluted in a larger volume, the phenomenon is reverted and the species is free in solution.

The main advantages of using CDs in drug delivery systems includes: the increase the biodisponibility, solubility enhancer, improve the stability of the drug, increase the therapeutic index, the efficacy/pharmacokinetics properties, and decrease the drug toxicity (Uekama et al., 1998).

The applicability of CDs includes: analytical chemistry as chromatographic separations (Li & Purdy, 2002), drug delivery systems (Arun et al., 2008), as masking agent in food

(Tamamoto et al., 2010), cosmetics (Schmann & Schollmeyer, 2002), in hydrogels (Hoarea &. Kohaneb, 2008) and in contact lenses (Santos et al., 2009).

3. Nuclear Magnetic Resonance spectroscopy

3.1 ^{1}H-Nuclear Magnetic Resonance spectroscopy

Nuclear Magnetic Resonance spectroscopy has been extensively employed in Chemistry and can be considered as one of the most complete spectroscopic techniques, due to its wide field of applications from structural elucidation of structures to investigations on intra/inter-molecular. Applications of NMR on CDs chemistry is so important that no other spectroscopic technique can provide the same wealth of chemical information on the supramolecular systems. Other spectroscopic techniques, like molecular UV-Vis absorption, fluorescence emission, circular dichroism, etc., are also suitable for thermodynamic study of the host-guest intermolecular interactions, but they give only indirect information on the molecular structure of the inclusion complexes.

The simplest experiment of NMR as an indicative of complexation is the observation of the difference in the proton chemical shifts between the free guest and host species and the suggested complex. There has been a long time since Demarco & Thakkar (Demarco & Thakkar, 1971) started studies on CDs complexes by observing the chemical shifts changes of the protons H3 and H5 inside the cavity of αCD when in presence of aromatic molecules due to the anisotropic effect of the aromatic ring. When there is a host-guest interaction, it leads to a change in the δ of the hydrogens due the complexation. This is a first evidence of the guest inclusion in the CD cavity (Schneider et al., 1998). The CDs protons are named according Figure 3.

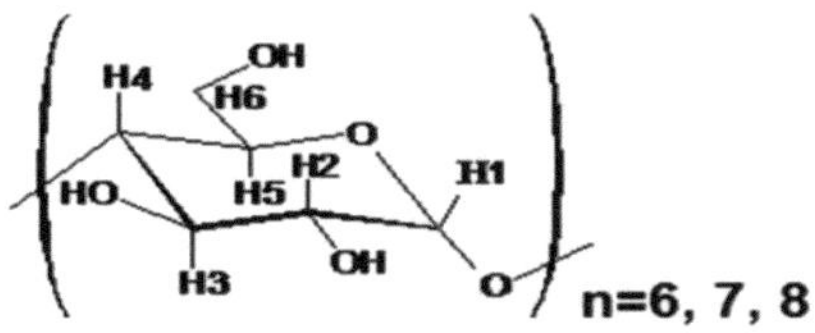

Fig. 3. NMR protons for α; β; γCD (n = 6; 7; 8, respectively)

The ^{1}H-NMR spectra of the three natural cyclodextrins are shown in Figure 4.

One can see that the differences among the spectra of the three CDs, due to the proton shielding, are smaller than 0.1 ppm. The characteristics of these spectra are discussed elsewhere (Schneider et al., 1998).

The stability of the inclusion complex and the orientation of the drug molecule can be inferred by this experiment. Greatbanks & Pickford (Greatbanks & Pickford, 1987) concluded that when Δδ H3 > Δδ H5, occurs partial inclusion of the guest inside the cavity and when Δδ H3 $\leq$ Δδ H5, a total inclusion takes place.

As an example, the stability of the inclusion complex between Minoxidil (MNX), a vasodilator drug also used for treatment of alopecia areata (Gorecki, 1988), and the natural CDs can be suggested by analyzing the differences between the protons chemical shifts of both species. Figure 5 shows the MNX structure and the protons assignment.

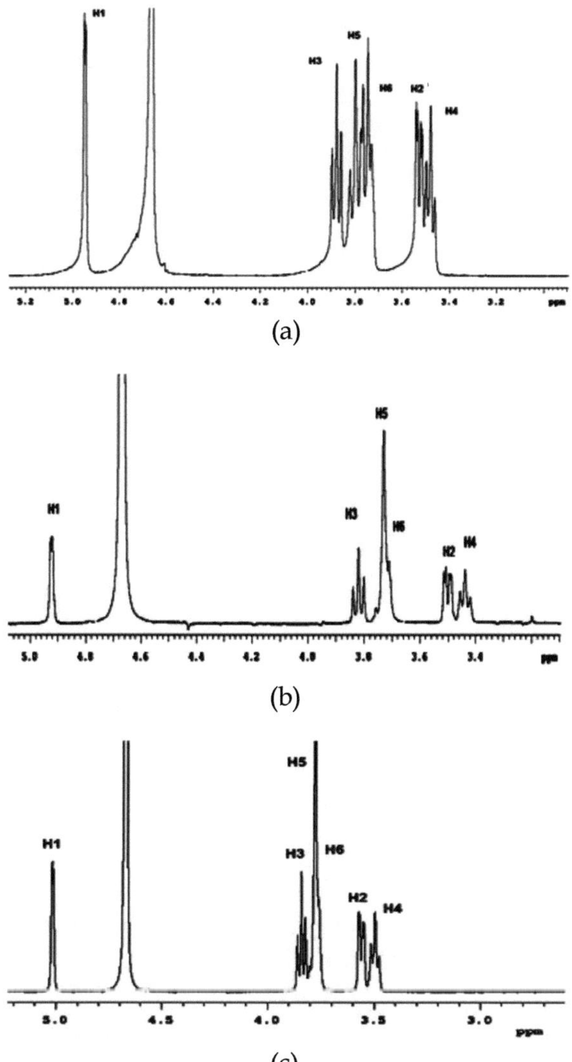

Fig. 4. ^{1}H-NMR spectra of the natural cyclodextrins (298 K; 500 MHz; D_2O; δ_{HOD} 4.67 ppm): (a) αCD; (b) βCD; (c) γCD

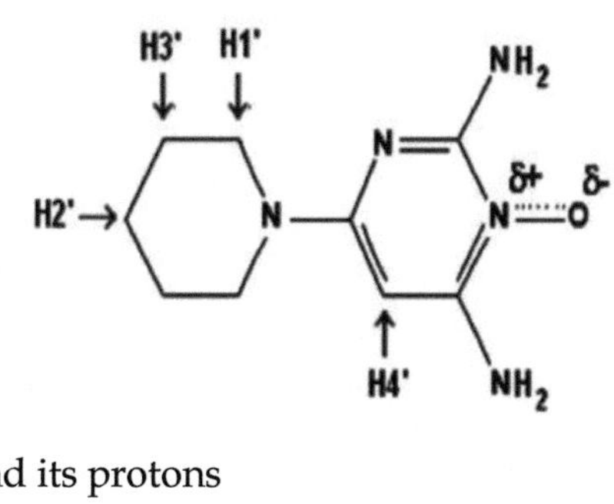

Fig. 5. Structure of MNX and its protons

Tables 2 and 3 summarized the data for this complex.

H	αCD	MNX: αCD		βCD	MNX: βCD		γCD	MNX: γCD	
	$\delta_{\alpha CD}$	$\delta_{\alpha CD:MNX}$	$\Delta\delta_{\alpha CD:MNX}$	$\delta_{\beta CD}$	$\delta_{\beta CD:MNX}$	$\Delta\delta_{\beta CD:MNX}$	$\delta_{\gamma CD}$	$\delta_{\gamma CD:MNX}$	$\Delta\delta_{\gamma CD:MNX}$
1	4.960	4.955	-0.005	4.960	4.965	0.005	5.015	5.015	---
2	3.530	3.540	0.010	3.545	3.550	0.005	3.560	3.555	-0.005
3	3.910	3.890	-0.020	3.830	3.820	-0.010	3.860	3.850	-0.010
4	3.490	3.480	-0.010	3.490	3.480	-0.010	3.495	3.490	-0.005
5	3.765	3.750	-0.015	3.720	3.710	-0.010	3.800	3.800	---

Table 2. CDs chemical shifts (δ) and their difference when in presence of MNX ($\Delta\delta = \delta_{complexed}-\delta_{free}$)

H	MNX	MNX:αCD		MNX:βCD		MNX:γCD	
	δ_{MNX}	$\delta_{\alpha CD:MNX}$	$\Delta\delta_{\alpha CD:MNX}$	$\delta_{\beta CD:MNX}$	$\Delta\delta_{\beta CD:MNX}$	$\delta_{\gamma CD:MNX}$	$\Delta\delta_{\gamma CD:MNX}$
1′	3.340	3.360	0.020	3.420	0.080	3.340	---
2′	1.535	1.550	0.015	1.570	0.035	1.535	---
3′	1.455	1.490	0.035	1.520	0.065	1.455	---

Table 3. MNX chemical shifts (δ) and their difference when in presence of CDs ($\Delta\delta=\delta_{complexed}-\delta_{free}$)

One can see that $\Delta\delta_{\beta CD:MNX} > \Delta\delta_{\alpha CD:MNX} > \Delta\delta_{\gamma CD:MNX}$. Therefore, the complexation between βCD and MNX is stronger than in α and γCD. Considering the values of Δδ for H3 and H5, there is a partial inclusion in α and γCD. For the complex βCD:MNX, the inclusion is total. These results were confirmed by other spectroscopic techniques.

Other drug that we had performed NMR studies with CDs is the anti-neoplasic 5-fluorouracil. No differences in the chemical shifts were observed. This lack of interaction was supposed to be due to the relatively high polarity and solubility of the drug in aqueous media (12.2 mg/mL) (Bayomi & Al-Badr, 1990).

Despite the chemical shift changes of ^{1}H from CD's inner cavity the characterization of inclusion complexes with NMR could be done. This same experimental evidence also could be observed for ^{1}H from the guest molecule inserted into the CD cavity. Moreover, this chemical shift analysis could be extended for other types of experiments, and the characterization of different properties around the complex supramolecular organization can be obtained easily.

One of the most employed NMR experiment based on chemical shift changes is NMR titration. In this experiment, NMR spectra are obtained for solutions containing a fixed concentration of guest [G_o], but the initial concentration of the CD [CD_O] is variable. Due to the chemical equilibrium of G:CD complex formation (equation 3.1), the increase on CD concentration in the solution will result in more population of the G:CD inclusion complex, consequently, it is expected more chemical shift changes in interacting host and guest nucleus as may be the higher CD concentration in the solution. Besides the CD concentration, the magnitude of equilibrium constant associated to the complex formation (K) will be directly related to the chemical shift changes, because it represents the thermodynamic tendency through the formation of G:CD complex, equation 3.2.

$$[G] + [CD] = [G{:}CD] \quad (3.1)$$

$$K = \{[G{:}CD]/([G]\,[CD]\} \quad (3.2)$$

[G] and [CD] are the concentration of free guest and CD in the equilibrium, respectively, which is defined, for a 1:1 complex, according to their respective mass balance (equations 3.3 and 3.4).

$$[G] + [G{:}CD] = G_O \quad (3.3)$$

$$[CD] + [G{:}CD] = CD_O \quad (3.4)$$

As the chemical shift changes in the experiment is defined as the molar weighted average of free and complexed G or CD molecules (equation 3.5), the correlation among the equations 3.2-3.5 can provide a non-linear math relationship between K and δobs, which leads to a thermodynamic application of NMR to cyclodextrin inclusion complexes (Fielding, 2000).

$$\delta exp = X_G\delta_G + X_{G:CD}\delta_{G:CD} \quad (3.5)$$

Examples of the linear relation between K and δ_{obs} are those reported by Mathur et al. (Mathur et al., 1963), Hannah & Ashbaugh (Hannah & Ashbaugh, 1964) and Foster & Fyfe (Foster & Fyfe, 1965a,b). Using the Benesi-Hildebrand and Scatchard linear models they investigated the thermodynamic properties of guest:CD inclusion complex using UV-Vis spectroscopy (equations 3.6 and 3.7).

$$1/\Delta\delta = 1/(K.\Delta\delta max.[CD_O]) + 1/\Delta\delta max \quad (3.6)$$

$$\Delta\delta/[CD_O] = -K.\Delta\delta + K.\Delta\delta max \quad (3.7)$$

Δδ = (δG – δexp), is the chemical shift change of guest proton as the concentration of the CD increase, and Δδmax = (δG – δG:CD), is the maximum possible chemical shift changes supposing all guest molecules are complexed with the CD. Equation 3.6 is known as the double reciprocal plot, and its deduction require an approximation that $[CD_O]$ must be at least 10 times higher than $[G_O]$. Besides, weak inclusion complexes implies significant uncertainly on Δδ, therefore, K estimation become prejudiced. Equation 3.7 is known as x-reciprocal plot, and is less often found in articles of NMR in CD complexes (Fielding, 2000).

Another application of Δδ is the determination of most stable molar stoichiometry of guest:CD in solution, which can be done through the Job plot experiment, that was initially developed for optical spectroscopy and adapted to NMR. Δδ is calculated in solution with different guest molar fraction r, and the stoichiometry relation is obtained for the r value that show the higher Δδ, which corresponds to the maximum population of inclusion complex in solution. If the complex most stable stoichometry is 1:1, Δδ will be maximum in the solution of r 0.5, while if guest:CD complex is 1:2, the higher Δδ will occur for r 0.33. The principle of this method is based on the mass balance of each specie guest, CD and guest:CD complex in equilibrium, that depend on the r value according to equations 3.8 and 3.9 (Loukas, 1997).

$$[G] = rM - [G{:}CD] \quad (3.8)$$

$$[CD] = M(1 - r) - n\,[G{:}CD] \quad (3.9)$$

where r is the guest molar fraction, M = [G] + [CD] and n is the number of CD molecules that encapsulate the guest. The maximum [G:CD] can be determined as a function of r calculating d[G:CD]/dr = 0 that gives $r = (n+1)^{-1}$. Therefore, for n = 1 (1:1 guest:CD complex) [G:CD] will be higher in the solution which r must be 0.5.

As the thermodynamic models for K prediction assumes a fixed stoichometry for the guest:CD complex, equations assuming different stoichometries can also be adjusted, which could lead to uncorrected predictions of guest:CD molar relation. Then, this experiment become very important for study of CDs inclusion complexes, as NMR allow any kind of guest to be investigated, because it does not depend on guest optical spectroscopy activity.

3.2 T_1 measurement

The T_1 measurement is directly related to the relaxation phenomenon, then it will be given a brief review about it. In NMR experiments, the irradiation of the resonance frequency disturbs the thermal equilibrium of the spin system, changing the population ratio and causing appearance of transverse field magnetic components (M_x and M_y). The relaxation occurs when the perturbation ceases until it reaches the equilibrium. It can be divided in two different processes:

1. The relaxation in the applied field direction is characterized by the *spin-lattice* or longitudinal relaxation time T_1 and will be discussed further,
2. The relaxation perpendicular to the field direction, which is characterized by the *spin-spin* or transverse relaxation time.

The time needed for the relaxation of nuclear system is very small which may be seconds, minutes or hours. For protons under high-resolution, T_1 is in the order of a second (Friebolin, 1993; Günther, 1994).

As discussed in the previous paragraph, immediately after exposing the spins to B_0 (the external magnetic field), they are in a non-equilibrium state because all spin states are equally populated and M_0 (initially M_z) = 0, i.e., the magnetization vector M_0 is rotated by $90°_{x'}$ pulse into the axis direction y', or by a $180°_{x'}$ pulse into the negative z direction, leading to $M_z = 0$. After a $180°_x$ pulse, its new value is $M_0 = - M_z$, as in Figure 6 (Friebolin, 1993).

The population ratio changes because the $90°_{x'}$ pulse equalizes the population of the two energy levels, whereas the $180°_{x'}$ pulse inverts the population ratio. Therefore, after the perturbation, the equilibrium condition is reached when $M_z = M_0$ and the rate at which it occurs is determined by the spin-lattice relaxation time T_1. This process was described by the Bloch's differential equation (Friebolin, 1993).

$$\frac{dM_z}{dt} = -\frac{M_z - M_0}{T_1} \tag{3.10}$$

where T_1^{-1} is the rate constant of the relaxation, which is a first-order process.

T_1 can be understood by a change in the energy in the spin system, as the energy absorbed form the pulse must be given up again, transferring to the lattice (or the surroundings), whose thermal energy increases. Intra and intermolecular interactions like dipole-dipole, spin rotation, anisotropy, etc., can contribute to the spin-lattice relaxation. This is recognized as a significant phenomenon related to the dynamic properties of molecules. The most used method to determine T_1 is the inversion recovery method (Günther, 1994), as seen in Figure 7.

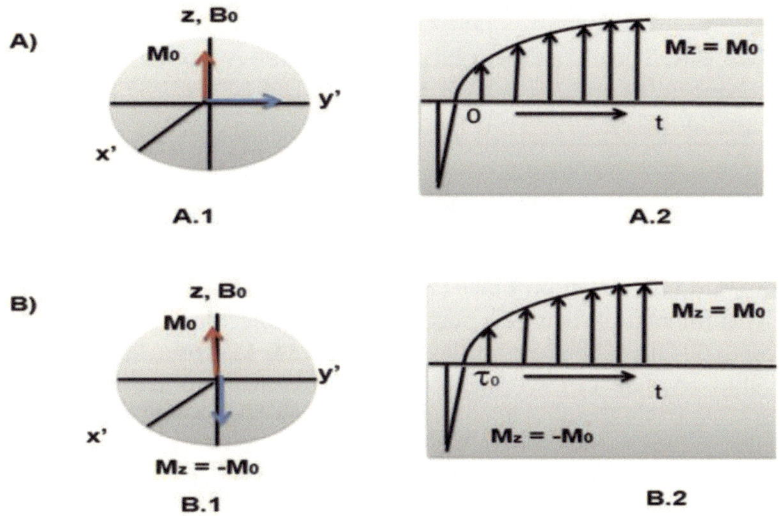

Fig. 6. The longitudinal component M_z in the rotating coordinate system x′; y′; z: A) after a $90°_{x'}$ pulse; B) after a $180°_{x'}$ pulse

Consider the macroscopic magnetization M_0 in the rotating coordinate system.

1. A 180° pulse at the beginning of the experiment brings the vector M_0 to the negative z direction,
2. The value of M_0 decreases due to the spin-lattice relaxation at time τ_1,
3. M_0 passes through zero at time τ_0,
4. M_0 begins to increase in the positive z-direction at time τ_2 reaching its final value.

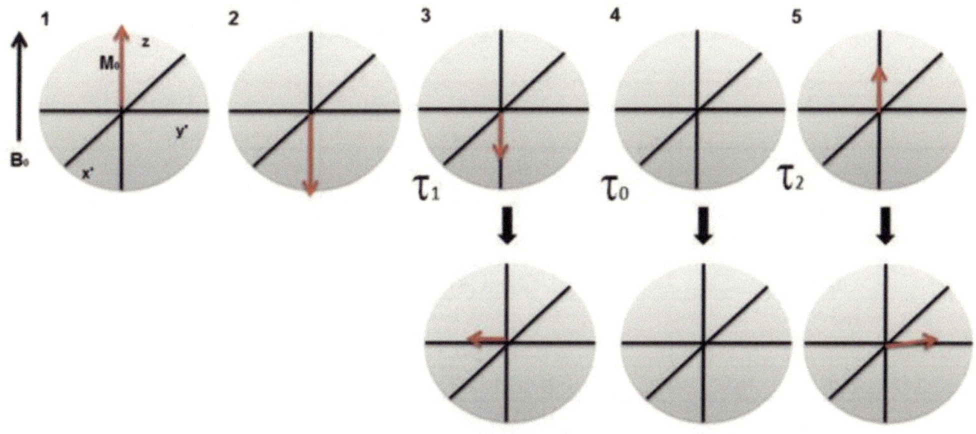

Fig. 7. The inversion-recovery experiment for T_1 measurement

The magnetization can be detected by two signals, applying 90° pulses at time τ_1 and τ_2 which align M_0 along the negative or positive y-direction, respectively, differing in phase by 180°. At time τ_0, there is no magnetization and no signal can be detected. Equation 3.11 is used to determine T_1 (Günther, 1994).

$$\tau_0 = T_1 \ln 2 = 0.693\, T_1 \tag{3.11}$$

In an alternative way, T_1 can be determined more accurately from a semi logarithmic plot of the intensity changes M_0 and M_z against τ, since it can be derived from equation 3.10 by integration (equation 3.12).

$$\ln(M_0 - M_Z) = \ln 2M_0 - \frac{\tau}{T_1} \tag{3.12}$$

Therefore, longitudinal relaxation times (T1) give information about the nucleus mobility in solution and the interaction between host and guest molecules by a qualitative analysis of the decreasing of T_1 values in the complexes (Lambert & Mazzola, 2004). Grillo et al. (Grillo et al., 2007) showed that T_1 lowering of the hydroxymethylnitrofurazone and dimethyl-βcyclodextrin system is a strong evidence of interactions between both molecules.

One of the inclusion compounds studied by this technique in our group was Dapsone:βCD, where the T_1 values for all hydrogens were obtained for each molecule and for the complex (data to be published). The values for each sample are summarized in Tables 4 and 5. The structure of Dapsone (DPS) is in Figure 8.

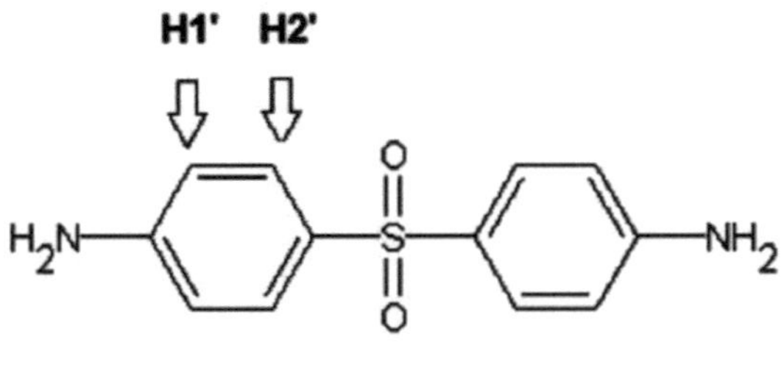

Fig. 8. Structure of Dapsone and the protons probed in NMR experiments

Proton	$T1_{DPS}$ (s)	$T1_{DPS:\beta CD}$ (s)
H1′	3.95 ± 0.54	1.02 ± 0.16
H2′	6.76 ± 3.07	1.73 ± 0.22

Table 4. Longitudinal relaxation times (T1, s) of DPS hydrogens in presence of βCD

Proton	$T1_{\beta CD}$ (s)	$T1_{DPS:\beta CD}$ (s)
H1	1.2 ± 0.1	0.73 ± 0.07
H3	1.56 ± 0.13	1.48 ± 0.07
H5	0.63 ± 0.03	0.39 ± 0.03
H4	0.91 ± 0.06	0.81 ± 0.04

Table 5. Longitudinal relaxation times (T1, s) of βCD hydrogens in presence of DPS

One observed that all T_1 values decrease for the inclusion compound. Note that the T_1 values obtained for the DPS hydrogens became at the same order as the T_1 values of βCD, indicating a strong host:guest interaction.

3.3 DOSY experiment (Diffusion Ordered SpectroscopY)

The molecular diffusion in solution is a phenomenon related to the molecular dynamics in biological and chemical systems, which can be probed by NMR. The diffusion coefficients D provide important information about the molecular organization and the phase structures. Typical D values in liquids (298-303 K) are from 10^{-12} m^2s^{-1} (polymers with high molecular weight) to 10^{-9} m^2s^{-1} (small molecules) (Stilbs, 1987).

Even though the molecular diffusion is not straightway related with interactions and spins energies, the relation of this property with the longitudinal (T_1) and transversal (T_2) times are better understood. Brownian motion perturbs the nuclei magnetic field, changes T_1 and T_2 (Price, 1997).

These studies started with the discovery of the spin echoes by Hahn in 1950. In this experiment, a pulse sequence $[90°\text{-}\tau\text{-}180°\text{-}\tau\text{-(echo)-}]_n$ is applied and it will result in a perfect refocus of the nuclei magnetization (spin echoes) only if there is any changes in the magnetic field gradient G applied during the time 2τ. However, the molecular diffusion does not allow G to keep totally homogeneous, decreasing the echoes amplitude in 2τ. The relation between the spin echoes and the diffusion coefficient D is given by equation 3.13 (Souza & Laverde, 2002).

$$\frac{A(2\tau)}{A(0)} = \exp\left[-\left(\frac{2\tau}{T2}\right) - \frac{2}{3}\gamma^2 G^2 D \tau^3\right] \tag{3.13}$$

The disadvantage in the Hahn equation is the difficulty in separate the contributions due to the transversal relaxation (T_2) and the molecular diffusion (D). This was solved by Carr and Purcell in 1954, where the pulse sequence $90°\text{-}\tau\text{-}[180°\text{-}\tau\text{-(eco)-}\tau\text{-}180°\text{-}\tau\text{-(eco)-}]_n$ can separate the D effect from the T_2 effect (equation 3.14).

$$\frac{A(t)}{A(0)} = \exp\left[-\left(\frac{t}{T2}\right)\right] \exp\left[-\frac{1}{3}(\gamma G \tau)^2 D\tau\right] \tag{3.14}$$

Even though the application of this sequence and the improvement on the echo amplitude with the Stimulated Spin Echo (STE), also discussed by Hahn in 1950, the application of static magnetic field gradients (G) resulted in the necessity to use high values of G to measure small values of D, which led to a increase in the echo and, consequently, a decrease in the noise/signal ratio, causing a difficulty in the detection (Souza & Laverde, 2002).

These difficulties were overcome with application of Pulsed Magnetic Field Gradients (PFG), with spin echoes (PFGSE) (Johnson, 1999) and stimulated spin echoes (PFGSTE) (Stilbs, 1987; Woessner, 1961; Tanner, 1970). Other advantages due to PFG are (Parella, 1998):

1. Reduction of the steps in the cycles phases to suppression of undesired artifacts,
2. Decrease of the signal acquisition time,
3. Noise reduction of the 2D experiment,

4. Improvement of the spectral processing,
5. Efficient suppression of undesired signals, like solvent and heteronuclear coupling.

The advantages of PFG application are (Souza & Laverde, 2002):

a. Separation of the echo attenuation caused by the D effect due to T_2, doing the experiment to a fix τ interval between the RF pulses and changing the area of the gradient pulse,
b. The spin echo is detected in a homogeneous magnetic field condition.

In 1992, Morris and Johnson (Morris & Johnson, 1992) developed an analytical technique based on PFGSE that made possible the distinction among the components of a mixture by the molecular diffusion of each chemical shift. This technique was named DOSY (Diffused Ordered Spectroscopy). In this experiment, D is obtained from the decay of the signal intensity I, which is a function of the area of the magnetic field gradient q ($q = \gamma g\delta$). It can be correlated with q and D by equation 3.15.

$$I(q, v) = \sum\left[An(v).exp\left[-Dn\left(\Delta - \frac{\delta}{3}\right)q^2\right]\right] \tag{3.15}$$

where An(v) is the NMR signal intensity when q=0; Dn is the diffusion coefficient of the component n and Δ is the monitoring time. The DOSY spectrum has two dimensions: the chemical shift in the x axis and Dn in the y axis. It is obtained applying a Laplace inverse transformation after the signal processing by Fourier transformation.

The DOSY experiment allows a global analysis of the sample dynamics, involving since small molecules to aggregates and supramolecular structures. Besides, this technique presents other advantages as impurity detection with no interference, evaluation of the species in equilibrium and selection of the desired specie to analysis.

The small sensibilities of NMR technique, superposition of the signals and similar D values interfere with the acquisition of a good DOSY spectrum. Also, this experiment requires a good stability of the signal, which can be impaired by phenomena as induced vortex currents in the sample, coupling between the gradient coil and the principal magnetic field and perturbation in the system of lock frequency and field. So, to try to minimize such effects, various pulse sequences were developed, each with advantages and disadvantages according to the characteristics of the sample components. The main examples of DOSY pulse sequences are: BPPSTE (Bipolar Pulser Pair STimulated Echo), BPPLED (Bipolar Pulse Pair Longitudinal Eddy currents Decay), GCSTE (Gradient Compensated STimulated Echo) e GCSTESL (Gradient Compensated Stimulated Echo Spin Lock) (Souza & Laverde, 2002).

The implementation of simple PFGSE experiments on cyclodextrins complexes was initiated with Stilbs in 1983 (Stilbs, 1987), and the group of Lin first studied this interaction by DOSY in 1995 (Lin et al., 1995). The formation of inclusion complex in a solution containing a drug and CD can be observed by reduction of its diffusion coefficient. The larger the difference between D in solution with CD compared to D obtained from solution without CD, the higher the fraction of drug inclusion complex.

The diffusion coefficient (D) depends on the size of the molecule and it can be calculated by equation 3.16.

$$D = \frac{\kappa T}{6\, \pi \eta\, r} \tag{3.16}$$

where κ is the Boltzmann constant, T is the absolute temperature, η is the dynamic viscosity, and r is the radius of the molecule. The population of the guest involved in this complexation process can be calculated from the diffusion coefficients observed for the species in the free and complexed forms, using the equations 3.17-3.19 (Lin et al., 1985; Rymdén et al., 1983).

$$D_{observed} = D_{free}\, p_{free} + D_{complexed}\, p_{complexed} \tag{3.17}$$

where:

$$p_{free} + p_{complexed} = 1 \tag{3.18}$$

and:

$$p_{free} = 1 - p_{complexed} \tag{3.19}$$

$D_{observed}$ is the diffusion coefficient of the active in the presence of CD; D_{free} is the diffusion coefficient of the active in the absence of CD; $p_{complexed}$ is the population fraction of completely complexed active, and $D_{complexed}$ is the diffusion coefficient of the completely complexed.

Substituting the equation 3.19 in the equation 3.17, and considering that the diffusion of the active totally complexed is the same as the CD totally complexed and that the diffusion observed to the CD partially complexed is very close to the same free diffusion:

$$D_{CD\ complexed} \approx D_{CD\ observed\ free} \approx D_{CD\ free} \tag{3.20}$$

Substituting the equation 3.8 in the equation 3.5, $p_{complexed}$ can be obtained as:

$$p_{complexed} = \frac{D_{free} - D_{complexed}}{D_{free} - D_{CDobserved}} \tag{3.21}$$

Knowing $p_{complexed}$ and the molar concentration of each species in solution, it is possible to obtain an estimative of the complex association constant (Ka), if some precautions are taken account as: association constants in the order of $10\text{-}10^4$ L/mol, the NMR observation and the solution concentration (Fielding, 2000). In our studies, one could observe that if the complex is sparkling soluble, more difficult is to acquire the DOSY data because the diffusion coefficients will have big errors.

The determination of association constants by DOSY provides an additional NMR method and an alternative of the chemical shift titration method (Simova & Berger, 2005). The K_a for a complex between the n mol of drug D and m mol of CD is (Rymdén et al., 1983).

$$n\, D + m\, CD \leftrightarrow Complex\ [DnCDm] \tag{3.22}$$

$$Ka = \frac{[\,Complex]}{[D]^n\, [CD]^m} = \frac{[Complex]}{([D]_0 - n[Complex])^n([CD]_0 - m[Complex])^m} \tag{3.23}$$

The equation 3.23 can be related with equation 3.21, then:

$$K_a = \frac{p_{complexed}}{(1 - p_{complexed})([CD]_0 - p_{complexed}\,[D]_0)} \tag{3.24}$$

Fraceto et al. (Fraceto et al., 2007) applied DOSY to study the interaction between charged tetracaine in βCD and p-sulphonic acid calix[6]arene, obtaining Ka 1,358 M^{-1} and 3,889 M^{-1},

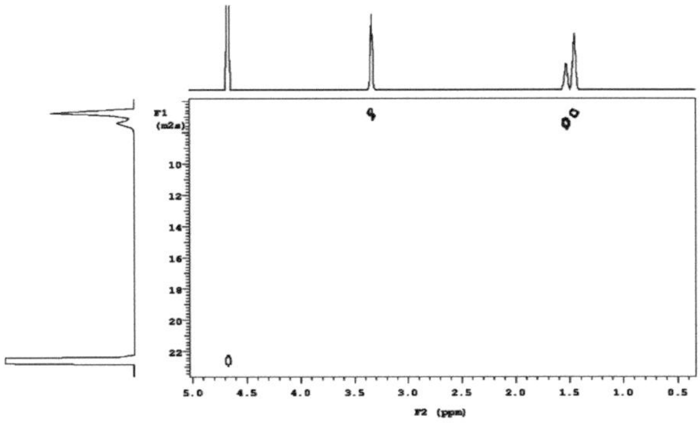

(a)

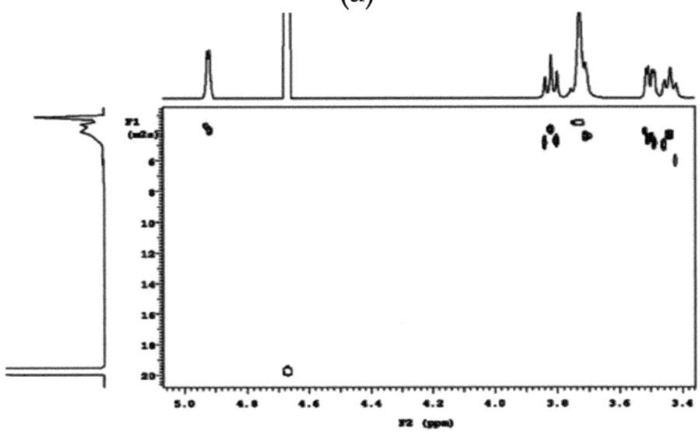

(b)

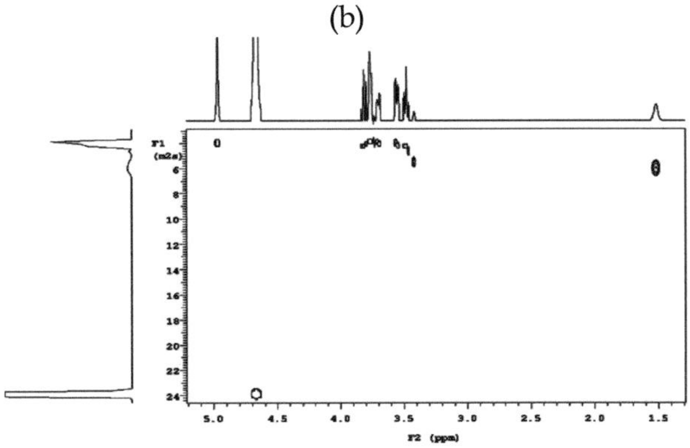

(c)

Fig. 9. ^{1}H-NMR DOSY spectra. (a) MNX; (b) βCD; (c) NMX-βCD 1:1, respectively (500 MHz; D_2O; δ_{HOD} 4.67 ppm) respectively, indicating a good stability of the complexes. Jullian et al. (Jullian et al., 2007) studied the interaction between (+) cathecin and natural and modified βCDs observing a stronger interaction with natural βCD than with hydroxipropil-βCD or dimethyl-βCD, with association constants of 21,800 M^{-1}, 13,580 M^{-1} and 3,500 M^{-1}, respectively.

Besides the applicability of this technique to measure diffusion coefficients and association constants, DOSY experiments with cyclodextrins can be used with other techniques to predict enantiomeric discrimination (Laverde et al., 2002), to predict drug diffusion with polymeric CD (Bakkour et al., 2006), to conclude by the formation of conjugates with CDs, as for example the conjugate between CD and folic acid, studied by Clementi et al. (Clementi et al., 2010), etc. In our group, the complexes of Minoxidil (MNX) and βCD was investigated by DOSY using the pulse sequence GCSTESL (*DOSY Gradient Compensated* was *Stimulated Echo with Spin Lock)*, 25 different amplitudes of pulse gradients in each experiment with the parameters pw = 6.1s; at = 3.3 s; d1 = 3.0 s; nt = 32; lb = 0.2 Hz. The spectra of MNX, βCD and MNX:βCD are shown in the Figure 9 and the data in Table 6.

Complex	D_{MNX} (/$10^{-10}m^2s^{-1}$)	D_{CD} (/$10^{-10}m^2s^{-1}$)	D_{OH} (/$10^{-10}m^2s^{-1}$)	$P_{complexed}$ (%)
MNX free	6.363 ± 0.019	---	22.538 ± 0.087	---
αCD	---	3.449 ± 0.021	23.366 ± 0.017	19.8
α 1:1	5.811 ± 0.014	3.581 ± 0.006	22.127 ± 0.111	
βCD	---	3.254 ± 0.024	21.943 ± 0.079	91.4
L β 1:1	3.565 ± 0.058	3.302 ± 0.021	23.935 ± 0.118	
γCD	---	3.154 ± 0.012	22.082 ± 0.105	17.5
L γ 1:1	5.778 ± 0.050	3.014 ± 0.033	23.172 ± 0.119	

Table 6. MNX diffusion coefficient (D_{MNX}) free and in the presence of CDs, diffusion coefficient of α, β and γCDs and diffusion coefficients of water (D_{OH}). Values of percentages of complexed MNX with CDs

It turns out that D of HOD, free CD and MNX are quite different. Considering the size of the species in solution, the values are consistent, because the smaller hydrodynamic radius, the greater is tis coefficient. As expected, βCD complexes are those with smaller diffusion coefficient and hence the largest population of complexed species, as the more complex the MNX is with the CDs, the lower its diffusion. Finally, it was also observed that these results have small errors.

DOSY was also employed to study the interaction between 5FU, a water soluble drug and the natural cyclodextrins. The diffusion coefficients data are in Table 7. It is evident that there are no interactions between the CDs and 5FU, as also observed by using other techniques.

Sample	$D_{5\text{-}FU}$ (/$10^{-10}m^2s^{-1}$)	D_{CD} (/$10^{-10}m^2s^{-1}$)	D_{OH} (/$10^{-10}m^2s^{-1}$)	$P_{complexed}$ (%)
5FU	9.216 ± 0.028	---	22.538 ± 0.087	---
αCD	---	3.449 ± 0.021	23.366 ± 0.017	0
α 1:1	9.347 ± 0.179	3.353 ± 0.146	22.871 ± 0.086	
βCD	---	3.254 ± 0.024	21.943 ± 0.079	0
L β 1:1	9.338 ± 0.295	3.356 ± 0.086	22.879 ± 0.087	

Table 7. Free 5FU diffusion coefficient (D_{5FU}) and in the presence of CDs, diffusion coefficient of α and βCDs and diffusion coefficients of water (D_{OH}). Values of percentages of complexed 5FU with CDs

Studies were done on the complex involving the anti-helmintic drug thiabendazole (TBZ) and βCD. TBZ is a poor water soluble drug derived from benzimidazole with wide pharmacological, fungicide and bactericide applicability (Tang et al., 2005). It is believed that the enhancement of its water solubility can be achieved through formation of inclusion complexes with βCD. The data are in Table 8.

Sample	D_{TBZ} (/$10^{-10}m^2s^{-1}$)	D_{CD} (/$10^{-10}m^2s^{-1}$)	D_{OH} (/$10^{-10}m^2s^{-1}$)	$P_{complexed}$ (%)
TBZ	4.614 ± 0.709	---	16.841 ± 0.271	---
βCD	---	2.513 ± 0.038	15.568 ± 0.230	18.4
L β 1:1	4.227 ± 0.636	2.243 ± 0.019	16.821 ± 0.400	

Table 8. Free TBZ diffusion coefficient (D_{TBZ}) free and in the presence of CDs, diffusion coefficient of βCD and diffusion coefficients of water (D_{OH}). Values of percentages of complexed TBZ with CDs

The values of D for free TBZ and for the drug in the 1:1 complex was not statistically different but the lower mean value for the complex indicates encapsulation of the molecules.

3.4 The NOE experiments for structural characterization of CDs inclusion complexes: NOESY and ROESY

When two nucleus, HI and HS, are closely situated (≈ 4 A), which can be in the same molecule or due to intermolecular forces, the local field existing in both nucleus will disturb each one, causing an dipole-dipole coupling that will have a null J-coupling (JIS = 0). However it will change the spin-lattice relaxation time (T1) in the inter-nucleus environment. The dipole-dipole coupling will cause splitting of the spin energy levels of both, HI and HS. When it occurs involving the nucleus of the same specie (as hydrogen nuclei), four new energy levels (αα, αβ, βα, ββ) , as in Figure 10 (Keeler, 2002).

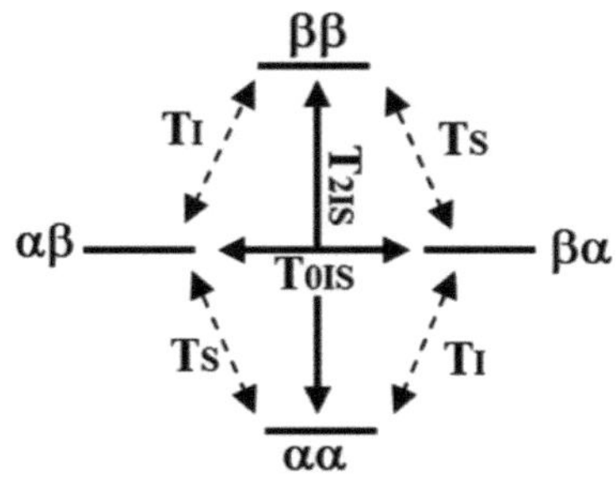

Fig. 10. Two homonuclear spin system energy levels diagram. T is respective transition occurrence probabilities. Spin states are shown for HI and HS nuclei, respectively

NOE can be defined as the change of the HI resonance intensity when HS resonance is perturbed. This can be probed applying a selective pulse into this nucleus (RF pulse applied has the same frequency as the HI Larmour frequency). Due to the dipolar coupling, this change is related to the population transition between the energy levels. While these transitions cannot be induced by another RF pulse, they can occur in the dipolar relaxation process. Initially, only αα and ββ spin energy levels are populated; however, when applying a selective pulse, all the levels become equally populated, but no change on resonance intensity in both HI and HS is observed. When the selective pulse in HS is ended, the re-equilibrium will occurs through dipolar relaxation, according to the transitions probability T0IS and T2IS or TI/TS, (the last ones are isolated from each nucleus and, therefore, will not cause NOE), during a specific time (*mixing time*). The relaxation through the transition probability T2IS will increase the HI resonance intensity (positive NOE), and the one that occurs through T0IS will result in decrease of HI resonance (negative NOE) (Neuhaus & Williamson, 1989).

NOE measurements can be done in both steady and dynamic states. In the steady-state, HS is irradiated with a weak and continuum RF field that does not affect HI spin, until its resonance become saturated. Then, the NOE enhancement over HI is measured as the difference of its resonance intensities under HS saturation and when this condition is not applied (system in equilibrium). In the dynamic NOE measurement (NOESY, Nuclear Overhauser Enhancement SpectroscopY) HS resonance will not be saturated during the mixing time, and the NOE enhancement will depend to both nuclei magnetization amplitudes after the evolution period t1 (Figure 2). The main difference in the NOESY experiment is that the NOE enhancement intensity will be describe as three different peaks in a 2D-spectrum which can discriminate HI-HS cross-peak correlation from peaks related to other changes on HS resonance. The pulse sequences for each experiment are those reported by Keeler (Keeler, 2002).

ROESY (Rotational Overhauser Enhancement SpectroscopY) experiment was firstly developed by Bothner-By et al. (Bothner-By et al., 1984), as an alternative methodology to study NOE, and it can be done in one or two dimensions. The 1D experiment was named CAMELSPIN (Cross-relaxation Apropriate for Mini-molecules EmuLated by SPIN-locking).

The main advantage of the ROESY experiment over the traditional NOESY is the use of the *spin-lock condition*, that is done applying of a strong, constant and coherent pulse at HS Larmour frequency throughout the *mixing time*. This pulse will saturate the HS resonance (magnetization vectors projections stays precessing in the XY plane), and then, the rOe (rotational Overhauser effect) will not only be enhanced due the longitudinal magnetization components interactions, but also due to the interactions of transversal ones. The main consequence will be a positive rOe condition over all molecules. The NOE signal will be enhanced even for molecules whose w.tc (w is the Larmour frequency and t_c is the rotational correlation time) product is small, in contrast to NOESY, wherein small t_c results on negative nOe (Neuhaus & Williamson, 1989). As this small w.t_c condition exist on NOE measurements of CD inclusion complexes, the ROESY experiment become suitable for structural study of these systems (Schneider et al., 1998).

Both NOESY and ROESY experiments have been widely applied for structural elucidation of guest:CD inclusion complexes, which are done through the internuclear NOE enhancement measures between the guest nuclei and the CD inner cavity nuclei H3, H5 and H6. Besides, NOE cross-peaks can be correlated to their respective internuclear distances (Evans, 1995; Pinto et al., 2005). Therefore more detailed information about the supramolecular organization of these systems can also be obtained beyond just qualitative structural analysis as with the changes in chemical shift.

NOE-based experiments are generally done in two-dimensions, as all cross-peak correlations can be seen in the spectrum, becoming easier the interpretation of the data. In the 1-D version, the experiment must be done separately by applying the selective pulses for each nucleus, obtaining the corresponding spectrum, which turn this experiment usually more time requesting. However 1D experiment has more sensibility, which can be necessary if detection of weak NOE interactions or complex limited solubility is involved.

The literature reports several NOESY and ROESY experiments, and some examples will be commented. An extent characterization of CDs inclusion complexes with different terpenes employing NMR based on ^{1}H and ^{13}C chemical shifts analyses ($\Delta\delta$) and 2D-ROESY was reported by Bergonzi et al. (Bergonzi et al., 2007).

Interactions involving the steroids prednisolone, ethinyloestradiol and estriol with βCD were studied by the NOE-based and chemical shift analysis NMR experiments (Bednarek et al., 2002). The authors could distinguish steroids affinities with βCD through their different penetration into the CD cavity.

Inclusion complex between the drug Tenoxican and βCD was also characterized by ROESY-2D experiment (Voulgari et al., 2007) and drug molecular dimerization was studied by NOESY, showing that further description of these systems can be obtained with different NMR different experiment.

Another very interesting application of NOE-based experiments on CDs inclusion complexes provides structure elucidation between enantiomers and CDs. With the 1D-ROESY experiment, interactions between Aminoglutethimide (Elbashir et al., 2009) and propranolol (Servais et al., 2010) enantiomers with CDs could have been separately characterized. This kind of study was also done with ROESY-2D experiment for vinca alkaloids enantiomers (Sohajda et al., 2010). In a recent work, de Paula et al. explored 1D-ROESY for studying interactions involved on ternary systems of Prilocaine-cyclodextrin-liposome (Cabeça et al., 2011) and propracaine-βCD-liposome (Cabeça et al., 2008), obtaining information on the topology of the inclusion complex inside the liposome membrane.

3.5 Solid state NMR

^{13}C-Cross Polarization Magic Angle Spinning (CPMAS) NMR is other technique used to study interactions between drugs and cyclodextrins (Schneider et al., 1998). Also CPMAS measurements provides a powerful non-invasive approach to the molecular analysis of starch-related structures, its cyclodextrin characterization provides information on the molecular organization at shorter distance scales (Gidley & Bociek, 1988). However, this study is more complex and fails when some drug characteristics are not obey, as it will be shown.

The spectra of solids in normal conditions are broad and unresolved, providing restricted information. This phenomenon happens because not only the indirect spin-spin interaction between nuclei through bonds takes place, but also the nuclear magnets can couple through the direct interaction of their nuclear dipoles, in order of 10^{2}–10^{4} Hz. This effect can be eliminated by applying a strong magnetic field perpendicular to the magnetic field B_0 (B_2). Other factor is the chemical shielding anisotropy, which are in the order of 103–104 Hz, due to the shielding of a specific nucleus in a time to record because the nuclei have to be allowed to relax for several minutes between pulses. This factor was solved by a process called Cross Polarization (CP). It takes advantage of the properties of the protons coupled to the carbons, as the double irradiation process (B_0 and B_2) is used to transfer some of the proton's faster relaxation and higher magnetization to the carbon atoms (Lambert & Mazzola, 2004; Saito et al., 2006).

When the protons move onto the x-axis by a 90° pulse, a continuous y field is applied, which intensity is controlled in the equipment, to keep the magnetization precessing in that axis (*spin locking*). As soon as the ^{13}C channel is turned on, the Hartmann-Hann condition is set, i.e. ^{13}C frequency become equal to the ^{1}H frequency. In this situation all nuclei precess at the same frequency and magnetization, turning the ^{13}C higher than in normal pulse experiments, enhancing the carbon resonances and the relaxation. Finally, at the maximum intensity, the magnetic field of the ^{13}C channel is turned off and the carbon magnetization is acquired (Lambert & Mazzola, 2004).

However, broad line widths and spectra of compounds with many non-equivalent nuclei are difficult to analyze due to the strong overlap even if the contributions of dipolar ^{1}H, ^{13}C coupling are practically eliminated. So, a technique is used to observe high resolution spectra, where the sample cell is rotated around the magic angle (MAS = Magic Angle Spinning). In this experiment, the rotor is rotated with a high spinning rate around an axis which makes the magic angle of $\theta = 54.7\,°$ with the axis of the external field B_o in order to vanish the chemical shift anisotropy. So, combining the MAS technique with the CP technique is possible to narrow the resonance lines and obtain the CPMAS spectra (Günter, 1994).

The confirmation of the inclusion complex between molecules and CDs is doing analyzing the differences in the chemical shifts and modification of the peaks between the free and complexed guest molecules. The appearance of multiple resonances for atoms C2, C3, C5, C4, and C6 of the glucopyranose units indicates the coexistence of different structural arrangements (Lima, 2001). Usually, the multiple resonances of the carbons of the glucose monomers tends to converge to a single peak in the inclusion compound, suggesting that the glucose units adopt a more symmetrical conformation in the complex (Lai et al., 2003). However, one has to take care in this analysis since this phenomenon can also be due to the freeze-drying process, which leads to amorphization of the sample, not indicating the host-guest interaction (Figure 11).

The imazalil :βCD complex was prepared using supercritical carbon dioxide and was characterized by CPMAS by Lai et al. The authors realized not only the conformation changing between the spectra of inclusion compound and physical mixture, but also changes in chemical shift, a marked broadening of all signals, and that several resonances of imazalil split up into multiple signals, indicative of a pronounced structural rearrangement of the imidazole and aryl rings (Lai et al., 2003) inside the CD cavity.

This technique is applied to confirm the inclusion between the CDs and polymers, as poly(ε-caprolactone) (Harada et al., 2007), comblike poly(ethylene oxide) grafted polymers (He et al., 2005) and poly(ε-lysine) (Huh et al., 2001). In these studies, they usually compared the spectrum of the complex with the physical mixture, showing that the CD molecule retain a less symmetrical cyclic conformation in the crystalline uncomplexed state, characterized by resolved C1 and C4 resonances of the glucose units, comparing with the CD in the complexed state, which has a symmetrical cyclic conformation.

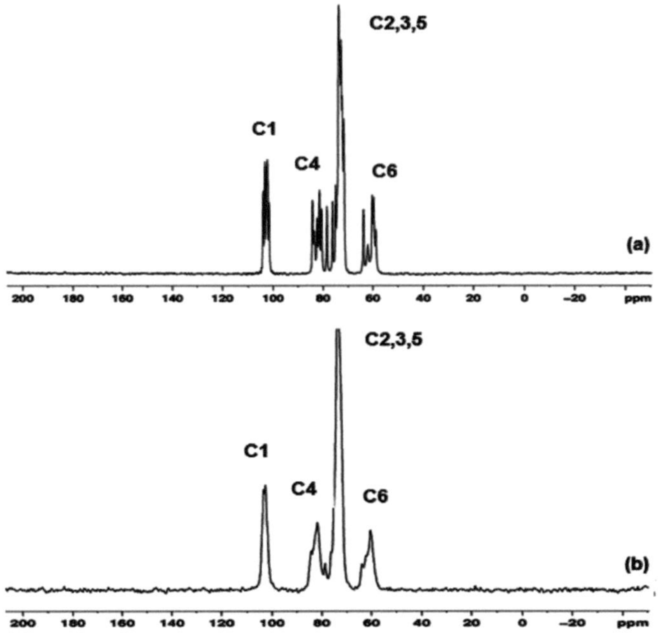

Fig. 11. ^{13}C- CPMAS NMR spectra. (a) natural; (b) freeze-dried βCD (10 kHz, 298 K)

One of the inclusion complex analyzed in our laboratory was Dapsona (DPS) and HP-hydroxypropyl-βCD. DPS (4,4'diaminodiphenylsulfone) is a very effective drug to treat leprosy and inflammatory conditions in *Pneumocystis carinii* pneumonia, toxoplasmosis and tuberculosis. However, the oral administration of this drug leads to serious side effects and treatment failures. It is believed that the complex DPS:HP-βCD would increase the wettability and the solubility of this drug for a supported and gradual release, maximizing its biodisponibility over time (Wozel et al., 1997; Chougule et al., 2008). The spectra of DPS, HP-βCD, the physical mixture and the inclusion compound are in the Figures 12-15.

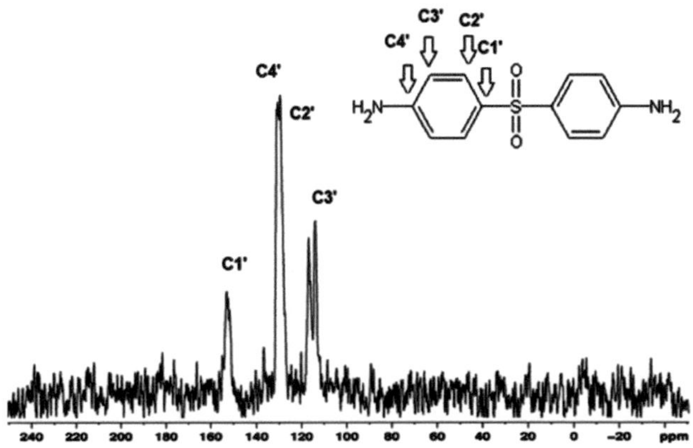

Fig. 12. ^{13}C- CPMAS NMR spectra of DPS (10 kHz, 298 K)

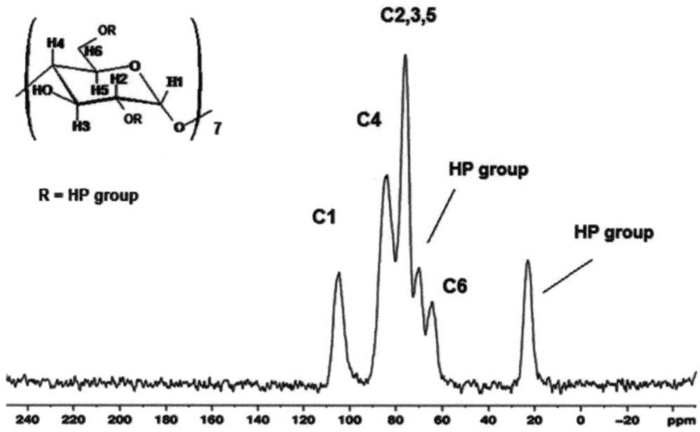

Fig. 13. ^{13}C- CPMAS NMR spectra of HP-βCD (10 kHz, 298 K)

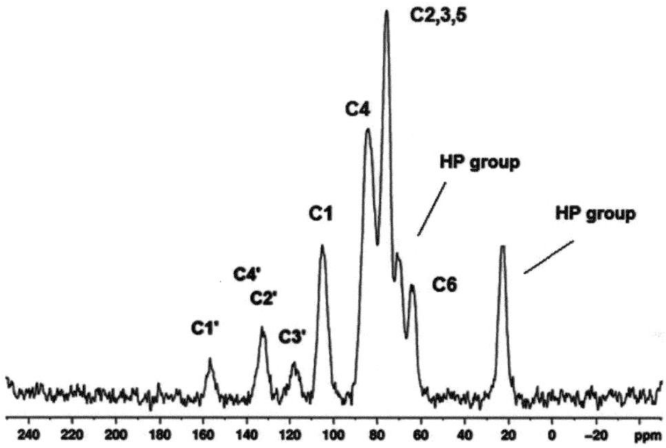

Fig. 14. ^{13}C- CPMAS NMR spectra of DPS :HP-βCD: (10 kHz, 298 K)

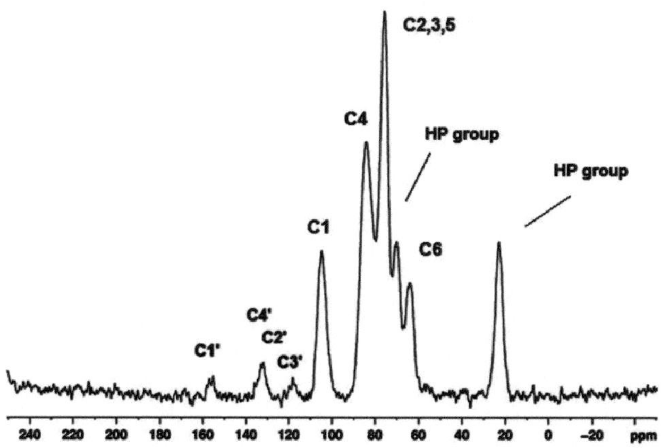

Fig. 15. ^{13}C- CPMAS NMR spectra of DPS and HP-βCD physical mixture (10 kHz, 298 K)

The ^{13}C chemical shifts for βCD, DPS, physical mixtures and complex are in the Tables 9-12.

C	$\delta_{HP\text{-}\beta CD}$	$\delta_{DPS:HP\text{-}\beta CD/PM}$	$\Delta(\delta_{DPS:HP\text{-}\beta CD} - \delta_{HP\text{-}\beta CD})$
C1	104.7	104.9	0.2
C2,3,5	76.3	76.3	0
C4	84	84.7	0.7
C6	64.3	64.3	0
HP-group	70.1; 23.2	70.3; 23.2	0.2; 0

Table 9. ^{13}C-CPMAS NMR chemical shifts of βCD and their change in the presence of DPS in the physical mixture ($\Delta\delta = \delta_{PM} - \delta_{free}$)

C	$\delta_{HP\text{-}\beta CD}$	$\delta_{DPS:HP\text{-}\beta CD}$	$\Delta(\delta_{DPS:\beta CD} - \delta_{HP\text{-}\beta CD})$
C1	104.7	105.3	0.6
C2,3,5	76.3	76.2	0.1
C4	84	84.5	0.5
C6	64.3	64.2	0.3
HP-group	70.1; 23.2	71.2; 22.9	1.1; 0.3

Table 10. ^{13}C-CPMAS NMR chemical shifts of HP-βCD and their change in the in the complex ($\Delta\delta = \delta_{complexed} - \delta_{free}$)

H	δ_{DPS}	$\delta_{DPS\ HP\text{-}\beta CD/PM}$	$\Delta(\delta_{DPS:HP\text{-}\beta CD/PM} - \delta_{HP\text{-}\beta CD})$
C1′	152.8	153.9	1.1
C2,4′	130	131.9	1.9
C3′	115.5	116	0.5

Table 11. ^{13}C-CPMAS NMR chemical shifts of DPS and their change in the presence of βCD in the physical mixture ($\Delta\delta = \delta_{PM} - \delta_{free}$)

H	δ_{DPS}	$\delta_{DPS:HP\text{-}\beta CD}$	$\Delta(\delta_{DPS:\beta CD} - \delta_{HP\text{-}\beta CD})$
C1′	152.8	156.9	4.1
C2,4′	130	133.1	3.1
C3′	115.5	118	2.5

Table 12. ^{13}C-CPMAS NMR chemical shifts of DPS and their variation in the presence of HP-βCD in the complex ($\Delta\delta = \delta_{complexed} - \delta_{free}$)

When DPS is complexed with HP-βCD Δδ is higher than in the physical mixture. Also, there is a peak broadening in the inclusion complex spectrum. As discussed before, both facts suggest that DPS is encapsulated into the cyclodextrin cavity and interacting with the hydroxypropyl group. Moreover, although it is observed a Δδ, one can clearly note that the spectrum of the physical mixture is a combination of the spectrum of HP-βCD and of DPS.

4. Experimental

4.1 Materials and methods

Dapsone was supplied by Ecofarma Farmácia Ltda.; Minoxidil by Galderma Brasil S.A.; Thiabendazole by EMS; α, β and γCD were supplied by Amaizo (American Maize-Products

Co.); hydroxypropyl-βCD and βCD were gifts from ISP Technologies, Inc.; ethyl alcohol 99.5% P.A. was purchased from LabSynth Ltda. Products for Laboratories; 99.9% deuterium oxide was purchased from Cambridge Isotope Laboratories, Inc.; Freeze-dryer FTS Systems; Bruker Avance II 300 MHz and Varian 500 MHz NMR spectrometers; rotary evaporator RE111, water bath 461 and vacuum pump Büchi Labortechnik AG.

4.2 Preparation of inclusion complex

The inclusion complexes were prepared by one of the two method, co-precipitation or freeze-drying, in an equimolar stoichoimetry.

4.3 Preparation of physical mixtures (PM)

Physical mixtures were prepared using the molar ratio of CD and drug by simply mixing the two compounds for 2 min.

4.4 NMR spectroscopy experiments

All experiments with liquid samples were run on a Varian INOVA-500 spectrometer (BO = 11 T), operating at 500 MHz for ^{1}H. The temperature was kept at 297.6 ± 0.1 K in all experiments. The chemical shifts were referenced against the HOD resonance (δ 4.67 ppm). The samples were prepared by dissolving of 2-4 mg of the FD complex in ≈ 0.6 mL of D_2O. The signal of the solvent was used to stop the magnetic field and the radio frequency. The data were acquired using standards Varian software in the following conditions and processed using the program VNMR of the equipment. To obtain the ^{1}H NMR spectra the conditions were: pw 6.1 s; at 3.3 s; d1 3.0 s; nt 32 scans; lb 0.2 Hz.

DOSY: The pulse sequence for DOSY was GCSTESL (DOSY Gradient Compensated Stimulated Echo with Spin Lock). In all analyses 25 different pulsed gradient amplitudes were: d1 6.1 s; at 3.3 s; nt 32 scans; lb 0.2 Hz.

T1 measurement: For ^{1}H-NMR, a 90° pulse was typically of 15 μs, and the recycling time was set to 15 s. Longitudinal relaxation times were obtained by the conventional inversion-recovery method.

ROESY: The ROESY experiment was carried out using the parameters: at 1.0 s; d1 3.0 s; nt 1024 scans; lb 1.0 Hz. The data was obtained applying a sequence of pulses 180° sel. - 90° sel. - spin lock-FID, mixing time of 500 ms. FIDs were acquired through the sequence of pulses 90° sel. - spin lock - FID. A modulator generated the selective pulses and automatically attenuated the power and duration of the pulse.

^{13}C-CPMAS: All spectra of ^{13}C-CPMAS of lyophilized samples, physical mixtures, drugs and CDs were run on a Bruker 300 MHz at 298 K and 10 kHz.

5. Conclusion

NMR is one of the most powerful techniques to investigate interactions between guest and cyclodextrins molecules as it gives extremely useful information on physico-chemical parameters, orientation of the guest molecule inside the cavity and the complex stability.

6. Acknowledgment

The authors gratefully acknowledge financial support from CAPES and CNPq, the ISP Technologies, Inc. for supplying βCD Sônia Fanelli and Anderson S. Pedrosa for assistance with the NMR work and Milene H. Martins for her cooperation with the Dapsone experiments.

7. References

Bakkour, Y., Vermeersch, G., Morcellet M., Boschini, F., Martel, B. & Azaroual, N. (2006). Formation of cyclodextrin inclusion complexes with doxycyclin-hydrate: NMR investigation of their characterization and stability. *Journal of Inclusion Phenomena and Macrocyclic Chemistry*, Vol. 54, N° 1-2, (April 2005), pp. 109–114, DOI 10.1007/s10847-005-5108-7

Bayomi, S.M. & Al-Badr, A.A. 5-Fluorouracil, In: *Analytical Profiles of Drug Substances.* Florey, K. (Ed.). (1990). Vol. 18, pp. 599-639, Academic Press, ISBN: 978-0-12-260819-3, New York, USA, DOI 10.1016/S0099-5428(08)60682-6

Bednarek, E., Bocian, W., Poznański, J., Sitkowski, J., Sadlej-Sosnowska, N. & Kozerski, L. (2002). Complexation of steroid hormones: prednisolone, ethinyloestradiol and estriol with β-cyclodextrin. An aqueous ^{1}H NMR study. *Journal of Chemical Society Perkin Transactions,* Vol. 2, Issue 5, (April 2002), pp. 999-1004, DOI 10.1039/B110435G

Bergeron, R.J. (1977). Cycloamyloses. *Journal of Chemical Education,* Vol. 54, Issue 4, (April 1977), pp. 204-207, DOI 10.1021/ed054p204

Bergonzi, M.C., Bilia, A.R., Di Bari, L., Mazzi, G. & Vincieri, F.F. (2007). Studies on the interactions between some flavonols and cyclodextrins. *Bioorganic & Medicinal Chemistry Letters,* Vol. 17, Issue 21, (November 2007), pp. 5744–5748, DOI 10.1016/j.bmcl.2007.08.067

Bothner-By, A.A., Stephens, R.L., Lee, J., Warren, C.D. & Jeanloz, R.W. (1984). Structure determination of a tetrasaccharide: transient nuclear Overhauser effects in the rotating frame. *Journal of American Chemical Society,* Vol. 106, Issue 3, (February 1984), pp. 811–813, DOI 10.1021/ja00315a069

Buschmann H.-J. & Schollmeyer E. (2002). Applications of cyclodextrins in cosmetic products: A review. *Journal of Cosmetic Science,* Vol. 53, (May/June 2002), pp. 185-191

Cabeça, S.A., Figueiredo, I.M., de Paula, E. & Marsaioli, A.J. (2011). Prilocaine–cyclodextrin–liposome: effect of pH variations on the encapsulation and topology of a ternary complex using ^{1}H NMR. *Magnetic Resonance in Chemistry,* Vol. 49, Issue 6, (June 2011), pp. 295-300, DOI 10.1002/mrc.2740

Cabeça, S.A., Fraceto, L.F., Marsaioli, A.J. & de Paula, E. (2007). Investigation of tetracaine complexation with beta-cyclodextrins and p-sulphonic acid calix[6]arenes by nOe and PGSE NMR. *Journal of Inclusion Phenomena and Macrocyclic Chemistry,* Vol. 57, N° 1-4, (February 2007), pp. 395–401, DOI 10.1007/s10847-006-9224-9

Casu, B., Reggiani, M., Gallo, G.G. & Vigenvani, A. (1966). Hydrogen bonding and conformation of glucose and polyglucoses in dimethyl-sulphoxide solution *Tetrahedron,* Vol. 22, Issue 9, (June 1966), pp. 3061-3083, DOI 10.1016/S0040-4020(01)82286-9

Casu, B., Reggiani, M., Gallo, G.G., Vigenvani, A. (1968). Conformation of O-methylated amylose and cyclodextrins. *Tetrahedron,* Vol. 24, Issue 2, (June 1968), pp. 803-821, DOI 10.1016/0040-4020(68)88030-5

Chen, G. & Jiang, M. (2011). Cyclodextrin-based inclusion complexation bridging supramolecular chemistry and macromolecular self-assembly. *Chemical Society Review,* Vol. 40, (February 2011), pp. 2254–2266, DOI 10.1039/c0cs00153h

Chougule, M., Padhi, B. & Misra, A. (2008). Development of spray dried liposomal dry powder inhaler of Dapsone. *AAPS PharmSciTech.*, Vol. 9, N° 1, (January 2008), pp. 47-55, DOI 10.1208/s12249-007-9024-6

Clementi, A., Aversa, M. C., Corsaro, C., Spooren, J., Stancanelli, R., O'Connor, C., McNamara, M. & Mazzaglia, A. (2010). Synthesis and characterization of a colloidal novel folic acid–β-cyclodextrin conjugate for targeted drug delivery, *Articles,* Paper 2, (January 2010), http://arrow.dit.ie/materart/2, accessed in August 2011

Connors, K.A. (1997). The stability of cyclodextrin complexes in solution. *Chemical Reviews,* Vol. 97, Issue 5, (August 1997), pp. 1325–1358, DOI 10.1021/cr960371r

Elbashir, A.A., Suliman, F.E.O., Saad, B. & Aboul-Enein, H.Y. (2009). Determination of aminoglutethimide enantiomers in pharmaceutical formulations by capillary electrophoresis using methylated-β-cyclodextrin as a chiral selector and computational calculation for their respective inclusion complexes. *Talanta,* Vol. 77, Issue 4, (February 2009), pp. 1388-1393, DOI 10.1016/j.talanta.2008.09.029

Evans, J.N.S. (1995). Biomolecular NMR spectroscopy. Oxford University Press, ISBN-10 0198547668, ISBN-13 978-0198547662, Oxford, England.

Fielding, L. (2000). Determination of association constants (K_a) from solution NMR data. *Tetrahedron,* Vol. 56, Issue 34, (May 2000), pp. 6151-6170, DOI 10.1016/S0040-4020(00)00492-0, ISSN 00404020

Foster, R. & Fyfe, C.A. (1965a). Interaction of electron acceptors with bases. Part 15.—Determination of association constants of organic charge-transfer complexes by n.m.r. spectroscopy. *Transactions of Faraday Society,* Vol. 61, (February 1965), pp. 1626-1631, DOI 10.1039/TF9656101626

Foster, R. & Fyfe, C.A. (1965b). Fluorine nuclear magnetic resonance determination of the association constant of an organic electron-donor–acceptor complex. *Chemical Communications (London),* Vol. 61, Issue 24, (November 1965), pp. 642-642, DOI 10.1039/C19650000642

Fraceto, L.F., Cabeça, S.A., de Paula, E. & Marsaioli, A.J. (2008). Topology of a ternary complex (propracaine–β-cyclodextrin–liposome) by STD NMR. *Magnetic Resonance in Chemistry,* Vol. 46, Issue 9, (September 2008), pp. 832–837, DOI 10.1002/mrc.2265

Friebolin, H. (1993). *Basic one- and two-dimensional NMR spectroscopy.* (2nd ed.). VHC, ISBN 1-56081-796-8, New York, USA.

Gidley, M.J. & Bociek, S.M. (1998). ^{13}C CPMAS NMR studies of amylose inclusion complexes, cyclodextrins, and the amorphous phase of starch granules: relationships between glycosidic linkage conformation and solid-state ^{13}C chemical shifts. *Journal of American Chemical Society,* Vol. 110, N° 12, (June 1998), pp. 3820–3829, DOI 10.1021/ja00220a016

Gorecki, D.K.J. Minoxidil, In: *Analytical Profiles of Drug Substances.* Florey, K. (Ed.). (1988). Vol. 17, pp. 185-219, Academic Press, ISSN: 0099-5428, New York, USA, DOI 10.1016/S0099-5428(08)60220-8

Greatbanks, D. & Pickford, R. (1987). Cyclodextrins as chiral complexing agents in water, and their application to optical purity measurements. *Magnetic Resonance in Chemistry,* Vol. 25, N° 3, (March 1987), pp. 208-215, DOI 10.1002/mrc.1260250306

Griffiths, D.W. & Bender, M.L. (1973). Orientational catalysis by cyclohexaamylose. *Journal of the American Chemical Society,* Vol. 95, (March 1973), pp. 1679-1680, DOI 10.1021/ja00786a064

Grillo, R., Melo, N.F.S., Moraes, C.M., Rosa, A.H., Royeda, J.A.F.R., Menezes, C.M.S., Ferreira, E.I.F. & Fraceto, L.F. (2007). Hydroxymethylnitrofurazone:dimethyl-β-cyclodextrin inclusion complex: a physical–chemistry characterization. *Journal of Biological Physics*, Vol. 33, N° 5-6, (December 2007), pp. 445-453, DOI 10.1007/s10867-008-9054-7

Günter, H. (1994). *NMR spectroscopy: basic principles, concepts and applications in chemistry.* (2nd ed.). John Wiley & Sons, ISBN 0-471-95199-4, Chichester, England

Hanna, M.W. & Ashbaugh, A.L. (1964). Nuclear Magnetic Resonance study of molecular complexes of 7,7,8,8-tetracyanoquinodimethane and aromatic donors. *Journal of Physical Chemistry*, Vol. 68, Issue 4, (April 1964), pp. 811–816, DOI 10.1021/j100786a018

Harada, A., Kawaguchi, Y., Nishiyama, T. & Kamachi, M. (1997). Complex formation of poly(ε-caprolactone) with cyclodextrin. *Macromolecular Rapid Communications*, Vol. 18, N° 7, (July 1997), pp. 535-539, DOI 10.1002/marc.1997.030180701

He, L., Huang, J., Chen, Y. & Liu, L. (2005). Inclusion complexation between comblike PEO grafted polymers and α-cyclodextrin. *Macromolecules*, Vol. 38, N° 8, (March 2005), pp. 3351–3355, DOI 10.1021/ma047748c

Hoarea, T.R. & Kohaneb, D.S. (2008). Hydrogels in drug delivery: progress and challenges. *Polymer*, Vol. 49, Issue 8, (April 2008), pp. 1993-2007, DOI 10.1016/j.polymer.2008.01.027

Huh, K.M., Ooya, T., Sasaki, S. & Yui, N. (2001). Polymer inclusion complex consisting of poly(ε-lysine) and alfa-cyclodextrin. *Macromolecules*, Vol. 34, N° 8, (March 2001), pp. 2402–2404, DOI 10.1021/ma0018648

Jullian, C., Miranda, S., Zapata-Torres, G., Mendizábal, F. & Olea-Azar, C. (2007). Studies of inclusion complexes of natural and modified cyclodextrin with (+) catechin by NMR and molecular modeling. *Bioorganic & Medicinal Chemistry*, Vol. 15, Issue 9, (May 2007), pp. 3217-3224, DOI 10.1016/j.bmc.2007.02.035

Keeler, J. (2005). *Understanding NMR Spectroscopy*. Wiley Inc., ISBN 13 978-0-470-01787-6 (P/B), Chichester, England.

Lai, S., Locci, E., Piras, A., Porcedda, S., Lai, A. & Marongiu, B. (2003). Imazalil–cyclomaltoheptaose (β-cyclodextrin) inclusion complex: preparation by supercritical carbon dioxide and ^{13}C CPMAS and ^{1}H NMR characterization. *Carbohydrate Research*, Vol. 338, Issue 21, (October 2003), pp. 2227-2232, DOI 10.1016/S0008-6215(03)00358-6

Lambert, J.B. & Mazzola, E.P. (2004). *Nuclear Magnetic Resonance Spectroscopy: an introduction to principles, applications, and experimental methods.* Pearson/Prentice Hall, ISBN 0130890669 9780130890665, Upper Saddle River, USA.

Laverde Jr., A., Conceição, G.J.A., Queiroz, S.C.N., Fujiwara, F.Y. & Marsaioli, A.J. (2002). An NMR tool for cyclodextrin selection in enantiomeric resolution by high-performance liquid chromatography. *Magnetic Resonance in Chemistry*, Vol. 40, Issue 7, (May 2002), pp. 433-442, DOI 10.1002/mrc.1043

Li, S. & Purdy, W.C. (1992). Cyclodextrins and their applications in analytical chemistry. *Chemical Review*, Vol. 92, N° 6, (September 1992), pp. 1457-1470, DOI 10.1021/cr00014a009

Lima, S., Gonçalves, I.S., Ribeiro-Claro, P., Pillinger, M., Lopes A.D., Ferreira, P., Teixeira-Dias, J.J.C., Rocha, J. & Romão C.C. (2001). Interactions of cationic and neutral molybdenum complexes with β-cyclodextrin host molecules. *Organometallics*, Vol. 20, N° 11, (May 2001), pp. 2191–2197, DOI 10.1021/om001088s

Lin, M., Jayawickrama, D.A., Rose, R.A., DelViscio, J.A. & Larive, C.K. (1995). NMR spectroscopic analysis of the selective complexation of the cis and trans isomers of phenylalanyl-proline by β-cyclodextrin. *Analytica Chimica Acta*, Vol. 307, Issues 2-3, (May 1995), pp. 449-457, DOI 10.1016/0003-2670(95)00006-L

Loukas, Y.L. (1997). Multiple complex formation of fluorescent compounds with cyclodextrins: efficient determination and evaluation of the binding constant with improved fluorometric studies. *The Journal of Physical Chemistry B*, Vol. 101, Issue 24, (June 1997), pp. 4863–4866, DOI 10.1021/jp9638189

Mathur, R., Becker, E.D., Bradley, R.B. & Li, N.C. (1963). Proton magnetic resonance studies of hydrogen bonding of benzenethiol with several hydrogen acceptors. *Journal of Physical Chemistry*, Vol. 67, Issue 10, (October 1963), pp. 2190–2194, DOI 10.1021/j100804a052

Morris, K.F. & Johnson Jr., C.S. (1992). Diffusion-ordered two-dimensional nuclear magnetic resonance spectroscopy. *Journal of the American Chemical Society*, Vol. 114, N° 8, (April 1992), pp. 3139–3141, DOI 10.1021/ja00034a071

Neuhaus, D. & Williamson, M. (2000). *The nuclear Overhauser effect in structural and conformation analysis.* Wiley-VHC, Inc., ISBN 0-471-24675-1, New York, USA.

Parella, T. (1998). Pulsed field gradients: a new tool for routine NMR. *Magnetic Resonance in Chemistry,* Vol. 36, Issue 7, (July 1998), pp. 467-495, DOI 10.1002/(SICI)1097-458X(199807)36:7<467::AID-OMR325>3.0.CO,2-S

Pinto, L.M.A., Fraceto, L.F., Santana, M.H.A., Pertinhez T.A., Oyama Jr., S. & de Paula, E. (2005). Physico-chemical characterization of benzocaine-β-cyclodextrin inclusion complexes. *Journal of Pharmaceutical and Biomedical Analysis,* Vol. 39, Issue 5, (October 2005), pp. 956-963, DOI 10.1016/j.jpba.2005.06.010

Price, W.S. (1997). Pulsed-field gradient nuclear magnetic resonance as a tool for studying translational diffusion: Part 1. Basic theory. *Concepts in Magnetic Resonance,* Vol. 9, Issue 5, (December, 1997), pp. 299–336, DOI 10.1002/ (SICI)1099-0534(1997)9:5<299::AID-CMR2>3.0.CO,2-U

Rasheed, A., Kumar C.K.A., Sravanthi V.V.N.S.S. (2008). Cyclodextrins as drug carrier molecule: A review. *Scienthia Pharmaceutica,* Vol. 76, (November 2008), pp. 567–598, DOI 10.3797/scipharm.0808-05

Rymdén, R., Carlfors, J. & Stilbs, P. (1983). Substrate binding to cyclodextrins in aqueous solution: A multicomponent self-diffusion study. *Journal of Inclusion Phenomena and Macrocyclic Chemistry,* Vol. 1, N° 2, (June 1983), pp. 159-167, DOI 10.1007/BF00656818

Saenger, W. (1980). Cyclodextrin inclusion compounds in research and industry. *Angewandte Chemie International Edition in English,* Vol.19, Issue 5, (April 1980), pp. 344–362, DOI 10.1002/anie.198003441

Saito, H., Ando, I. & Naito, A. (2006). *Solid state NMR spectroscopy for biopolymers: principles and applications.* Springer, ISBN: 10 1-4020-4302-3, Dordrecht, The Netherlands.

Santos, J.-F.R., Alvarez-Lorenzo, C., Silva, M., Balsa, L., Couceiro, J., Labandeira J.J.T., Concheiro, A. (2009). Soft contact lenses functionalized with pendant cyclodextrins for controlled drug delivery. *Biomaterials,* Vol. 30, Issue 7, (March 2009), pp. 1348–1355, DOI 10.1016/j.biomaterials.2008.11.016

Schneider, H.-J, Hacket, F, Rüdiger, V. & Ikeda, H. (1998). NMR studies of cyclodextrins and cyclodextrin complexes. *Chemical Reviews,* Vol. 98, Issue 5, (July 1998), pp. 1755-1785, DOI 10.1021/cr970019t

Servais, A.-C., Rousseau, A., Fillet, M., Lomsadze, K., Salgado, A., Crommen, J. & Chankvetadze, B. (2010). Capillary electrophoretic and nuclear magnetic resonance studies on the opposite affinity pattern of propranolol enantiomers towards various cyclodextrins. *Journal of Separation Science,* Vol. 33, Issue 11, (June 2010), pp. 1617-1624, DOI 10.1002/jssc.201000040

Simova, S. & Berger, S. (2005). Diffusion measurements vs. chemical shift titration for determination of association constants on the example of camphor-cyclodextrin complexes. *Journal of Inclusion Phenomena and Macrocyclic Chemistry,* Vol. 53, N° 3, (February 2005), pp. 163-170, DOI 10.1007/s10847-005-2631-5

Sohajda, T., Varga, E., Iványi, R., Fejõs, I., Szente, L., Noszál, B. & Béni, S. (2010). Separation of vinca alkaloid enantiomers by capillary electrophoresis applying cyclodextrin derivatives and characterization of cyclodextrin complexes by nuclear magnetic resonance spectroscopy. *Journal of Pharmaceutical and Biomedical Analysis,* Vol. 53, Issue 5, (December 2010), pp. 1258-1266, DOI 10.1016/j.jpba.2010.07.032

Souza, A.A. & Laverde Jr., A. (2002). Aplicação da espectroscopia de ressonância magnética nuclear para estudos de difusão molecular em líquidos: a técnica DOSY. *Quimica Nova*, Vol. 25, N° 6, (February 2002), pp. 10220-1026, ISSN 1678-7064

Steed, J.W. & Atwood, J.L. (2002). *Supramolecular Chemistry.* John Wiley & Sons Ltd, ISBN 978-0-470-51234-0 (Pbk), Chichester, England.

Stilbs, P. (1987). Fourier transform pulsed-gradient spin-echo studies of molecular diffusion. *Progress in Nuclear Magnetic Resonance Spectroscopy,* Vol. 19, Issue 1, (1987), pp. 1-45, DOI 10.1016/0079-6565(87)80007-9

Szejtli, J. (1988). *Cyclodextrin Technology.* Kluwer Academic Publishers, ISBN 979-90-4818427-9, Dordrecht, The Netherlands.

Szejtli, J. (1998). Introduction and general overview of cyclodextrin chemistry. *Chemical Reviews,* Vol. 98, (January 1998), pp. 1743-1753, DOI S0009-2665(97)00022-8

Tamamoto, L.C., Schmidt, S.J. & Lee, S.-Y. (2010). Sensory properties of ginseng solutions modified by masking agents. *Journal of Food Science,* Vol. 75, Issue 7, (September 2010), pp. S341–S347, DOI 10.1111/j.1750-3841.2010.01749.x

Tang, B., Wang, X., Liang, H., Jia, B. & Chen, Z. (2005). Study on the supramolecular interaction of thiabendazole and β-cyclodextrin by apectrophotometry and its analytical application. *Journal of Agricultural and Food Chemistry,* Vol. 22, N° 53, (October 2005), pp. 8452–8459, DOI 10.1021/jf051683a

Tanner, J.E. (1970). Use of the stimulated echo in NMR diffusion studies. *Journal of Chemical Physics,* Vol. 52, N° 5, (March 1970), pp. 2523-2525, DOI 10.1063/1.1673336

Thakkar, A.L. & Demarco, P.V. (1971). Cycloheptaamylose inclusion complexes of barbiturates: correlation between proton magnetic resonance and solubility studies. *Journal of Pharmaceutical Science,* Vol. 60, Issue 4, (April 1971), pp. 652–653, DOI 10.1002/jps.2600600444

Uekama, K., Hirayama, F. & Irie, T. (1998). Cyclodextrin drug carrier systems. *Chemical Reviews,* Vol. 98, Issue 5, (June 1998), pp. 2045–2076, DOI 10.1021/cr970025p

Voulgari, A., Benaki, D., Michaleas, S. & Antoniadou-Vyza, E. (2007). The effect of β-cyclodextrin on tenoxicam photostability, studied by a new liquid chromatography method, the dependence on drug dimerisation. *Journal of Inclusion Phenomena and Macrocyclic Chemistry,* Vol. 57, Issues 1-4, (April 2007), pp. 141–146, DOI 10.1007/s10847-006-9206-y

Woessner, D.E. (1961). Effects of diffusion in Nuclear Magnetic Resonance spin-echo experiments. *Journal of Chemical Physics,* Vol. 34, N° 6, (June 1961), pp. 2057-2061, DOI 10.1063/1.1731821

Wozel, G., Blasum, C., Winter, C. & Gerlach, B. (1997). Dapsone hydroxylamine inhibits the LTB4-induced chemotaxis of polymorphonuclear leukocytes into human skin: results of a pilot study. *Inflammatory Research,* Vol. 46, N° 10, (October 1997), pp. 420-422, DOI 10.1007/s000110050215

Yorozu, T., Hoshino, M., Imamura, M. & Shizuka, H. (1982). Photoexcited inclusion complexes of .beta.-naphthol with alpha-, beta-, and gamma-cyclodextrins in aqueous solutions. *Journal of Physical Chemistry,* Vol. 86, N° 22, (October 1982), pp. 4422–4426, DOI 10.1021/j100219a030